INTRACYTOPLASMIC SPERM INJECTION

The Revolution in Male Infertility

INTRACYTOPLASMIC SPERM INJECTION

The Revolution in Male Infertility

*Edited by Sean P. Flaherty
and Colin D. Matthews*

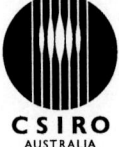

CSIRO Cataloguing-in-Publication Entry

Intracytoplasmic sperm injection: the revolution in male infertility.
Edited by Sean P. Flaherty and Colin D. Matthews.

Includes bibliographic references.
ISBN 0 643 05763 3.

1. Infertility, Male.   2. Fertilization *in vitro*.
I. Flaherty, Sean P.   II. Matthews, Colin D.   III. CSIRO.

599.0166

Reprinted from *Reproduction, Fertility and Development* Volume 7, Number 2 (1995)

© CSIRO Australia 1995

Sean P Flaherty
Reproductive Medicine Laboratories, Department of Obstetrics and Gynaecology,
The University of Adelaide, The Queen Elizabeth Hospital, Woodville, South Australia.

Colin D Matthews
Reproductive Medicine Laboratories, Department of Obstetrics and Gynaecology,
The University of Adelaide, The Queen Elizabeth Hospital, Woodville, South Australia.

Individual papers should be cited in the following format, or as near to this format as is consistent with the requirements of other journals:

Flaherty, S. P., Payne, D., Swann, N. J., and Matthews, C. D. (1995). Assessment of fertilization failure and abnormal fertilization after intracytoplasmic sperm injection (ICSI). In 'Intracytoplasmic Sperm Injection: the Revolution in Male Infertility'. *Reproduction, Fertility and Development* **7**, 197–210.

Contents

Papers from a Symposium on Intracytoplasmic Sperm Injection, held on 2–4 October 1994 at The Kooralbyn Hotel-Resort, Queensland, Australia.

Introduction *Sean P. Flaherty and Colin D. Matthews*	1
The potential of intracytoplasmic sperm injection (ICSI) to transmit genetic defects causing male infertility. *David M. de Kretser*	3
Cell cycle factors in the human oocyte and the intracytoplasmic injection of spermatozoa. *Robert G. Edwards*	9
Spermatids as male gametes. *Atsuo Ogura and Ryuzu Yanagimachi*	21
Comparative intracytoplasmic sperm injection (ICSI) in human and domestic species. *James W. Catt and Sally L. Rhodes*	27
Intracytoplasmic sperm injection (ICSI) *versus* high insemination concentration (HIC) for human conception *in vitro*. *Simon Fishel, Franco Lisi, Leonardo Rinaldi, Rosella Lisi, Judy Timson, Steven Green, Jenny Hall, Steven Fleming, Alison Hunter, Ken Dowell and Simon Thornton*	35
Sperm preparation for intracytoplasmic injection: methods and relationship to fertilization results. *Harold Bourne, Nadine Richings, De Yi Liu, Gary N. Clarke, Offer Harari and H. W. Gordon Baker*	43
Intracytoplasmic sperm injection: instrumentation and injection technique. *Dianna Payne*	51
Assessment of fertilization failure and abnormal fertilization after intracytoplasmic sperm injection (ICSI). *Sean P. Flaherty, Dianna Payne, Nicholas J. Swann and Colin D. Matthews*	63
Development and implementation of intracytoplasmic sperm injection (ICSI). *Gianpiero D. Palermo, Jacques Cohen, Mina Alikani, Alexis Adler and Zev Rosenwaks*	77

(continued)

Intracytoplasmic sperm injection—clinical results from the Reproductive Medicine Unit, Adelaide.
Dianna Payne and Colin D. Matthews — 85

Factors affecting success with intracytoplasmic sperm injection.
M. J. Tucker, P. C. Morton, G. Wright, P. E. Ingargiola, A. E. Jones and C. L. Sweitzer — 95

The use of intracytoplasmic sperm injection for the treatment of severe and extreme male infertility.
Harold Bourne, Nadine Richings, Offer Harari, William Watkins, Andrew L. Speirs, W. Ian H. Johnston and H.W. Gordon Baker — 103

Clinical results from intracytoplasmic sperm injection at Monash IVF.
Robert I. McLachlan, Giuliana Fuscaldo, Hwan Rho, Christine Poulos, Julie Dalrymple, Peter Jackson and Carol A. Holden — 113

Clinical intracytoplasmic sperm injection (ICSI) results from Royal North Shore Hospital.
James W. Catt, John P. Ryan, Ian L. Pike, Chris O'Neill and Douglas M. Saunders — 121

Microfertilization techniques: the Swedish experience.
Lars Hamberger, Anita Sjögren, Kersti Lundin, Brita Söderlund, Lars Nilsson, Christina Bergh, Ulla-Britt Wennerholm, Matts Wikland, Peter Svalander, Ann H. Jakobsson and Ann-Sofie Forsberg — 129

Intracytoplasmic sperm injection (ICSI): the Brussels experience.
Herman Tournaye, Jian Liu, Zsolt Nagy, Hubert Joris, Ari Wisanto, Maryse Bonduelle, Josiane Van der Elst, Catherine Staessen, Johan Smitz, Sherman Silber, Paul Devroey, Inge Liebaers and André Van Steirteghem — 135

Fertilizing capacity of epididymal and testicular sperm using intracytoplasmic sperm injection (ICSI).
Sherman J. Silber, Paul Devroey, Herman Tournaye and André C. Van Steirteghem — 147

Technical Discussion. — 161

Final Discussion. — 165

List of First Authors

Harold Bourne
Reproductive Biology Unit, Royal Women's Hospital, 132 Grattan Street, Carlton, Vic. 3053, Australia.

James W. Catt
Human Reproduction Unit, Royal North Shore Hospital, St Leonards, NSW 2065, Australia.

David M. de Kretser
Institute of Reproduction and Development, Monash University, Clayton, Vic. 3168, Australia.

Robert G. Edwards
Churchill College, Cambridge CB3 0DS, UK and The London Women's Clinic, 113 and 115 Harley Street, London W1N 1DG, UK.

Simon Fishel
NURTURE (Nottingham University Research and Treatment Unit in Reproduction), Department of Obstetrics and Gynaecology, Queen's Medical Centre, Nottingham NG7 2UH, UK.

Sean P. Flaherty
Reproductive Medicine Laboratories, Department of Obstetrics and Gynaecology, The University of Adelaide, The Queen Elizabeth Hospital, Woodville, SA 5011, Australia.

Lars Hamberger
Department of Obstetrics and Gynaecology, University of Göteborg, S-41345 Göteborg, Sweden.

Robert I. McLachlan
Monash IVF, 185–187 Hoddle Street, Richmond, Vic. 3121, Australia.

Atsuo Ogura
Department of Veterinary Science, National Institute of Health, 23-1 Toyama 1-Chome, Shinjuku-ku, Tokyo 162, Japan.

Gianpiero Palermo
The Centre for Reproductive Medicine and Infertility, The New York Hospital–Cornell Medical Centre, 505 East 70th Street, New York, NY 10021, USA.

Dianna Payne
Reproductive Medicine Laboratories, Department of Obstetrics and Gynaecology, The University of Adelaide, The Queen Elizabeth Hospital, Woodville, SA 5011, Australia.

Sherman J. Silber
St Luke's Hospital, 224 South Woods Mill Road, Suite 730, St Louis, MO 63017, USA.

Herman Tournaye
Centre for Reproductive Medicine, University Hospital and Medical School, Dutch-speaking Brussels Free University, Laarbeeklaan 101, Brussels B-1090, Belgium.

Michael J. Tucker
Reproductive Biology Associates, 5505 Peachtree Dunwoody Road, Suite 400, Atlanta, GA 30342, USA.

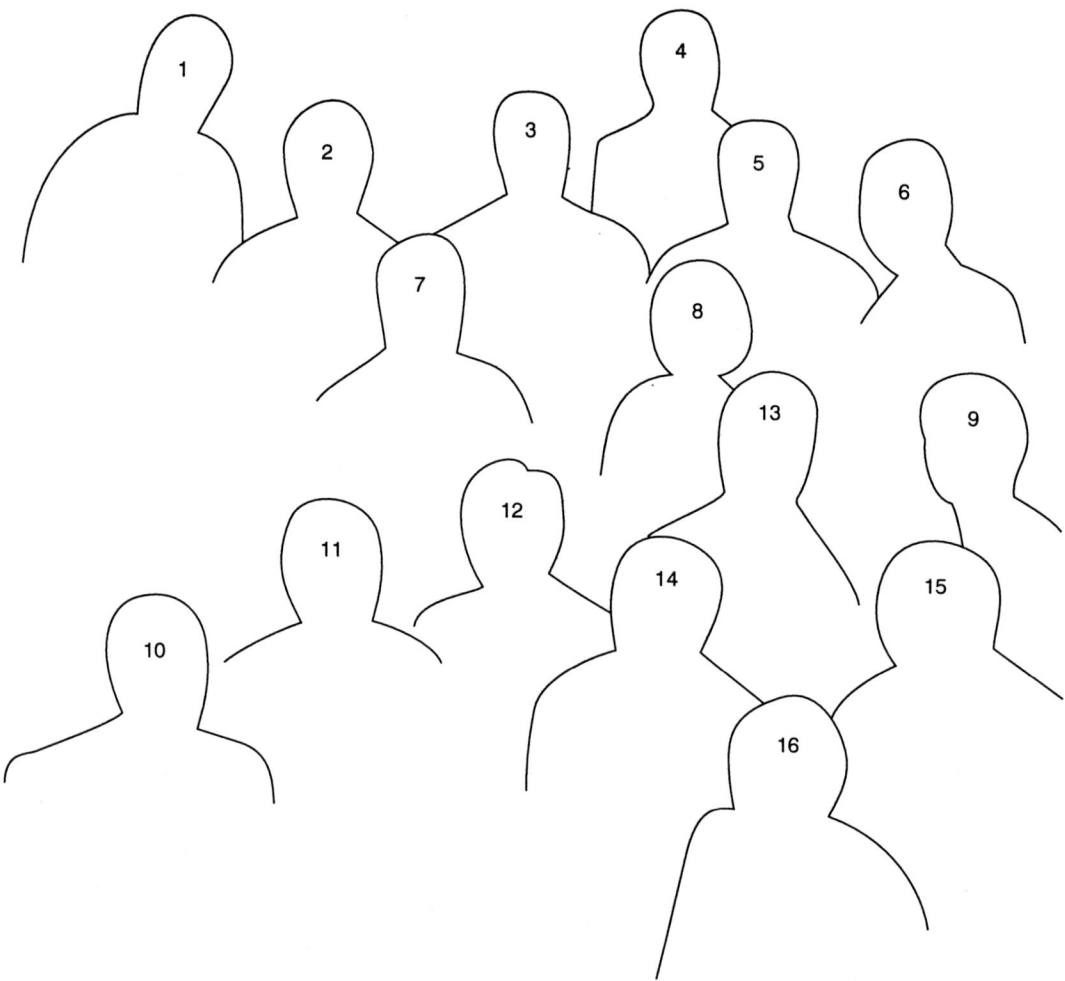

Participants in a Symposium on Intracytoplasmic Sperm Injection, held on 2–4 October 1994 at the Kooralbyn Hotel-Resort, Queensland, Australia.

1. Simon Fishel; 2. Herman Tournaye; 3. Michael Tucker; 4. Robert McLachlan; 5. Gianpiero Palermo; 6. Lars Hamberger; 7. Robert Edwards; 8. Dianna Payne; 9. Harold Bourne; 10. Atsuo Ogura; 11. David de Kretser; 12. Sean Flaherty; 13. James Catt; 14. Colin Matthews; 15. Alan Trounson; 16. Sherman Silber.

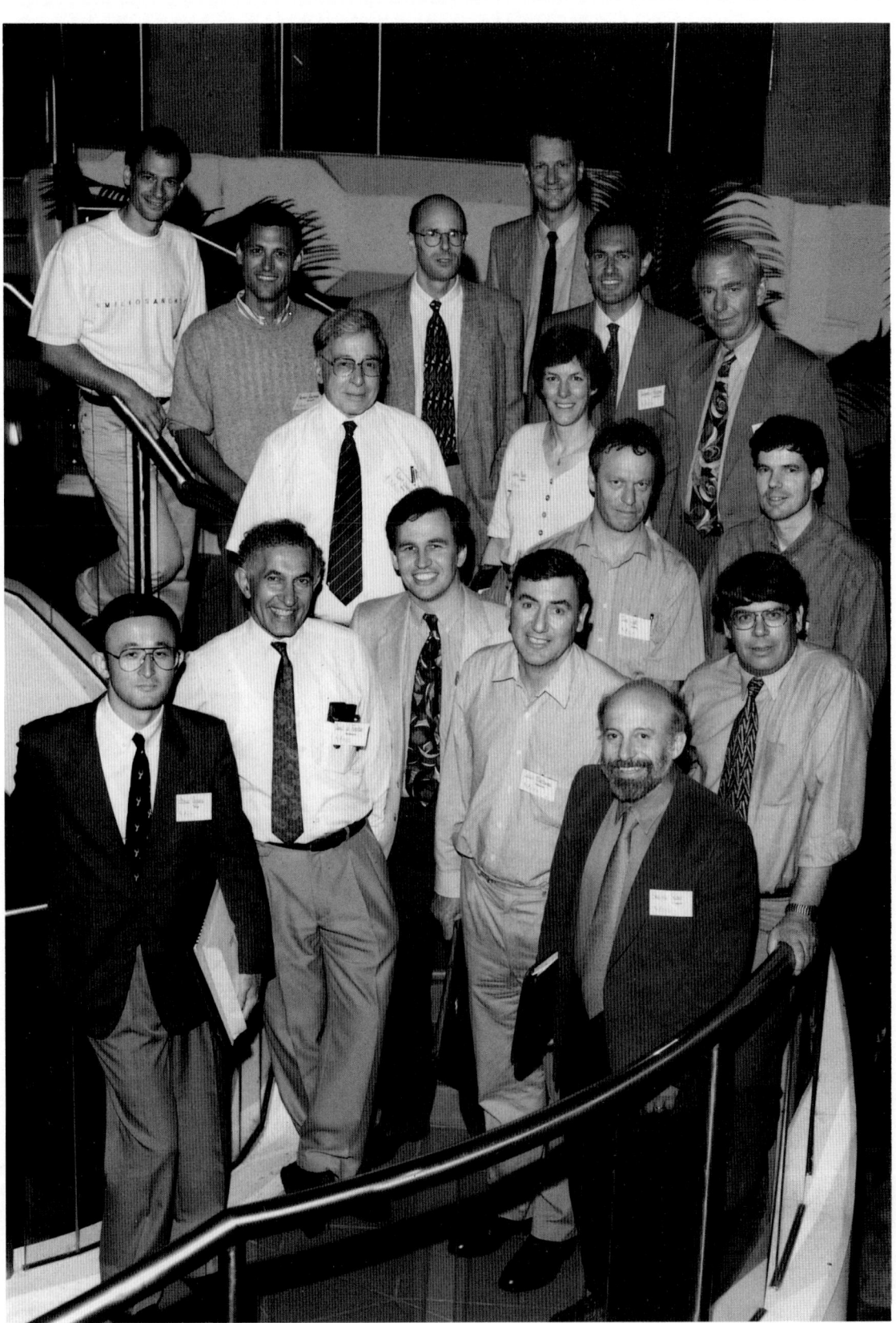

PRECISION GLASS INSTRUMENTS
for ICSI and other micromanipulative procedures

PRECISION INSTRUMENTS *for all micromanipulative applications - ICSI, Assisted Hatching, Embryo Biopsy, Fragment Removal, Cutting and Drilling.*

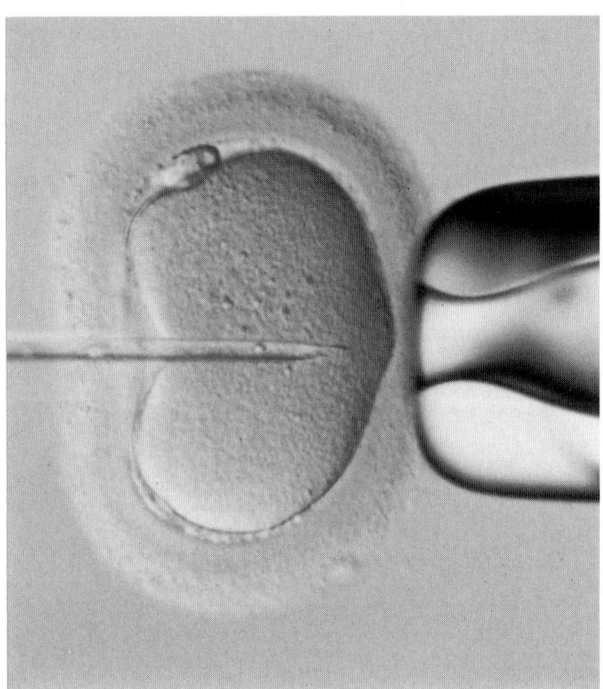

STANDARD SIZE *pipettes to suit most systems.*

CUSTOM MANUFACTURE *to your specifications.*

TRIAL PIPETTES *for you to evaluate in your own unit at no cost.*

COMPETITIVE PRICING *ensures quality instruments at reasonable prices.*

For information and brochure, please call or write to:

Precision Glass Instruments

Reproductive Medicine Laboratories, The University of Adelaide,
The Queen Elizabeth Hospital,
Woodville Road, Woodville, South Australia 5011

International phone: 61 8 222 6379 International fax: 61 8 268 7978
World Wide Service

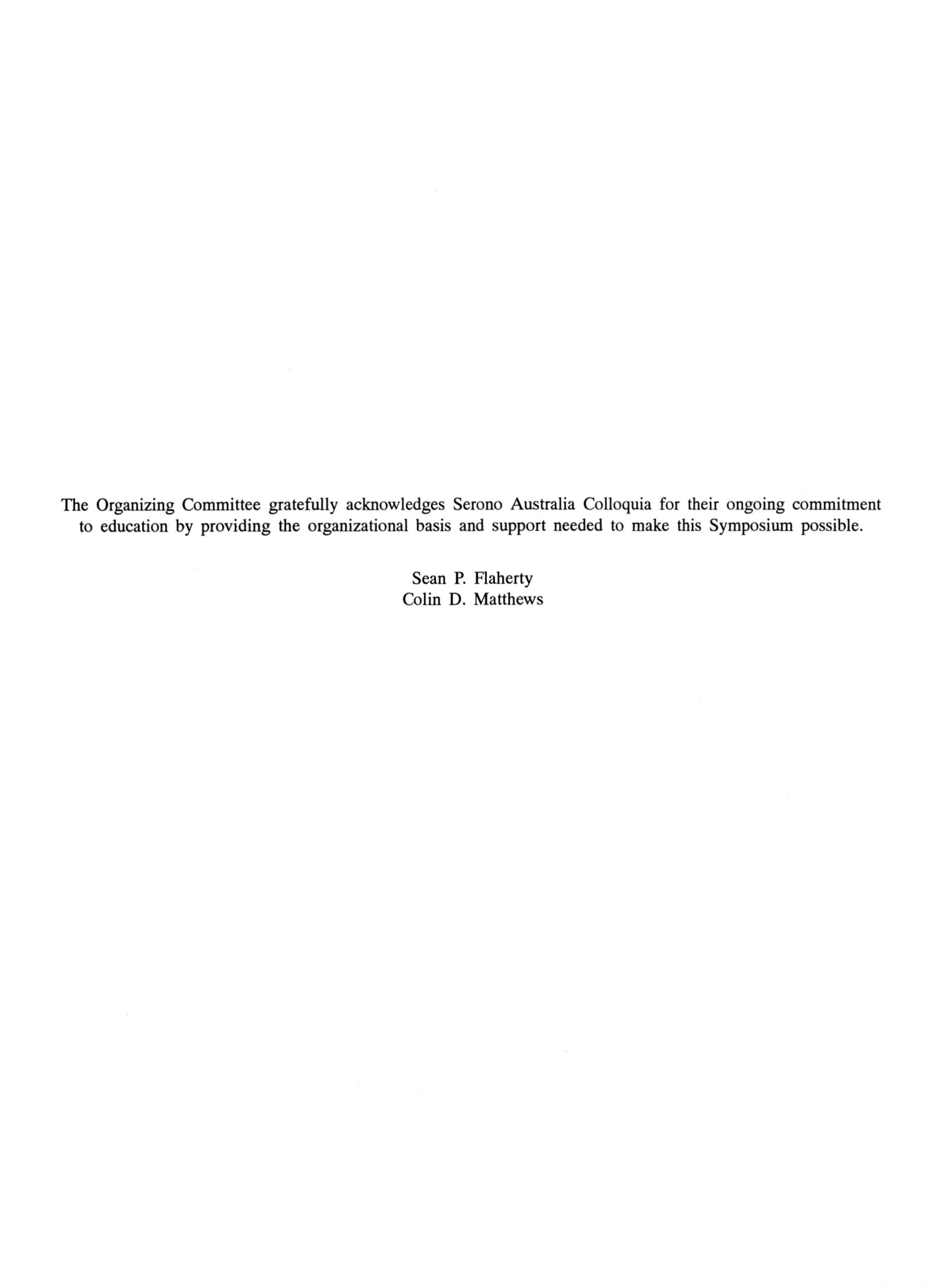

The Organizing Committee gratefully acknowledges Serono Australia Colloquia for their ongoing commitment to education by providing the organizational basis and support needed to make this Symposium possible.

Sean P. Flaherty
Colin D. Matthews

Introduction

Sean P. Flaherty and Colin D. Matthews

*Department of Obstetrics and Gynaecology, The University of Adelaide,
The Queen Elizabeth Hospital, Woodville, SA 5011, Australia.*

Since its introduction in 1992, intracytoplasmic sperm injection (ICSI) has revolutionized the treatment of male factor infertility. This issue is a compilation of papers presented at an International Symposium on ICSI. The purpose of the Symposium was to bring together acknowledged experts on ICSI to discuss the important technical, clinical and ethical aspects of ICSI, and to document, for the first time, clinical ICSI results from around the world. In all, the presentations comprise over 1000 ICSI pregnancies.

Male factor infertility has, for many years, been treated by intrauterine insemination and routine *in vitro* fertilization (IVF) with limited success. The introduction of micromanipulative techniques such as zona drilling, partial zona dissection (PZD) and subzonal insemination (SUZI) to facilitate fertilization led to improved fertilization rates in some cases, but overall the results were disappointing. The principal limitations were low fertilization rates and high polyspermy rates, leading to few embryos suitable for transfer. ICSI represents the first really effective and universally applicable technique for treating severe male factor infertility.

The technical aspects of ICSI are covered in detail in this issue. From these presentations, it is clear that good quality instruments (pipettes), immobilization of sperm before injection and rupture of the oolemma are crucial for the success of ICSI. Polyvinylpyrrolidone (PVP) can be used to slow down the sperm so that they can be more easily captured and manoeuvred into the injection pipette, but it is not essential for success. Furthermore, a brief exposure of oocytes to HEPES-buffered culture medium during injection is not detrimental to embryo development and implantation. Given these optimized technical considerations, fertilization rates of 60–70% can be routinely obtained with ICSI, and units which are not achieving these rates should re-examine their injection technique. An important point is that, unlike routine IVF, sperm morphology does not significantly affect fertilization or implantation rates after ICSI. Embryos which result from ICSI have a similar morphological profile to routine IVF embryos and survive freezing and thawing at similar rates. Moreover, implantation rates per embryo of 20% or more can be obtained after ICSI.

An important consideration with any new technique is the confirmation that it is both effective and safe. The clinical results from ICSI vouch for its efficacy, and many units around the world are now commencing studies to follow-up the babies born after ICSI to confirm that it is safe. The Brussels group leads the way with a comprehensive follow-up programme, which to date includes over 400 ICSI babies. Although the initial results are reassuring and indicate that the incidence of malformations after ICSI is comparable to routine IVF, vigilance is still required, and we encourage clinical units to collaborate in large scale, long-term follow-up studies.

IVF using epididymal sperm met with some success, but the results have always been inferior to those obtained using ejaculated sperm. ICSI has changed that, and has opened the way for successful treatment of epididymal blockages and congenital absence of the vas deferens (CAVD). Outstanding fertilization, pregnancy and implantation rates are now being obtained in many centres with ICSI using epididymal sperm. Furthermore, ICSI can be performed using testicular sperm, thus creating a viable treatment option for those men who have intratesticular blockages or hypospermatogenesis. Sperm can be isolated from tissue obtained by needle biopsy or standard excision of a piece of testicular tissue. However, one of the new and exciting areas of ICSI research will relate to the injection or electrofusion of round spermatids or spermatid nuclei. This technology has been successfully applied to a number of animal species, but careful consideration must be given before it is applied clinically to the human. And with the application of ICSI to these extreme male factor cases and those with known spermatogenic anomalies, some of which are likely to be associated with genetic mutations, comes the responsibility of identifying deletions and gene mutations which could be passed on to the offspring. CAVD is a point in case, since many men with CAVD carry one or more cystic fibrosis mutations, and careful screening of the male and female partners and subsequent genetic counselling is required.

There is no question that ICSI has revolutionized the treatment of severe male factor infertility, and its introduction has given many couples the chance of biological parenthood which they would otherwise not have had. The only criterion for success with ICSI is the presence of a few motile or live sperm somewhere in the male reproductive tract which can be recovered for injection. ICSI overcomes all the limitations of earlier micromanipulative techniques such as PZD and SUZI, and in doing so, renders them obsolete. Furthermore, the application of ICSI to the human has also led to a re-evaluation of the potential uses of ICSI in domestic and endangered species, and it is opening the way for new research into the control of the cell cycle and activation in human oocytes.

The Potential of Intracytoplasmic Sperm Injection (ICSI) to Transmit Genetic Defects Causing Male Infertility

David M. de Kretser

*Institute of Reproduction and Development, Monash University,
Clayton, Vic. 3168, Australia*

Extra keywords: Y chromosome, spermatogenesis.

Introduction

Spermatogenesis is a complex process which results in the production of spermatozoa with the capacity to pass through the female genital tract, interact with the ovum during the process of fertilization and provide the genetic material from the paternal source to fuse with that from the female to form an embryo (Yanagimachi 1988). With the development of assisted reproductive technologies (ART), particularly intracytoplasmic sperm injection (ICSI), many of the components of spermatozoa are rendered redundant making it possible for genetic material carried by an 'incompetent' spermatozoon, to participate in fertilization. This capacity raises the possibility that genetic abnormalities resulting in defective spermatozoa (Bhasin *et al.* 1994) which, without ICSI, could not fertilize an ovum, could transmit these abnormalities to a future male offspring.

The present review examines our knowledge of spermatogenesis, its control mechanisms and the types of testicular pathology likely to require ICSI, and assesses the potential for the transfer of genetic abnormalities which could result in infertility to the children resulting from this ART.

Major Steps in Spermatogenesis

Testicular Development

Normal testicular development is essential for normal spermatogenesis and requires the delineation of the mesodermal anlagen of the testis, the migration of the primordial germ cells from the yolk sac, the multiplication of both primitive germ cells and immature Sertoli cells and the normal emergence and function of the foetal generation of Leydig cells (reviewed by Wartenburg 1989).

Multiplication of Sertoli Cells

There is increasing evidence that the number of Sertoli cells limits the ultimate sperm output of the testis, and the concept that each Sertoli cell can 'nurse' a fixed number of germ cells is gaining acceptance (Orth *et al.* 1988). Since Sertoli cells cease dividing at the completion of puberty in man (Cortes *et al.* 1987), the hormonal milieu during this phase is important. The fact that patients with Kallmann's syndrome less frequently attain normal sperm counts has been attributed to the failure of the testis of these patients, who lack follicle-stimulating hormone (FSH) and luteinizing hormone (LH) stimulation, to exhibit normal Sertoli cell replication (Sheckter *et al.* 1988).

Mitotic Replication of Spermatogonia

The mitotic replication of gonocytes initially, and subsequently spermatogonia, at key stages of the spermatogenic cycle (Clermont 1972) is crucial to maintaining a population of stem cells from which groups of Type B spermatogonia commence meiosis (de Kretser and Kerr 1994).

Meiosis

The two meiotic cell divisions represented by the conversion of primary spermatocytes to secondary spermatocytes and the division of the latter to form spermatids, result in the formation of cells with a haploid chromosomal complement.

Spermiogenesis

The spermatid, which results from the second meiotic division and initially is round in shape, depends on a haploid genome for the generation of the complex series of cytological events which transform it into a spermatozoon (de Kretser and Kerr 1994). This process encompasses the following.

(a) Nuclear condensation and movement to an eccentric position.

(b) Formation of the acrosome.

(c) Flagellar formation including the development of the core of microtubules, the axoneme, from one of the centrioles. This process also includes formation of the outer dense fibres (ODF), the fibrous sheath and the mitochondrial helix, which characterize the midpiece and principal piece of the tail.

(d) Commencement of membrane specialization over selected regions of the spermatid, particularly over the head.

(e) Shedding of excess cytoplasm as the residual body as a terminal event during spermiation.

Epididymal Maturation

It is well recognized that the process resulting in the production of fertile sperm continues in the epididymis with numerous changes associated with the acquisition of motility and the capacity for fertilization (Eddy and O'Brien 1994). It is likely that the latter involves a continued evolution of changes in the membrane of the sperm but the mechanisms are unknown.

Consideration of Testicular Pathology Resulting in Infertility and the Potential for the Transmission of Genetic Defects by ICSI

Testicular biopsy represents a common investigation in patients with infertility, and over many years, the appearance of the testis in such patients has been well characterized. These patterns and their implications for ICSI are considered below.

Normal Spermatogenesis

This appearance in a testicular biopsy most commonly accompanies an obstructive lesion in the epididymis, vas deferens (vasectomy) or the ejaculatory duct (Meacham *et al.* 1993). Even with the use of microsurgery, correction of obstructive lesions is difficult and many failures result. This poor outcome, as well as congenital absence of the vas (CAV), are indications for the use of epididymal or testicular sperm in ICSI (Silber *et al.* 1990, 1995). Although spermatozoa obtained from post-infective obstructions are unlikely to transmit any genetic defects, patients with CAV will transmit a mutation of the cystic fibrosis gene (Anguiano *et al.* 1992; Gervais *et al.* 1993). To date, although these men do not show the respiratory component of cystic fibrosis, over 50% demonstrate the common $\Delta F508$ mutation of cystic fibrosis and it is likely that the others will show a less common mutation. Consequently, the female partners of these men should be screened for cystic fibrosis gene mutations.

The other group with obstructive azoospermia causing concern are those with Young's syndrome, the linkage of bronchiectasis and epididymal obstruction (Handelsman *et al.* 1984; Wilton *et al.* 1990). The description of twins with Young's syndrome has raised the possibility of a genetic defect and a possible linkage to cystic fibrosis (Teichtahl *et al.* 1987). However, we have been unable to show an increase in the frequency of cystic fibrosis gene mutations in patients with Young's syndrome (Friedman *et al.* 1995; de Kretser, unpublished data). Furthermore, the declining incidence of Young's syndrome (Hendry *et al.* 1993) and its linkage to Pink's disease, an illness which has disappeared and was attributed to the presence of mercury in infant teething powders, raises the possibility that the syndrome represents the outcome of neonatal mercury poisoning.

Normal spermatogenesis in the testis is also associated with the condition of epididymal necrozoospermia which presents with severe loss of motility, many abnormally-shaped sperm in the ejaculate and a high percentage of dead sperm (Wilton *et al.* 1988). This condition is characterized by an improvement in semen quality if epididymal storage is limited by the use of a frequent ejaculation regime. The cause of the hostile epididymal environment is unknown, but patients with this disorder may progress to ICSI, perhaps even requiring the recovery of normal testicular sperm to achieve fertilization.

The final condition in which the production of normal sperm in the testis may result in infertility requiring ICSI, is the poorly characterized failure of sperm binding to the zona pellucida (Oehninger 1992). This may result from abnormal sperm surface proteins, failure to undergo capacitation, or the failure of the acrosome reaction, all of which may result in fertilization failure. Since the mechanisms are unknown, the possibility of transmitting a genetic infertility trait must remain a consideration.

Normal Spermatogenesis but 'Abnormal' Sperm

One important abnormality, likely to be caused by an as yet undetermined genetic abnormality, is the occurrence of sperm without an acrosome. This is a well recognized condition which results in the inability to fertilize the ovum (Aitken *et al.* 1990) but it is likely that ICSI will circumvent the need for the acrosome. Patients with this abnormality (globozoospermia) have sperm with a characteristically globular head shape which can be recognized by careful assessment of sperm morphology.

Disorders of sperm motility are common and are frequently associated with normal spermatogenesis as assessed by light microscopy and normal sperm morphology. However, axonemal defects which cause the loss of sperm and ciliary motility, are due to losses of specific proteins such as the ATPase, dynein (Eliasson *et al.* 1977; Eddy and O'Brien 1994). Structurally, the dynein ATPase is represented by the dynein arms in the axoneme and its absence is likely to represent a genetic defect. This, and the absence of nexin links in the axoneme, cause total sperm immotility, and men with this condition will require ICSI to achieve fertilization. Many of these patients, but not all, exhibit features of Kartagener's syndrome such as bronchiectasis and dextrocardia (Eliasson *et al.* 1977) and may be identified by these symptoms.

Other defects in sperm motility might arise from abnormal development of the outer dense fibres, the fibrous sheath or the mitochondrial helix of the midpiece (Zamboni 1987). The basis of these disorders is unknown, but potentially they may arise from mutations in genes encoding for structural proteins which form these organelles. The recent cloning of one of the major proteins of the outer dense fibres will allow study of the genetic basis of such disorders (Burfeind *et al.* 1993).

The process of chromatin condensation during spermiogenesis is likely to involve carefully controlled cellular events and the reverse process of male pronuclear decondensation before syngamy is also likely to prove to be chemically controlled. Abnormalities in the process of chromatin condensation may result in sperm with abnormal morphology, and it is well recognized that the sperm morphology is a good predictor of the likelihood of fertilization (Kruger *et al.* 1988). Should these morphological defects prove to be genetically based, then the use of ICSI may result in propagation of these defects to future generations.

Hypospermatogenesis

This biopsy category, in which all stages of spermatogenesis are present but simply reduced in numbers, is the spermatogenic pattern that represents the basis of most cases of oligozoospermia. In many instances the reduction in spermatogenesis is due to a variety of causes (Baker 1994). However, in approximately 40–50% of cases, the cause is unknown and it is possible that in some of these men, there may be a genetic basis for hypospermatogenesis. The use of ART and particularly ICSI, is substantial in this group of patients, especially if sperm counts are $<5\times10^6$ mL^{-1} (Van Steirteghem *et al.* 1993). Should infertility in these patients be due to genetic mechanisms, then ICSI does represent a mechanism by which offspring could be afflicted by the same problem. Recent studies suggest that micro deletions in the long arm of the Y chromosome are found in 5–20% of patients with azoospermia or severe oligozoospermia (Ma *et al.* 1993; Vogt *et al.* 1995).

Germ Cell Arrest

The cessation of spermatogenesis at a specific stage of spermatogenesis is often observed in the biopsies of patients with azoospermia or severe oligozoospermia ($<1\times10^6$ mL^{-1}). This arrest most frequently occurs at the spermatogonial or primary spermatocyte stage, wherein germ cells fail to successfully complete meiosis. Although a number of molecules have been implicated in the meiotic process, the precise mechanisms which enable successful production of haploid spermatids are not known. ICSI is not an option in this group of patients, as successful production of haploid germ cells has not been achieved. Rarely, germ cell arrest occurs during spermiogenesis after the completion of meiosis, and the potential use of spermatids for ICSI has been raised (Ogura and Yanagimachi 1995). Under these circumstances, there is the potential to propagate underlying genetic defects to offspring.

Germ Cell Aplasia

In these patients, the seminiferous tubules are composed of Sertoli cells only. This biopsy appearance can result from a multiplicity of aetiological agents, for example, cyclophosphamide treatment which destroys all developing germ cells. However, in a proportion of these patients, failure of germ cell migration into the testis or their replication during fetal development may cause this pattern. Recent data arising from studies of mouse mutant models has shown that stem cell factor (SCF) (also known as mast cell growth factor), is crucial in germ cell migration and replication processes which involve the receptor for SCF which is encoded for by the proto-oncogene *c-kit* (Zsebo *et al.* 1990; Yoshinaga *et al.* 1991).

There is also increasing evidence that non-obstructive azoospermic patients may have deletions in the long arm of the Y chromosome which result in infertility (Vogt *et al.* 1995). Recent data from a study of a number of patients with Y deletions has identified two Y-specific genes which the authors proposed may be candidates for the putative azoospermia factor (Ma *et al.* 1993). These genes encode for proteins which have significant homology to other RNA binding proteins and it has been shown that the expression of these genes is restricted to the testis. These and other studies place these genes and the putative azoospermia gene (AZF) to interval 6 on the long arm of the Y chromosome. Since the AZF gene causes azoospermia due to the loss of germ cells from the testis, its transmission to future generations by ICSI will not arise unless it is also associated with severe oligozoospermia (Vogt *et al.* 1995).

Another genetic cause of germ cell aplasia is the sex chromosome disorder characterized by Klinefelter's syndrome (47XXY), in which the extra X chromosome results in conditions that do not permit the survival of germ cells in the testis (Paulsen *et al.* 1968).

Seminiferous Tubule Hyalinization

In this biopsy appearance, all germ cells and Sertoli cells are undeveloped and the seminiferous tubules are represented by a fibrotic hyalinized outline. This pathological appearance may result from many aetiological factors such as mumps orchitis, torsion of the testis or cryptorchidism. It can also result from chromosomal disorders such as Klinefelter's syndrome. As with germ cell aplasia, this pathological state does not permit ICSI since all the germ cells are destroyed.

Immature Testis

This is usually observed in patients with delayed puberty due to pathology arising in the hypothalamus or pituitary which leads to inadequate gonadotrophin stimulation of the testis. A group of these patients will have a genetic basis for their disorder, namely Kallmann's syndrome, where the *kalig-1* gene has been cloned (Ballabio *et al.* 1989). The cloning of this gene has led to the recognition that adhesion molecules are crucial for the migration of gonadotrophin-releasing hormone (GnRH)-secreting neurons to the hypothalamus during development (Franco *et al.* 1991). However, the screening of a large number of patients with Kallmann's syndrome has shown detectable deletions in only a small proportion, raising the possibility of other mechanisms.

In many of these patients, administration of GnRH or FSH and LH leads to spermatogenesis and successful fertilization, but in some instances, the sperm output may be limited and therefore requires the use of ICSI. In such instances, transmission of this genetically determined disorder might be enhanced.

References

Aitken, R. J., Kerr, L., Bolton, V., and Hargreave, T. (1990). Analysis of sperm function in globozoospermia: implications for the mechanism of sperm zona interaction. *Fertil. Steril.* **54**, 701–7.

Anguiano, A., Oates, R. D., Amos, J. A., Dean, M., Gerrard, B., Stewart, C., Maher, T. A., White, M. B., and Milunsky, A. (1992). Congenital bilateral absence of the vas deferens. A primarily genital form of cystic fibrosis. *J. Am. Med. Assoc.* **267**, 1794–7.

Baker, H. W. G. (1994). Male Infertility. In 'Endocrinology'. (Ed. L. J. de Groot.) pp. 2404–33. (W. B. Saunders: Philadelphia.)

Ballabio, A., Bardoni, B., Carrozzo, A., Andria, G., Bick, D., Campbell, L., Hamel, B., Ferguson-Smith, M. A., Gimelli, G., Fraccano, M., Maraschio, P., Zuffordi, O., Guioli, S, and Camerino, G. (1989). Contiguous gene syndromes due to deletions in the distal short arm of the human X chromosome. *Proc. Natl Acad. Sci. USA* **86**, 10001–5.

Bhasin, S., de Kretser, D. M., and Baker, H. W. G. (1994). Pathophysiology and natural history of male infertility. *J. Clin. Endocrinol. & Metab.* **79**, 1525–9.

Burfeind, P., Belgardt, B., Szpirer, C., and Hoyer-Fender, S. (1993). Structure and chromosomal assignment of a gene encoding the major protein of rat sperm outer dense fibres. *Eur. J. Biochem.* **216**, 497–505.

Clermont, Y. (1972). Kinetics of spermatogenesis in mammals. Seminiferous epithelium cycle and spermatogonial renewal. *Physiol. Rev.* **52**, 198–236.

Cortes, D., Muller, J., and Skakkebaek, N. E. (1987). Proliferation of Sertoli cells during development of the human testis assessed by stereological methods. *Int. J. Androl.* **10**, 589–96.

de Kretser, D. M., and Kerr, J. B. (1994). The cytology of the testis. In 'The Physiology of Reproduction'. 2nd Edn. (Eds E. Knobil and J. D. Neill.) pp. 1177–290. (Raven Press: New York.)

Eddy, E. M., and O'Brien, D. A. (1994). The spermatozoon. In 'The Physiology of Reproduction'. 2nd Edn. (Eds E. Knobil and J. D. Neill.) pp. 29–77. (Raven Press: New York.)

Eliasson, R., Mossberg, B., Camner, P., and Afzelius, B. A. (1977). The immotile cilia syndrome. A congenital ciliary abnormality as an etiologic factor in chronic airway infection and male sterility. *New Engl. J. Med.* **297**, 1–6.

Franco, B., Guioli, S., Pragliola, A., Incerti, B., Bardoni, B., Tonlorenzi, R., Carrozzo, R., Maestrini, E., Pieretti, M., Taillon-Miller, P., Brown, C. J., Willard, H. F., Lawrence, C., Persico, M. G., Camerino, G., and Ballabio, A. (1991). A gene deleted in Kallmann's syndrome shares homology with neural cell adhesion and axonal path-finding molecules. *Nature (Lond.)* **353**, 529–36.

Freidman, K. J., Teichtahl, H., de Kretser, D. M., Temple-Smith, P. D., Southwick, G. J., Silverman, L. M., Highsmith, W. E., Boucher, R. C., and Knowles, M. R. (1995). Screening Young syndrome patients for CFTR mutations. *Am. Rev. Resp. Dis.* (In press.)

Gervais, R., Dumur, V., Rigot, J. M., Lafitte, J. J., Roussel, P., Claustres, M., and Demaille, J. (1993). High frequency of the R117H cystic fibrosis mutation in patients with congenital absence of the vas deferens. *New Engl. J. Med.* **328**, 446–7.

Handelsman, D. J., Conway, A. J., Boylan, L. M., and Turtle, J. R. (1984). Young's syndrome. Obstructive azoospermia and chronic sinopulmonary infections. *New Engl. J. Med.* **310**, 3–9.

Hendry, W. F., A'Hern, R. P., and Cole, P. J. (1993). Was Young's syndrome caused by exposure to mercury in childhood? *Br. Med. J.* **307**, 1579–82.

Kruger, T. F., Acosta, A. A., Simmons, K. F., Swanson, R. J., Matta, J. F., and Oehninger, S. (1988). Predictive value of abnormal sperm morphology in *in vitro* fertilization. *Fertil. Steril.* **49**, 112–17.

Ma, K., Inglis, J. D., Sharkey, A., Bickmore, W. A., Hill, R. E., Prosser, E. J., Speed, R. M., Thomson, E. J., Jobling, M., Taylor, K., Wolfe, J., Cooke, H. J., Hargreave, T., and Chandley, A. C. (1993). A Y chromosome gene family with RNA-binding protein homology: candidates for the azoospermia factor AZF controlling human spermatogenesis. *Cell* **75**, 1287–95.

Meacham, R. B., Hellerstein, D. K., and Lipschultz, L. I. (1993). Evaluation and treatment of ejaculatory duct obstruction in the infertile male. *Fertil Steril.* **59**, 393–7.

Oehninger, S. (1992). Diagnostic significance of sperm–zona pellucida interaction. *Reprod. Med. Rev.* **1**, 57–81.

Ogura, A., and Yanagimachi, R. (1995). Spermatids as male gametes. In 'Intracytoplasmic Sperm Injection: the Revolution in Male Infertility'. *Reprod. Fertil. Dev.* **7**, 155–9.

Orth, J. M., Gunsalus, G. L., and Lamperti, A. A. (1988). Evidence from Sertoli cell-depleted rat indicates that spermatid number in adults depends on numbers of Sertoli cells produced during perinatal development. *Endocrinology* **122**, 787–94.

Paulsen, C. A., Gordon, D. L., Carpenter, R. W., Gandy, H. M., and Drucker, W. D. (1968). Klinefelter's syndrome and its variants: a hormonal and chromosomal study. *Recent Prog. Horm. Res.* **24**, 321–63.

Sheckter, C. B., McLachlan, R. I., Tenover, J. S., Matsumoto, A. M., Burger, H. G., de Kretser, D. M., and Bremner, W. J. (1988). Stimulation of serum inhibin concentrations by gonadotrophin releasing hormone in men with idiopathic hypogonadotropic hypogonadism. *J. Clin. Endocrinol. & Metab.* **67**, 1221–4.

Silber, S. J., Ord, T., Balmaceda, J., Patrizio, P., and Asch, R. H. (1990). Congenital absence of the vas deferens. The fertilizing capacity of human epididymal sperm. *New Engl. J. Med.* **323**, 1788–92.

Silber, S. J., Devroey, P., Tournaye, H., and Van Steirteghem, A. C. (1995). Fertilizing capacity of epididymal and testicular sperm using intracytoplasmic sperm injection (ICSI). In 'Intracytoplasmic

Sperm Injection: the Revolution in Male Infertility'. *Reprod. Fertil. Dev.* **7**, 281–93.

Teichtahl, H., Temple-Smith, P. D., Johnson, J. L., Southwick, G. J., and de Kretser, D. M. (1987). Obstructive azoospermia and chronic sinobronchial disease (Young's syndrome) in identical twins. *Fertil. Steril.* **47**, 879–81.

Van Steirteghem, A. C., Nagy, Z., Joris, H., Liu, J., Staessen, C., Smitz, J., Wisanto, A., and Devroey, P. (1993*b*). High fertilization and implantation rates after intracytoplasmic sperm injection. *Hum. Reprod. (Oxf.)* **8**, 1061–6.

Vogt, P. H., Edelmann, A., Hirschmann, P., and Kohler, H. R. (1995). The azoospermia factor (AZF) of the human Y chromosome in Yq11: function and analysis in spermatogenesis. *Reprod. Fertil. Dev.* **7**. (In press.)

Wartenberg, H. (1989). Differentiation and development of the testes. In 'The Testis'. (Eds H. G. Burger and D. M. de Kretser.) pp. 67–118. (Raven Press: New York.)

Wilton, L. J., Temple-Smith, P. D., Baker, H. W. G., and de Kretser, D. M. (1988). Human male infertility caused by degeneration and death of sperm in the epididymis. *Fertil. Steril.* **49**, 1052–8.

Wilton, L. J., Teichtahl, H., Temple-Smith, P. D., Johnson, J. L., Southwick, G. J., Burger, H. G., and de Kretser, D. M. (1990). Young's syndrome (obstructive azoospermia and chronic sinobronchial infection): a quantitative study of axonemal ultrastructure and function. *Fertil. Steril.* **55**, 144–51.

Yanagimachi, R. (1988). Mammalian fertilization. In 'The Physiology of Reproduction'. 2nd Edn. (Eds E. Knobil and J. D. Neill.) pp. 189–317. (Raven Press: New York.)

Yoshinaga, K., Nishikawa, S., Ogawa, M., Hayashi, S., Kunisada, T., Fujimoto, T., and Nishikawa, S. (1991). Role of *c-kit* expression in mouse spermatogenesis: identification of spermatogonia as a specific site of *c-kit* expression and function. *Development* **113**, 689–99.

Zamboni, L. (1987). The ultrastructural pathology of the spermatozoon as a cause of infertility: the role of electron microscopy in the evaluation of semen quality. *Fertil. Steril.* **48**, 711–34.

Zsebo, K. M., Williams, D. A., Geissler, E. N., Broudy, V. C., Martin, F. H., Atkins, H. L., Hsu, R.-Y., Birkett, N. C., Okino, K. H., Murdock, D. C., Jacobsen, F. W., Langley, K. E., Smith, K. A., Takeishi, T., Cattanach, B. M., Galli, S. J., and Suggs, S. V. (1990). Stem cell factor is encoded in the Sl locus of the mouse and is the ligand for the *c-kit* tyrosine kinase receptor. *Cell* **63**, 213–24.

Manuscript received 8 March 1995

Open Discussion

Sherman Silber (St Louis):

I don't believe that we can say that we know the cause of male factor infertility in most cases. By and large, if we look at men with oligoasthenozoospermia with poor or no fertilization, other than a few cases such a cryptorchidism, Klinefelter's syndrome or Duchenne muscular dystrophy which in themselves are genetic, we have no idea what causes male factor infertility. So it is possible that there is a genetic cause for every case of male factor infertility. In collaboration with David Page's group, we have fairly reliably identified a deletion in the same location on Yq for men with maturation arrest and men with Sertoli cell only syndrome. That study hasn't been done yet for hypospermatogenesis cases. I think there is strong evidence that most cases of male factor infertility will be genetic and that with ICSI, there is a good chance of transmitting that to the male offspring. But my answer to that is so what, because we will still have ICSI. I just present that as an opposing point of view.

de Kretser:

In our ongoing collaborative studies, we have also identified a number of Y chromosome deletions in patients with azoospermia. That gene may not be the cause of all cases of male infertility, but it is going to be one of the causes.

With the availability of ICSI, there is a tendency that the male should not even be examined and I'd like to state that it is wrong. I have found at least three or four testicular carcinomas in patients that presented to me with male infertility. And I would hate to have missed that on a simple physical examination, no matter how crude it might be. Nobody treats a sore throat without looking at the throat and I would make a plea that nobody treats male infertility without examining the patient.

Ultimately our knowledge will only increase with careful assessment. We cannot just assume that Y_q deletions are going to cause all male infertility because there may be deletions in other genes such as stem cell factor and *c-kit*. And as we identify more and more of the mechanisms, that's when we'll be able to state what is the actual defect and cause.

Silber:

Obviously you have to do a physical exam on every patient. Blood should also be drawn from these men and the DNA should be stored so that it can be studied later with more sophisticated methods to make sure we're not limiting our ability to find out whether most of these conditions are genetic.

Lars Hamberger (Göteborg):

With respect to the transfer of genetic diseases to the next generation using ICSI, the selection of patients is crucial. We have successfully used acrosomeless sperm for ICSI, a condition which as far as we know is not linked to anything else, and if we can treat them today then in 20 years we can probably treat the boy that will be born. However, immotile cilia syndrome is a different matter because it is associated with other defects. Similarly, the risk may be considerable with some of the translocations that we could probably treat with ICSI. So I don't think we can say that all genetic risks are the same, although we can treat the first generation with ICSI.

de Kretser:

I agree that it's very difficult to sit here and determine policy, and I fully agree that if we can treat an acrosomal defect today by ICSI it's probably going to be even more successful when the offspring are considering having children. I also agree that where you have translocations which are likely to cause greater disruption to the development of the fetus and to that particular individual or the offspring, that's when we should be much more cautious. But again, identifying those translocations is not always easy.

Hamberger:

Another problem is that, even if you have a careful discussion with the couple and they agree to have prenatal diagnosis, they don't always do so when they become pregnant. Several couples have refused in our programme.

Cell Cycle Factors in the Human Oocyte and the Intracytoplasmic Injection of Spermatozoa

Robert G. Edwards

*Churchill College, Cambridge CB3 0DS, UK and The London Women's Clinic,
113 and 115 Harley Street, London W1N 1DG, UK.
Address for correspondence: Bourn Hall, Bourn, Cambridgeshire CB3 7TR, UK.*

Extra keywords: activation, MPF, calcium, fertilization.

Introduction

Intracytoplasmic injection of spermatozoa into oocytes (ICSI) has transformed the treatment of male infertility (Van Steirteghem *et al.* 1993). Recent clinical results using ICSI are presented in detail elsewhere (Hamberger *et al.* 1995; Palermo *et al.* 1995; Payne and Matthews 1995; Tournaye *et al.* 1995). A high percentage of two-pronuclear eggs form after ICSI, which is surprising since it apparently bypasses the closely-knit interactions which normally occur during fertilization, including sperm–egg fusion, membrane hyperpolarization, calcium discharges and activation of the egg. However, success with ICSI may have been a narrow victory, since many oocytes display a disordered activation.

The present review relates the principles of the cell cycle to oocyte growth and maturation, and to the events which occur during normal fertilization and ICSI. This is reviewed in greater detail by Edwards and Brody (1995).

The Cell Cycle and Oocyte Growth and Maturation

Formation and Growth of the Oocyte

Numerous studies on invertebrates, mice and other mammals have shown that oocytes have an unusual cell cycle. Normally, the cell cycle is composed of several phases. The end of mitosis (M) signifies the onset of the G1 interphase. G1 lasts until DNA synthesis (S) begins (Fig. 1). A second interphase, G2, then intercedes until the cell enters mitosis. The phases of the cell cycle are regulated at various control points. START represents the beginning of the S phase. ENTRY organizes the M phase and EXIT terminates it by triggering the metaphase to anaphase transition. Each control point involves movements in intracellular free calcium (Ca^{2+}), which regulate the oncogenes encoding $p34^{cdc2}$ and cyclin.

In the fetal ovary, primary oocytes pass through G1 and S via START and ENTRY of meiosis 1. They arrest immediately afterwards (probably at EXIT) as a germinal vesicle (GV) forms at dictyotene (a nucleated stage of diplotene) and this introduces an elongated G2 phase. The follicle pool is thereby established in the neonatal ovary, and oocyte growth is arrested at diplotene as primordial follicles form. The GV persists in oocytes until just before ovulation, when the luteinizing hormone (LH) surge activates the preovulatory follicle.

The meiotic cycle remains arrested in prophase I as follicles and oocytes begin to grow and leave the pool. Growing oocytes of many species, including man, synthesize and store ribosomal, transfer and poly (A) RNA, especially ribosomal RNA (Davidson 1986). Growing oocytes also incorporate or synthesize amino acids, ribonucleotides, ribonucleosides and proteins such as α- and β-tubulin, β- and γ-actin and approximately 400 others (Wassarman 1988). The Golgi complex produces cortical granules, probably via multivesicular bodies and granular endoplasmic reticulum. The zona pellucida forms from pools of fibrillar material between the oocyte and its surrounding cells. The three zona glycoproteins ZP1, ZP2 and ZP3 represent 7–8% of the total protein in the oocyte (Liang *et al.* 1990).

Meiotic Competence and Oocyte Maturation

The growing follicle cannot respond to gonadotrophins until the oocyte is almost fully grown. Nor can oocytes undergo germinal vesicle breakdown (GVBD) and resume meiosis in response to the LH surge until they have acquired 'meiotic competence', when nucleolar transcription ends and they synthesize the proteins needed for maturation. Meiotic competence is the beginning of the G2 to M transition, and involves the initial step in the re-activation of meiosis (Edwards and Brody 1995). Competence involves an initial chromosomal condensation, re-organization of phosphorylation centres and microtubules, and perhaps the activation of protein kinase A or C. Phosphorylation may be evoked by the action of maturation (mitosis or meiosis) promoting factor (MPF), and phosphorylation inhibitors have been shown to reverse the onset of meiotic competence (Wickramasinghe and Albertini 1992). As these changes occur, oocytes exhibit prominent nucleoli, a fine fibrillar nuclear structure, many mitochondria and a scattered endoplasmic reticulum (Wassarman 1988). Competent oocytes can respond to the ovulatory LH

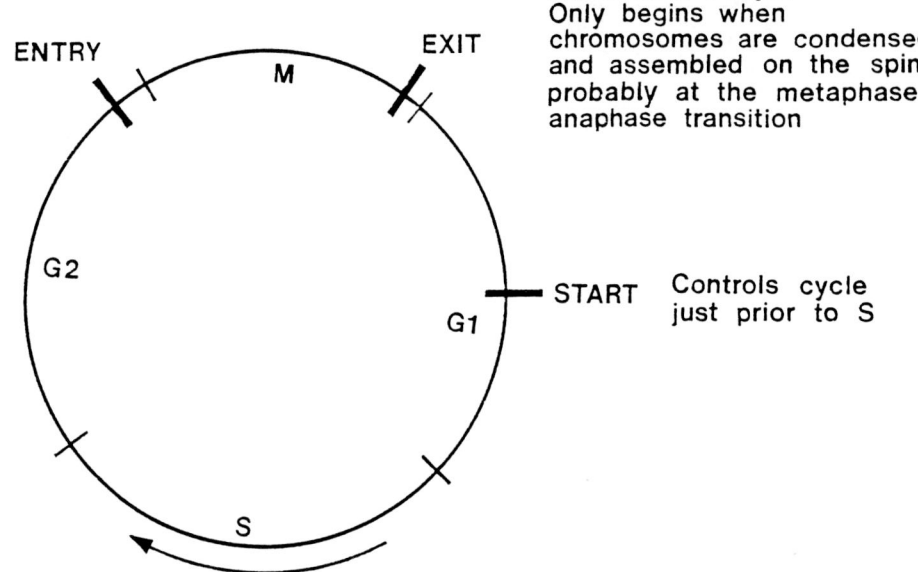

Fig. 1. The proliferative cell cycle and its relationship to oocyte growth and maturation. The labels relate to the situation in the mammalian oocyte as it passes through the various stages of meiosis I and II.

surge, and their maturation begins as MPF and the cyclins interact with various oncogene products to induce GVBD.

The onset of maturation in mice is signalled by brief calcium discharges (transients) from intracellular stores, which last for 6 h and are apparently essential to sustain the maturation process (Carroll and Swann 1992). GVBD may also involve the release of calcium from oocyte stores which are mobilized via the phosphoinositide pathway, although this conclusion has been contested (Tombes *et al.* 1992; Homa *et al.* 1993). GVBD and maturation also require synthesis of peptides after maturation has begun (Fulka *et al.* 1988). Gap junctions, cyclic adenosine 3′,5′-monophosphate (cAMP), growth factors and steroids are also involved in oocyte maturation. cAMP is believed to be involved in the G2 to M transition in mitotic cells (Dekel and Beers 1980). Maturation is associated with reductions in the cAMP level in follicles and perhaps in oocytes (Channing *et al.* 1983; Yoshimura and Wallach 1987), and factors which raise the cAMP level in oocytes can arrest the onset of maturation. The role of the phosphoinositide pathway in oocyte maturation has received considerable attention, in view of observations that repetitive injections of inositol 1,4,5-trisphosphate ($InsP_3$) can activate the eggs of several mammals (Miyazaki 1991). $InsP_3$ or Ca^{2+} may be transported in pulses into oocytes from cumulus cells responding to the LH surge (Homa *et al.* 1993).

Maturing oocytes of mammals and other orders initially pass through diakinesis and metaphase I which last for a few hours, and then through anaphase I and telophase I, each of which require 1–2 h. The first polar body is extruded as the G1 phase is bypassed, and meiosis proceeds very quickly to metaphase I in ovulatory oocytes. The cell cycle is arrested again, and maturation is only completed when metaphase II arrest is overcome at sperm entry.

Disorders in cell cycle activity can cause anomalies during maturation and at fertilization (Table 1). A delay in GVBD and a block at metaphase I occur in many oocytes of a particular strain of mice and this leads to the ovulation of semi-mature or diploid oocytes (Eppig and Wigglesworth 1994). These blocks may occur at the G2 to M transition point and at the metaphase

Table 1. Cell cycle factors which disturb oocyte maturation and fertilization

Oocytes of some mouse strains do not reach metaphase II
Oocytes fail to stop at metaphase II when the *c-mos* protein is inactivated by gene knock-out
Inadequate stimuli may lead to metaphase III
A male pronucleus may be associated with meiotic chromosomes
Gynogenetic eggs may contain a sperm head or a delayed male pronucleus
Delayed fertilization is associated with more meiotic irregularities
Disorders in spindle orientation and chromosome movement may lead to androgenetic human eggs and hydatidiform moles

to anaphase transition point at ENTRY and EXIT. An abnormally oriented metaphase-II spindle would result in all the metaphase-II chromosomes being incorporated into, or ejected from the egg. The total expulsion of metaphase-II chromosomes from human oocytes before fertilization may result in human androgenic embryos and hydatidiform moles (Edwards *et al.* 1992). Male and female pronuclei develop asynchronously in some human eggs inseminated *in vitro*, resulting in one pronucleus entering metaphase while the other is still in G1 or G2 (Schmiady and Kentenich 1993).

Regulation of the Cell Cycle by Proto-oncogenes

A series of proto-oncogenes regulate the cell cycle. They code for signal transduction proteins, membrane-binding proteins and protein kinases. Some of these proteins are transcribed *de novo*, whereas others are produced after post-translational modification (Solomon *et al.* 1990). Protein kinases are essential for regulation of the cell cycle. The oncogene *cdc2*, first identified in yeast, produces a 34 kDa serine–threonine kinase ($p34^{cdc2}$) which complexes with cyclins and other compounds to regulate kinase activity in mammalian cells (Lowndes *et al.* 1992). Kinases influence specific stages of the mitotic cell cycle, for example S and the G2 to M transition. They probably impose START, ENTRY and EXIT.

Active MPF is a protein dimer serine–threonine kinase composed of cyclin B and $p34^{cdc2}$ (Hunt 1989). Cyclin B is phosphorylated at ENTRY and is destroyed at EXIT (Whitaker and Patel 1990). The cdc2 protein is a substrate for tyrosine kinases in mammalian cells. Maturation involves the action of cAMP-dependent protein kinases A and C, and phosphatases such as phosphatase I. The resulting phosphoproteins evoke the activation of $p34^{cdc2}$ (Shuttleworth *et al.* 1990). In pig oocytes, MPF is a phosphoprotein with a molecular weight of 34 kDa and may be a H1 histone kinase related to cdc2. It is phosphorylated by $p34^{cdc2}$ kinase, and its conversion from a latent to an active form by dephosphorylation invokes the formation of MPF and cyclins (Dunphy and Newport 1988; Draetta *et al.* 1989).

Cyclins are stabilized by cytostatic factor (CSF) after cell division or polar body extrusion, and accumulate as degradation ceases. Oocytes may stockpile cyclins in a complex with $p34^{cdc2}$, which may be the MPF precursor (pre-MPF). Cyclins are not essential for all meiotic stages, and oocytes can proceed to metaphase II if cyclin RNA is destroyed by antisense nucleotides (Yew *et al.* 1992). Cyclins may be synthesized 8–16 h after the onset of maturation while the GV is still intact (Moor *et al.* 1990).

Other relevant proto-oncogenes include *cdc32* which may interact with microtubules and stimulate maturation by phosphorylating microtubule organizing centres and by organizing the spindle (Albertini 1992). *c-kit* may affect oocyte maturation via cell signalling since its mRNA increases during oocyte maturation. The *c-kit* protein is a tyrosine kinase receptor structurally related to CSF-1 (*c-fms*) and the platelet-derived growth factor (PDGF) receptor. *c-fms* mRNA also increases during oocyte maturation (Arceci *et al.* 1992). Its ligand is SLT (Steel factor or kit ligand, KL), a growth factor which has extracellular, transmembrane and cytoplasmic domains. *c-myc* encodes a nuclear protein which binds to DNA and regulates ENTRY, the S-phase and cell proliferation. *c-fos* apparently regulates gene expression, and *c-abl* encodes a protein kinase in many cell types. *c-mos* is involved in the imposition of metaphase II arrest (Grootegoed 1989).

The protein p39mos, the product of the gene *c-mos*, is probably a cytostatic factor which imposes metaphase II arrest. It causes metaphase II arrest in mouse oocytes. It must be inactivated if metaphase is to proceed to anaphase II, and this is achieved soon after sperm entry into the oocyte. The activity of the *c-mos* gene and the production of p39mos in mouse oocytes can also be suppressed by gene knock-out or by the injection of antisense *c-mos* oligonucleotides into oocytes. This results in ovulated oocytes which fail to stop at metaphase II (O'Keefe *et al.* 1989; Colledge *et al.* 1994; Hashimoto *et al.* 1994). A 357-bp fragment of a sequence similar to *c-mos* has been identified in human eggs by applying reverse transcriptase and DNA amplification to *c-mos* mRNA extracted from the eggs (Pal *et al.* 1994). The mos protein may interact with and stabilize cyclin B (a substrate for mos protein kinase) or with MPF. This property confers its cytostatic actions at metaphase II in oocytes. It is apparently inactivated immediately after sperm binding to the oocyte. An understanding of its role in mammalian eggs is essential for studies on ICSI.

The Biology of Fertilization

The Mature Oocyte

The second meiotic spindle in mature oocytes is barrel-shaped and is oriented radially with its long axis perpendicular to the plasma membrane. It has neither asters nor centrioles (Fleming and Johnson 1988) and its foci of pericentriolar material enlarge to form an extensive cortical mesh after fertilization (Maro *et al.* 1985). Tubulin polymerization is modulated locally by each meiotic chromosome, so that the microtubules are confined to the spindle.

A thin sub-cortical mesh of microfilaments project to the oolemma, and a dense ring of actin forms at the site of extrusion of the second polar body (Maro *et al.* 1985; Pickering *et al.* 1988). Round mitochondria form complexes with smooth endoplasmic reticulum, whereas rough endoplasmic reticulum is sparse. Cortical granules, which mediate the block to polyspermy, have migrated during maturation to the oocyte periphery (Szollosi et al. 1986). Long, slender microvilli on the oolemma are approximately 200 nm in diameter and 3 μm long.

The Activation of Metaphase II Oocytes at Sperm Entry

Capacitated spermatozoa bind to the zona pellucida, undergo the acrosome reaction and then pass through it. ZP3 is the primary sperm receptor whereas ZP2 maintains sperm binding during zona penetration by interacting with the inner acrosomal membrane. The plasma membrane over the equatorial segment and post-acrosomal region of the acrosome-reacted spermatozoon fuses with the oolemma (Yanagimachi 1988).

The adhesion peptides integrin and disintegrin may have primary roles in gamete fusion, and fusion could depend on an RGD (Arg-Gly-Asp) sequence on the sperm surface and integrins on the oolemma. The acrosomal adhesion protein PH-30 might also be involved (Bronson and Fusi 1990; Blobel et al. 1992). A membrane glycoprotein which is an isoform of CD46 may have a more direct role in fusion since it is expressed on human oocytes and acrosome-reacted spermatozoa. It might also protect spermatozoa from proteolytic damage (Taylor et al. 1994). After the initiation of fusion, the spermatozoon becomes immotile and its plasma membrane is incorporated into the oocyte membrane. Fusion may activate G proteins and InsP$_3$, leading to the activation of membrane phospholipases (Moore et al. 1993).

Membrane hyperpolarization is an initial response to sperm–egg fusion and it is immediately followed by a propagating wave of Ca^{2+} release in the egg. These two events are not necessarily related, however, since a cytosolic protein released from the fertilizing spermatozoon may diffuse into the oocyte or pass through an aqueous pore to gain access to the ooplasm. This protein might be a primary agent in an activation system which is separate and occurs simultaneously with regulatory systems controlled by signal transduction. The sperm protein could generate InsP$_3$ or induce oscillatory Ca^{2+} release (Swann 1990; Homa et al. 1993), and it could be the sole stimulus of Ca^{2+} spiking, since the binding of RGD sequences to integrins on the egg does not invoke Ca^{2+} release (Swann et al. 1994). This putative sperm protein is sometimes called an 'oscillogen', and a similar protein stimulates the cortical reaction in sea urchin eggs (Dale et al. 1985; Swann et al. 1994). Ryanodine receptors similar to those in the heart, which control Ca^{2+}-induced Ca^{2+} release (CICR), could have a role in the control of Ca^{2+} spiking in mammalian eggs (Swann 1992). It is also worth noting that many artificial stimuli which induce some aspects of activation in mammalian oocytes do not induce Ca^{2+} spikes which are typical of those evoked at fertilization.

Ca^{2+} and Egg Activation

Ca^{2+} itself evokes a massive CICR discharge, which is recognizable as repetitive Ca^{2+} transients (spikes) over a period of several hours after fertilization (Cuthbertson and Cobbold 1985; Swann 1990; Whitaker and Patel 1990). The oscillations begin 20–35 min after the insemination of human eggs. Their amplitude initially reaches 2·25 μM [Ca^{2+}]$_i$, but decreases with time, and each oscillation lasts for 100–120 s (Taylor et al. 1992; Homa et al. 1993).

Ca^{2+} release from intracellular stores might be facilitated by the periodic generation of InsP$_3$ and G proteins or by the oscillogen released from the fertilizing spermatozoon (Taylor 1994). Calcium fluxes begin from an initiation locus and then spread around the egg periphery. They may sustain the actions of the integrins, retraction of oocyte microvilli and the exocytosis of cortical granules.

Ca^{2+} spiking might also initiate destruction of the mos protein and other proteins by activating the enzyme calpain, a cysteine protease found in *Xenopus* but not yet in mammals (Watanabe et al. 1989). Other calcium-dependent proteases could independently neutralize MPF or the cyclins (Watanabe et al. 1991). Cyclins can be degraded more rapidly than p39mos in a process requiring less Ca^{2+} and calmodulin. Ca^{2+} might therefore stimulate MPF, re-initiate the cell cycle and activate metaphase II. Cyclic adenosine diphosphate (cADP) ribose or cyclic guanidine 3′,5′-monophosphate (cGMP) may be involved in these processes (Berridge 1993).

The Block to Polyspermy, Pronucleus Formation and the First Cleavage Division

Meanwhile, microfilaments integrate the sperm head into the ooplasm and cortical granules fuse with the oolemma and release their contents into the perivitelline space. Cortical granules confer a block to polyspermy as their contents interact with and modify ZP2 and ZP3 (Yanagimachi 1988). Peptide spread from the swollen sperm head activates K$^+$ channels in the oolemma (Babcock et al. 1992).

The G2 phase in the spermatid nucleus is modified as histones are replaced by protamines during spermiogenesis. Within minutes of sperm–egg fusion, the cell cycle factors which hold oocytes at metaphase are destroyed, and simultaneously, protamines in the sperm nucleus are replaced by histones. It is possible that protamines or the condensed nature of sperm DNA offer some protection against the M factors in the oocyte. The systems in the egg and the sperm head are thus finely balanced. The mos protein may have evolved for this purpose, enabling oocytes to be held at metaphase II ready for fertilization, with protamines protecting the sperm nucleus until it is inactivated.

The second polar body is extruded shortly after sperm–egg fusion. The sperm head swells and enlarges, the chromatin decondenses, the nuclear envelope disintegrates and disulfide bonds between protamines are reduced (Yanagimachi 1988; Tesarik 1992). Nucleohistones synthesized by the egg replace nuclear sperm protamines as the pronucleus forms under the influence of local growth factors (Thibault et al. 1987). Remnants of the inner acrosomal membrane are ingested in a phagocytic-like process, and the midpiece and principal piece of the sperm tail disintegrate in the ooplasm. The sperm centriole probably organizes the cleavage spindle during the first and later cell divisions, as in many other invertebrate and vertebrate eggs (Sathananthan et al. 1991).

The female pronucleus, which is usually smaller than the male pronucleus, is formed from telophase chromosomes some time after the male pronucleus. The transition from telophase to a female pronucleus resembles the transition from M to G2 in somatic cells. A general rise in Ca^{2+}, rather than Ca^{2+} spiking, might be essential for pronucleus formation (Tesarik 1994).

The genes that regulate meiosis and oocyte maturation regulate the successive mitotic cell cycles in cleavage stage embryos. The $p34^{cdc2}$-cyclin B complex forms pre-MPF which regulates the onset of the M phase during the first and later cleavage divisions. Cyclin B inactivates $p34^{cdc2}$ by phosphorylating some of its specific tyrosine and threonine residues. The complex is abruptly activated as these residues are dephosphorylated, to initiate the M phase (Jessus and Beach 1992). Mitosis begins as $p34^{cdc2}$ activity is abolished and the cyclin subunit is destroyed by a protease.

Artificial Activation of Mammalian Eggs

The activation of the egg at fertilization can be partially or wholly mimicked using artificial stimuli. Some of these stimuli are clearly traumatic, such as pricking the eggs with a fine needle or exposing them to high or low temperatures. A knowledge of these phenomena and stimuli will help us to understand the events during ICSI, which also involves a series of traumatic incidents for the oocyte. Such artificial stimuli can activate mammalian oocytes, even though they induce a monotonic release of Ca^{2+} rather than an oscillatory discharge.

Exposure of oocytes to moderate or high Ca^{2+} concentrations, Ca^{2+} ionophores or alcohol also offer simple means of activating oocytes from many mammals (Cran and Esper 1990; Miyazaki 1991; Winston et al. 1991; Swann 1992). However, certain concentrations of Ca^{2+} ionophore evoke an incomplete activation, which can impair the transition from metaphase II to anaphase and telophase. Consequently, meiotic chromosomes re-form on the spindle, and enter a third meiotic stage called metaphase III (Kubiak 1989). Extrusion of the second polar body is delayed in human oocytes exposed to ionophores, indicating that the activation stimulus is delayed (Taylor et al. 1993).

More complex forms of activation have been applied to mammalian eggs, and reveal some of the consequences of artificial activation. These stimuli include single or repetitive injections of Ca^{2+} or $InsP_3$. Varying strengths and patterns of repeated calcium injections evoke partial or complete activation including polar body extrusion and pronucleus formation (Vincent et al. 1992; Vitullo and Ozil 1992). Aged oocytes require more cytosolic Ca^{2+} for full activation, and delayed fertilization may compromise polar body extrusion (Homa et al. 1993).

Ca^{2+} chelators block Ca^{2+} oscillations, chromosome movements to anaphase, the exocytosis of cortical granules and the formation of pronuclei (Kline and Kline 1992). Ca^{2+} oscillations at fertilization are inhibited by monoclonal antibodies against the $InsP_3$ receptor (Miyazaki et al. 1992) and heparin may also inhibit the $InsP_3$ receptor (Carroll and Swann 1992).

Various forms of electrical stimulation can also be used to activate mammalian eggs (Ozil 1990). Controlled electric pulses of $1 \cdot 8$ V cm^{-1} for 900-μs intervals every 4 min will activate mouse oocytes provided that 12 μM $CaCl_2$ is included in the culture medium. Activated oocytes which display Ca^{2+} spiking have an extended period of embryonic growth, whereas less optimal conditions and an absence of spiking invoke incomplete maturation (Vitullo and Ozil 1992). A single electrical pulse of $0 \cdot 75$ kV cm^{-1} for 30–100 μs suffices for pig oocytes; a lower voltage fails to activate them and higher voltages prevent second polar body extrusion (Prochazka et al. 1992). Electrical stimulation is as effective as exposure to Ca^{2+} or alcohol, but oocytes often have to be stimulated individually.

What Happens During ICSI?

Integration of Cell Cycles in the Egg and Sperm Head

The successive stages of fertilization after ICSI seem to proceed at the same rate as, or more quickly than, normal fertilization (Table 2; Nagy et al. 1994). Nevertheless, pronuclei form asynchronously in 25% of

Table 2. Timing of second polar body extrusion and pronucleus formation after intracytoplasmic sperm injection (ICSI)

From Nagy et al. (1994). PB, polar body; PN, pronuclei

Time post-ICSI	Eggs with second PB	Eggs with PN
2 h	21/93 (23%)	0
4 h	63/93 (68%)	0
6 h	73/93 (80%)	31/93 (33%)[A]
8 h	—	85/93 (91%)[B]
20 h	—	83/93 (89%)[C]

[A] 16 oocytes with 2 PN, 15 with 1 PN.
[B] 75 oocytes with 2 PN, 10 with 1 PN.
[C] 63 oocytes with 2 PN, 1 with 1 PN, and 19 entering syngamy.

Table 3. Potential cell cycle disorders after injection of spermatozoa or spermatids

ICSI, intracytoplasmic sperm injection; IVF, *in vitro* fertilization

Female pronucleus associated with an unchanged sperm head
Swollen sperm head or pronucleus associated with metaphase II in the oocyte
Delayed extrusion of the second polar body
Formation of more digynic tripronuclear eggs than with IVF
Asynchronous formation of pronuclei
Appearance of a third pronucleus after two have already formed
Disappearance of the spermatid nucleus after injection into the oocyte
Small size of male pronuclei after spermatid injection
Asynchronous entry of pronuclei into syngamy after ICSI

human oocytes after ICSI, and their disappearance at syngamy is virtually always asynchronous. These events seem to be at variance with the pronuclear events observed after conventional *in vitro* fertilization (IVF) (Edwards *et al.* 1992). Approximately 7% of the eggs have three pronuclei after ICSI and these eggs are apparently digynic in origin (Table 3). A pronucleus forms long after the other(s) in some of these eggs. The frequency of asynchrony seems to be greater than after IVF, in which most three-pronuclear eggs are diandric (Edwards *et al.* 1992).

Some of these anomalies seem to be predicted by the method of sperm injection during ICSI, and perhaps especially since ICSI involves the fusion of a sperm nucleus in its G2 phase with an oocyte in the M phase. Two cells undergoing fusion should preferably be at the same stage of the cell cycle, otherwise the M-phase cell might drive the G1-cell into a premature mitosis containing single chromatids. A G2-cell which is fused with a cell at M-phase would be driven to a premature mitosis involving double chromatids. Such disorders also arise during IVF, resulting in one or two sets of prematurely condensed chromosomes (PCC) or in eggs with a single pronucleus and metaphase chromosomes (Schmiady and Kentenich 1993).

Potential Artificial Stimuli to the Oocyte during ICSI

ICSI clearly disturbs the normal course of events. Membrane hyperpolarization cannot occur normally, so the persisting MPF–p39mos complex could impair the growth of the sperm nucleus or drive it to a precocious metaphase. On the other hand, some manipulations during ICSI may partially stimulate the oocyte and destroy the MPF–p39mos complex. For instance, the deep deformation of the oocyte before the injection pipette penetrates into the ooplasm could evoke stress responses and this in turn could release heat-shock proteins, since these proteins are transcribed in pronuclear eggs and cleaving embryos.

Piercing the oolemma with the injection pipette might induce Ca^{2+} discharges and activate the egg. Only one modest Ca^{2+} discharge, judged insufficient to induce activation, was observed during the injection of human eggs, and repetitive Ca^{2+} spiking did not occur (Tesarik *et al.* 1994). Oocytes might receive further stimuli as the injection pipette is moved slightly to permit ooplasm to enter it and so confirm that it is in the ooplasm. Injecting the spermatozoon in a bolus of fluid followed by withdrawal of the pipette might provide further stimuli. Slightly raised concentrations of Ca^{2+} in the medium do not seem to modify the results of ICSI (Edwards and Van Steirteghem 1993). Nevertheless, the oocyte receives a series of successive stimuli during ICSI, and each one or a combination of several, could partially activate the oocyte. Some of the accompanying Ca^{2+} discharges are minor and may be delayed (Tesarik *et al.* 1994), although these anomalies may have been partly due to the use of 48-h-old eggs.

Although Ca^{2+} fluxes have not been observed during sperm injection, sham ICSI with medium alone can activate some metaphase-II human oocytes, resulting in polar body extrusion and pronucleus formation (Dozortsev *et al.* 1995; Flaherty *et al.* 1995). Hence, there may be variations in the magnitude of the Ca^{2+} discharges which depend on the species, the ICSI technique, or the response of individual oocytes from the same cohort. In molecular terms, the degree of stimulation may be decided by the effects of the injection pipette on MPF and the activation of calpain. A slight Ca^{2+} stimulus might fail to activate some oocytes, drive others to meiosis III and induce pronucleus formation in a few.

Role of the Spermatozoon in Egg Activation during ICSI

The successive stimuli that the egg receives during ICSI may be reinforced by the presence of a spermatozoon in the injection pipette. Oocyte enzymes might modify the sperm membrane sufficiently to release a sperm oscillogen, which in turn might trigger oocyte activation. However, it is also recognized that $InsP_3$ and other secondary messenger systems must be activated at fertilization. A combination of the effects of the pipette and the sperm protein may provide sufficient stimuli to activate oocytes after ICSI, without necessarily stimulating membrane hyperpolarization or cortical granule discharge.

Many human oocytes display a non-oscillatory Ca^{2+} release over a period of several hours, which may be delayed by some time after ICSI (Tesarik *et al.* 1994). Despite the monotonic Ca^{2+} release, some of the oocytes activated normally. These observations need to be repeated since polar body extrusion and pronucleus formation are not usually delayed after ICSI (Table 2; Nagy *et al.* 1994).

Alternatively, a modified form of membrane fusion might occur during ICSI which could activate the oocytes. Perhaps a very brief contact occurs between the sperm and oocyte plasma membranes during injection. It has also been reported that a more prolonged contact between the spermatozoon and the oolemma during ICSI might provide time for an activating stimulus to the oocyte (Tesarik 1994), although in most cases the spermatozoon is injected into the cytoplasm and would not contact the oolemma. Capacitation and the acrosome reaction could occur in the bolus of medium within the oocyte, resulting in modification of the equatorial segment. A process analogous to normal fertilization might therefore arise if the equatorial segment were to fuse with a membranous organelle such as the endoplasmic reticulum.

Oocytes display variable responses to the intracytoplasmic passage of the injection pipette and to the injected spermatozoon (Table 3). Some remain in metaphase II, others might proceed to metaphase III or form a female pronucleus. Assuming that the spermatozoon is not ejected into the perivitelline space, the oocyte will form a male pronucleus, produce prematurely condensed sperm chromosomes or fail to be activated. Various combinations of sperm and egg responses to ICSI have been described by Flaherty *et al.* (1995).

Fate of Various Types of One-cell Embryos Formed after ICSI

Some injected spermatozoa are expelled into the perivitelline space, apparently via the channel made by the pipette. The potential consequences of this include a metaphase-II egg, a metaphase-III egg, or an activated egg which has a female pronucleus and an intact spermatozoon in the perivitelline space. Such conditions would result in gynogenetic haploid or diploid embryos. It is also possible that a spermatozoon expelled into the perivitelline space could undergo the acrosome reaction there, then fuse with the oolemma. Some eggs with two normal pronuclei after ICSI might be formed by this mechanism. Spermatozoa which are located in the perivitelline space after ICSI might never have entered the ooplasm, since considerable force is needed to penetrate the oolemma.

The succession of sperm-dependent Ca^{2+} transients in some oocytes after ICSI indicates that they received a normal activating stimulus, whereas almost half of them had a delayed discharge commencing 4–12 h after sperm injection and some oocytes displayed non-oscillatory patterns typical of parthenogenetically-activated oocytes (Tesarik *et al.* 1994). Many eggs with two or more pronuclei have apparently passed through a near-normal activation process and are fully capable of growth to full-term fetuses. Pronuclear development appears to be normal. We will not know which activating systems are involved until we have acquired more data on the nature of hyperpolarization and the ultrastructural events which occur in human oocytes after ICSI. This knowledge could change current concepts on the significance of the successive events which occur during normal fertilization.

What is the significance of the other mechanisms which are normally involved in fertilization? For example, are the cortical granules discharged after ICSI? If the granules are not discharged, they may spontaneously release their enzymes during cleavage and harden the zona pellucida. Blastocyst hatching may not be affected, however, since the small hole made in the zona pellucida during injection might assist the hatching process.

The mishaps seen during ICSI might be averted by preliminary activation of the oocytes. Simple stimuli should suffice as described above. Metaphase II arrest could then be terminated before ICSI is performed, and this simple procedure could avert many anomalies in the eggs after ICSI and thus improve the efficiency of the procedure.

The Potential for Injecting Spermatids into Oocytes

The injection of spermatids raises slightly different questions about the need to control the cell cycle. The spermatid nucleus is less condensed and its protamine conversion is less advanced than in the nucleus of a mature spermatozoon. Therefore, it could quickly form a male pronucleus after injection if conditions are propitious, for example, if the oocyte is in the G2 phase. However, a spermatid's histone-dominated nucleus would be at a disadvantage if it were driven precociously to metaphase by the ooplasm of a non-activated oocyte; under these circumstances, nuclei of round spermatids would be more vulnerable than those of elongating spermatids. It is not known if the putative oscillogen protein is present in spermatids, or if the simple injection of these eggs would suffice to activate them.

Oocyte activation before ICSI may thus be more important with spermatids than with spermatozoa (Edwards *et al.* 1994) and, if so, activation should be performed an hour or so before spermatid injection. Exposure of human oocytes to Ca^{2+} ionophores or alcohol probably offers the simplest protocol. Electrofusion induces activation and fusion simultaneously, and this may not give enough time for the MPF–mos protein complex to be inactivated. It is currently unclear whether injecting a spermatid into an oocyte will produce normal gamete fusion without the need for artificial activation.

Mouse and rabbit offspring have been born after the incorporation of round spermatids into oocytes. Mouse spermatids were electrofused with oocytes after exposure to a single DC fusion pulse of 3000 V cm^{-1} for 10 μs, followed by an AC exposure of 2 MHz, 20 V cm^{-1} for 30 μs on either side of the DC pulse (Ogura et al. 1993, 1994; Ogura and Yanagimachi 1995). Round spermatid nuclei from rabbits have also been successfully injected into rabbit oocytes (Sofikitis et al. 1994). Hamster spermatid nuclei formed nucleoli by 2 h after fusion and later synthesized DNA. However, the male pronuclei were very small in most (90–95%) of these electrofused hamster oocytes (Ogura et al. 1993; Ogura and Yanagimachi 1993, 1995). This unusual form of pronuclear growth may be another example of imbalance between the cell cycles of the oocyte and spermatid (Table 3). Nevertheless, the birth of mouse and rabbit offspring indicates that these pronuclear anomalies can be tolerated. It has been shown that a single pronucleus formed in two non-activated human eggs after elongated spermatids were injected into them, but a small male pronucleus may have been overlooked (J. J. Tarín, personal communication).

With spermatid injection, the centriole must be included with the nucleus to regulate normal cleavage of the embryo (Sathananthan et al. 1991; Palermo et al. 1994). The centriole is probably included automatically with the entire spermatid during electrofusion. Intact spermatids could be injected or they could be first disrupted by loading them into a narrow pipette and then injecting the entire contents of the cell. Round spermatids are transcriptionally active and process nucleic acids (Hecht 1986; Cebra-Thomas et al. 1991), but gene expression would not be a problem since it would be reversed once the spermatid was in the ooplasm.

Other Possible Consequences of Spermatid Injection

The injection of spermatids or spermatozoa might disturb the fine architecture of the oocyte. Passing a pipette into and out of the oocyte could perturb the microtubular system which is associated with the metaphase-II spindle. As such, chromosomal segregation would be disturbed, leading to the formation of complex monosomic or trisomic embryos. Disturbing the microfilament system might also disorientate the spindle, so that all the chromosomes consequently move into either the egg or into the second polar body. The one-pronuclear egg and digynic three-pronuclear eggs observed after ICSI could have arisen in this way (Table 3). Transposition of the spindle to the centre of the oocyte would result in immediate cleavage, and the oocyte would divide into two equal halves instead of into a large egg and a small second polar body. No examples of this have been reported after ICSI. Some oocytes might contain neither chromosomes nor pronuclei. This would arise from a misoriented spindle which caused all the egg chromosomes to be expelled into the polar bodies, combined with the ejection of the spermatozoon from the egg.

Disturbances in chromosome movement on the spindle, or pronuclear fragmentation, would result in many small pronuclei in the oocyte. This condition is rare after ICSI. Parthenogenesis may occur, with the formation of one or two female pronuclei, and these could be mistakenly classified as fertilized eggs. There appears to be no risk of re-incorporating the first polar body during ICSI or electrofusion.

Conclusions

Cell cycle factors regulate meiosis, oocyte maturation and the initial steps of fertilization. Evidence from IVF shows that an imbalance of these factors in the oocyte and in the sperm nucleus may cause various disturbances at fertilization. Such disorders could occur with increasing frequency after the injection of spermatozoa or spermatids into oocytes. Some oocytes may be activated by the injection process during ICSI. More information is needed about Ca^{2+} discharges, membrane hyperpolarization, second messenger systems and oocyte activation after ICSI. The role of a sperm cytosolic protein (oscillogen) in oocyte activation must be resolved, since it could be a major factor in the success of ICSI. Chromosome movements on the spindle and spindle orientation could be disturbed during ICSI.

References

Albertini, D. F. (1992). Regulation of meiotic maturation in the mammalian oocyte: interplay between exogenous cues and the microtubule cytoskeleton. *Bioessays* **14**, 97–103.

Arceci, R. J., Pampfer, S., and Pollard, J. W. (1992). Expression of CSF-1/c-fms and SF/c-kit mRNA during preimplantation mouse development. *Dev. Biol.* **151**, 1–8.

Babcock, D. F., Bosma, M. M., Battaglia, D. E., and Darszon, A. (1992). Early persistent activation of sperm K$^+$ channels by the egg peptide speract. *Proc. Natl Acad. Sci. USA* **89**, 6001–5.

Berridge, M. J. (1993). Inositol trisphosphate and calcium signalling. *Nature (Lond.)* **361**, 315–25.

Blobel, C. P., Wolsberg, T. G., Turck, C. W., Myles, D. G., Primakoff, P., and White, J. M. (1992). A potential fusion peptide and an integrin ligand domain in a protein active in sperm–egg fusion. *Nature (Lond.)* **356**, 248–52.

Bronson, R. A., and Fusi, F. (1990). Evidence that an arg-gly-asp adhesion sequence plays a role in mammalian fertilization. *Biol. Reprod.* **43**, 1019–25.

Carroll, J., and Swann, K. (1992). Spontaneous cytosolic calcium oscillations driven by inositol trisphosphate occur during *in vitro* maturation of mouse oocytes. *J. Biol. Chem.* **267**, 11196–201.

Cebra-Thomas, J. A., Decker, C. L., Snyder, L. C., Pilder, S. H., and Silver, L. M. (1991). Allele- and haploid-specific product generated by alternative splicing from a mouse t complex responder locus candidate. *Nature (Lond.)* **349**, 239–41.

Channing, C. P., Liu, C.-Q., Jones, G. S., and Jones, H. (1983). Decline of follicular oocyte maturation inhibitor coincident with maturation and achievement of fertilizability of oocytes recovered at midcycle of gonadotropin-treated women. *Proc. Natl Acad. Sci. USA* **80**, 4184–8.

Colledge, W. H., Carlton, M. B. L., Udy, G. B., and Evans, M. J. (1994). Disruption of c-mos causes parthenogenetic development of unfertilized mouse eggs. *Nature (Lond.)* **370**, 65–8.

Cran, D. G., and Esper, C. R. (1990). Cortical granules and the cortical reaction in mammals. *J. Reprod. Fertil.* (Suppl.) **42**, 177–88.

Cuthbertson, K. S., and Cobbold, P. H. (1985). Phorbol ester and sperm activate mouse oocytes by inducing sustained oscillations in cell Ca^{2+}. *Nature (Lond.)* **316**, 541–2.

Dale, B., De Felice, L. J., and Ehrenstein, G. (1985). Injection of a soluble sperm fraction into sea-urchin eggs triggers the cortical reaction. *Experientia* **41**, 1068–70.

Davidson, E. H. (1986). 'Gene Activity in Early Development.' (Academic Press: Orlando.)

Dekel, N., and Beers, W. H. (1980). Development of the rat oocyte *in vitro*: inhibition and induction of maturation in the presence or absence of the cumulus oophorus. *Dev. Biol.* **75**, 247–54.

Dozortsev, D., Rybouchkin, A., De Sutter, P., Qiam, C., and Dhont, M. (1995). Human oocyte activation following intracytoplasmic injection: the role of the sperm cell. *Hum. Reprod. (Oxf.)* **10**, 403–7.

Draetta, G., Luca, F., Westendorf, J., Brizuela, L., Ruderman, J., and Beach, D. (1989). Cdc2 protein kinase is complexed with both cyclin A and B: evidence for proteolytic inactivation of MPF. *Cell* **56**, 829–38.

Dunphy, W. G., and Newport, J. W. (1988). Unraveling of mitotic control mechanisms. *Cell* **55**, 925–8.

Edwards, R. G., and Van Steirteghem, A. C. (1993). Intracytoplasmic sperm injections (ICSI) and human fertilization: does calcium hold the key to success? *Hum. Reprod. (Oxf.)* **8**, 988–9.

Edwards, R. G., and Brody, S. L. (1995). 'Principles and Practice of Assisted Human Reproduction.' (Saunders: Philadelphia.) (In press.)

Edwards, R. G., Crow, J., Dale, S., Macnamee, M. C., Hartshorne, G. M., and Brinsden, P. (1992). Pronuclear, cleavage and blastocyst histories in the attempted preimplantation diagnosis of the human hydatidiform mole. *Hum. Reprod. (Oxf.)* **7**, 994–8.

Edwards, R. G., Tarin, J. J., Dean, N., Hirsch, A., and Tan, S. L. (1994). Are spermatid injections into human oocytes now mandatory? *Hum. Reprod. (Oxf.)* **9**, 2217–19.

Eppig, J. J., and Wigglesworth, K. (1994). Atypical maturation of oocytes of strain I/LnJ mice. *Hum. Reprod. (Oxf.)* **9**, 1136–42.

Flaherty, S. P., Payne, D., Swann, N. J., and Matthews, C. D. (1995). Assessment of abnormal fertilization and fertilization failure after intracytoplasmic sperm injection (ICSI). In 'Intracytoplasmic Sperm Injection: the Revolution in Male Infertility'. *Reprod. Fertil. Dev.* **7**, 197–210.

Fleming, T. P., and Johnson, M. H. (1988). From egg to epithelium. *Ann. Rev. Cell Biol.* **4**, 459–85.

Fulka, J. Jr, Flechon, J. E., Motlik, J., and Fulka, J. (1988). Does autocatalytic amplification of maturation-promoting factor (MPF) exist in mammalian oocytes? *Gamete Res.* **21**, 185–92.

Grootegoed, J. A. (1989). Proto-oncogenes and spermatogenesis. *Int. J. Androl.* **12**, 251–3.

Hamberger, L., Sjögren, A., Lundin, K., Söderlund, B., Nilsson, L., Bergh, C., Wennerholm, U.-B., Wikland, M., Svalander, P., Jakobsson, A. H., and Forsberg, A.-S. (1995). Microfertilization techniques: the Swedish experience. In 'Intracytoplasmic Sperm Injection: the Revolution in Male Infertility'. *Reprod. Fertil. Dev.* **7**, 263–8.

Hashimoto, N., Watanabe, N., Furoto, Y., Tememoto, H., Sagata, N., Yokoyama, M., Okazaki, K., Nagayoshi, M., Takeda, N., Ikawa, Y., and Aizawa, S. (1994). Parthenogenetic activation of oocytes in c-mos-deficient mice. *Nature (Lond.)* **370**, 68–71.

Hecht, N. B. (1986). Regulation of gene expression during mammalian spermatogenesis. In 'Experimental Approaches to Mammalian Embryonic Development'. (Eds J. Rossant and R. A. Pedersen). pp. 151–93. (Cambridge University Press: Cambridge.)

Homa, S. T., Carroll, J., and Swann, K. (1993). The role of calcium in mammalian oocyte maturation and egg activation. *Hum. Reprod. (Oxf.)* **8**, 1274–81.

Hunt, T. (1989). Maturation promoting factor, cyclin and the control of M-phase. *Curr. Opin. Cell Biol.* **1**, 268–74.

Jessus, C., and Beach, D. (1992). Oscillation of MPF is accompanied by periodic association between cdc25 and cdc2-cyclin B. *Cell* **68**, 323–32.

Kline, D., and Kline, J. T. (1992). Repetitive calcium transients and the role of calcium in exocytosis and cell cycle activation in the mouse egg. *Dev. Biol.* **149**, 80–9.

Kubiak, J. Z. (1989). Mouse oocytes gradually develop the capacity for activation during the metaphase II arrest. *Dev. Biol.* **136**, 537–45.

Liang, L.-P., Chamow, S. M., and Dean, J. (1990). Oocyte-specific expression of mouse ZP-2: developmental regulation of the zona pellucida genes. *Mol. Cell. Biol.* **10**, 1507–15.

Lowndes, N. F., McInerny, C. J., Johnson, A. L., Fantes, P. A., and Johnston, L. H. (1992). Control of DNA synthesis genes in fission yeast by the cell cycle gene cdc10+. *Nature (Lond.)* **355**, 449–53.

Maro, B., Johnson, M. H., Pickering, S. J., and Louvard, D. (1985). Changes in the distribution of membranous organelles during mouse early development. *J. Embryol. Exp. Morphol.* **90**, 287–309.

Miyazaki, S. (1991). Repetitive calcium transients in hamster oocytes. *Cell Calcium* **12**, 205–16.

Miyazaki, S., Yazuki, M., Nakada, K., Shirakawa, H., Nakanishi, S., Nakade, S., and Mikoshiba, K. (1992). Block of Ca^{2+} wave and Ca^{2+} oscillation by antibody to the inositol 1,4,5-trisphosphate receptor in fertilized hamster eggs. *Science* **257**, 251–5.

Moor, R. M., Mattioli, M., Ding, J., and Nagai, T. (1990). Maturation of pig oocytes *in vivo* and *in vitro*. *J. Reprod. Fertil.* (Suppl.) **40**, 197–210.

Moore, G. D., Kopf, G. S., and Schultz, R. M. (1993). Complete mouse egg activation in the absence of sperm by stimulation of an exogenous G protein-coupled receptor. *Dev. Biol.* **159**, 669–78.

Nagy, Z. P., Liu, J., Joris, H., Devroey, P., and Van Steirteghem, A. C. (1994). Time-course of oocyte activation, pronucleus formation and cleavage in human oocytes fertilized by intracytoplasmic sperm injection. *Hum. Reprod. (Oxf.)* **9**, 1743–8.

Ogura, A., and Yanagimachi, R. (1993). Round spermatid nuclei injected into hamster oocytes form pronuclei and participate in syngamy. *Biol. Reprod.* **48**, 219–25.

Ogura, A., and Yanagimachi, R. (1995). Spermatids as male gametes. In 'Intracytoplasmic Sperm Injection: the Revolution in Male Infertility'. *Reprod. Fertil. Dev.* **7**, 155–9.

Ogura, A., Yanagimachi, R., and Usui, N. (1993). Behaviour of hamster and mouse round spermatid nuclei incorporated into mature oocytes by electrofusion. *Zygote* **1**, 1–8.

Ogura, A., Matsuda, J., and Yanagimachi, R. (1994). Birth of normal young after electrofusion of mouse oocytes with round spermatids. *Proc. Natl Acad. Sci. USA* **91**, 7460–2.

O'Keefe, S. J., Wolfes, H., Kiessling, A. A., and Cooper, G. M.

(1989). Microinjection of antisense c-mos oligonucleotide prevents meiosis II in the maturing mouse egg. *Proc. Natl Acad. Sci. USA* **86**, 7038–42.

Ozil, J.-P. (1990). The parthenogenetic development of rabbit oocytes after repetitive pulsatile electrical stimulation. *Development* **109**, 117–27.

Pal, S. K., Torry, D., Serta, R., Crowell, R. C., Seibel, M. M., Cooper, G. M., and Kiessling, A. A. (1994). Expression and potential function of the c-mos proto-oncogene in human eggs. *Fertil. Steril.* **61**, 496–503.

Palermo, G., Munné, S., and Cohen, J. (1994). The human zygote inherits its mitotic potential from the male gamete. *Hum. Reprod. (Oxf.)* **9**, 1220–5.

Palermo, G. D., Cohen, J., Alikani, M., Adler, A., and Rosenwaks, Z. (1995). Development and implementation of intracytoplasmic sperm injection (ICSI). In 'Intracytoplasmic Sperm Injection: the Revolution in Male Infertility'. *Reprod. Fertil. Dev.* **7**, 211–18.

Payne, D., and Matthews, C. D. (1995). Intracytoplasmic sperm injection—clinical results from the Reproductive Medicine Unit, Adelaide. In 'Intracytoplasmic Sperm Injection: the Revolution in Male Infertility'. *Reprod. Fertil. Dev.* **7**, 219–27.

Pickering, S. J., Johnson, M. H., Braude, P. R., and Houliston, E. (1988). Cytoskeletal organization in fresh, aged and spontaneously activated human oocytes. *Hum. Reprod. (Oxf.)* **3**, 978–89.

Prochazka, R., Kanka, J., Sutovsky, P., Fulka, J., and Motlik, J. (1992). Development of pronuclei in pig oocytes activated by a single electric pulse. *J. Reprod. Fertil.* **96**, 725–34.

Sathananthan, A. H., Kola, I., Osborn, J., Trounson, A., Ng, S.-C., Bongso, A., and Ratnam, S. S. (1991). Centrioles in the beginning of human development. *Proc. Natl Acad. Sci. USA* **88**, 4806–10.

Schmiady, H., and Kentenich, H. (1993). Cytological studies of human zygotes exhibiting developmental arrest. *Hum. Reprod. (Oxf.)* **8**, 744–51.

Shuttleworth, J., Godfrey, R., and Colman, A. (1990). p40MO15, a cdc2-related protein kinase involved in negative regulation of meiotic maturation of *Xenopus* oocytes. *EMBO J.* **9**, 3233–40.

Sofikitis, N., Zavos, P., Koutselinis, A., Mourtzinis, D., Loutradis, D., and Glanzounis, G. (1994). Achievement of pregnancy after injection of round spermatid (RS) nuclei into rabbit oocytes and embryo transfer: a possible mode of treatment for men with spermatogenic arrest at the spermatid stage. *J. Urol.* **151**, 311A. [Abstr.]

Solomon, M. J., Glotzer, M., Lee, T. H., Philippe, M., and Kirschner, M. W. (1990). Cyclin activation of p34cdc2. *Cell* **63**, 1013–24.

Swann, K. (1990). A cytosolic sperm factor stimulates repetitive calcium increases and mimics fertilization in hamster eggs. *Development* **110**, 1295–302.

Swann, K. (1992). Different triggers for calcium oscillations in mouse eggs involve a ryanodine-sensitive calcium store. *Biochem. J.* **287**, 79–84.

Swann, K., Homa, S., and Carroll, J. (1994). An inside job: the results of injecting whole sperm into eggs supports one view of signal transduction at fertilization. *Hum. Reprod. (Oxf.)* **9**, 978–80.

Szollosi, D., Mandelbaum, J., Plachot, M., Salat-Baroux, J., and Cohen, J. (1986). Ultrastructure of the human preovulatory oocyte. *J. In Vitro Fertil. Emb. Transfer* **3**, 232–42.

Taylor, A. S., Winston, N. J., Braude, P. R., and Johnson, M. H. (1993). The development and DNA content of human parthenogenetic embryos derived from activated failed fertilized oocytes. *Hum. Reprod. (Oxf.)* **8** (Suppl. 1), 63. [Abstr.]

Taylor, C. T. (1994). Calcium signals and human oocyte activation: implications for assisted conception. *Hum. Reprod. (Oxf.)* **9**, 980–4.

Taylor, C. T., Lawrence, Y. M., Kingsland, C. R., Biljan, M. M., and Cuthbertson, K. (1992). Oscillations in intracellular free calcium induced by spermatozoa in human oocytes at fertilization. *Hum. Reprod. (Oxf.)* **8**, 2174–9.

Taylor, C. T., Biljan, M. M., Kingsland, C. R., and Johnson, P. M. (1994). Inhibition of human spermatozoon–oocyte interaction *in vitro* by monoclonal antibodies to CD46 (membrane cofactor protein). *Hum. Reprod. (Oxf.)* **9**, 907–11.

Tesarik J. (1992). Metabolism of human preimplantation embryos. In 'Preconception and Preimplantation Diagnosis of Human Genetic Disease'. (Ed. R. G. Edwards.) pp. 43–79. (Cambridge University Press: Cambridge.)

Tesarik, J. (1994). How the spermatozoon awakens the oocyte: lessons from intracytoplasmic sperm injection. *Hum. Reprod. (Oxf.)* **9**, 977–8.

Tesarik, J., Sousa, M., and Testart, J. (1994). Human oocyte activation after intracytoplasmic sperm injection. *Hum. Reprod. (Oxf.)* **9**, 511–18.

Thibault, C., Szollosi, D., and Gerard, M. (1987). Mammalian oocyte maturation. *Reprod. Nutr. Dev.* **27**, 865–96.

Tombes, R. M., Simerly, C., Borisy, C., and Schatten, G. (1992). Meiosis, egg activation, and nuclear envelope breakdown are differentially reliant on Ca^{2+}, whereas germinal vesicle breakdown is Ca^{2+}-independent in the mouse oocyte. *J. Cell Biol.* **117**, 799–811.

Tournaye, H., Liu, J., Nagy, Z., Joris, H., Wisanto, A., Bonduelle, M., Van der Elst, J., Staessen, C., Smitz, J., Silber, S., Devroey, P., Liebaers, I., and Van Steirteghem, A. (1995). Intracytoplasmic sperm injection (ICSI): the Brussels experience. In 'Intracytoplasmic Sperm Injection: the Revolution in Male Infertility'. *Reprod. Fertil. Dev.* **7**, 269–79.

Van Steirteghem, A. C., Nagy, Z., Joris, H., Liu, J., Staessen, C., Smitz, J., Wisanto, A., and Devroey, P. (1993). High fertilization and implantation rates after intracytoplasmic sperm injection. *Hum. Reprod. (Oxf.)* **8**, 1061–6.

Vincent, C., Cheek, T. R., and Johnson, M. H. (1992). Cell cycle progression of parthenogenetically activated mouse oocytes to interphase is dependent on the level of internal calcium. *J. Cell Sci.* **103**, 389–96.

Vitullo, A. D., and Ozil, J.-P. (1992). Repetitive calcium stimuli drive meiotic resumption and pronuclear development during mouse oocyte activation. *Dev. Biol.* **151**, 128–36.

Wassarman, P. M. (1988). The mammalian ovum. In 'The Physiology of Reproduction'. (Eds E. Knobil and J. D. Neill.) pp. 69–102. (Raven Press: New York.)

Watanabe, N., Vande-Woude, G. F., Ikawa, Y., and Sagata, N. (1989). Specific proteolysis of the c-mos proto-oncogene product by calpain on fertilization of *Xenopus* eggs. *Nature (Lond.)* **342**, 505–11.

Watanabe, N., Hunt, T., Ikawa, Y., and Sagata, N. (1991). Independent inactivation of MPF and cytostatic factor (mos) upon fertilization of *Xenopus* eggs. *Nature (Lond.)* **352**, 247–8.

Whitaker, M., and Patel, R. (1990). Calcium and cell cycle control. *Development* **108**, 525–42.

Wickramasinghe, D., and Albertini, D. F. (1992). Centrosome phosphorylation and the developmental expression of meiotic competence in mouse oocytes. *Dev. Biol.* **152**, 62–74.

Winston, N., Johnson, M., Pickering, S., and Braude, P. (1991). Parthenogenetic activation and development of fresh and aged human oocytes. *Fertil. Steril.* **56**, 904–12.

Yanagimachi, R. (1988). Mammalian fertilization. In 'The Physiology of Reproduction'. 2nd Edn. (Eds E. Knobil and J. D. Neill.) pp. 189–317. (Raven Press: New York.)

Yew, N., Mellini, M. L., and Vande-Woude, G. F. (1992). Meiotic initiation by the mos protein in *Xenopus. Nature (Lond.)* **355**, 649–52.

Yoshimura, Y., and Wallach, E. E. (1987). Studies on the mechanisms of mammalian ovulation. *Fertil. Steril.* **47**, 22–34.

Manuscript received 10 April 1995

Open Discussion

Sherman Silber (St Louis):

In some poor responders, we find a majority of metaphase I or germinal vesicle eggs. Can you say whether this is due to a poor response to the human chorionic gonadotrophin (hCG) or if more follicle-stimulating hormone (FSH) stimulation for a longer time would have made the follicles more responsive to hCG?

Edwards:

When you collect oocytes from a patient who has been given hCG, remember that all your patients have been given hCG.

There are three classes of oocyte. First, some oocytes never reach meiotic competence and they will be collected as germinal vesicle oocytes which do not appear to be capable of fertilization. Second, there are oocytes which have had a very delayed onset in maturation. For example, when you inject hCG you can't expect every follicle to be ready to respond to hCG at the same time, and if you look at the steroid concentrations in follicles you find that there are different follicles at different stages of growth when you inject hCG. So the metaphase I eggs are probably perfectly normal eggs which had a late start. The third class are metaphase II eggs. There are going to be some anomalies in the human system. I would say that the poor responders may include some people who failed to produce the right systems at the right times, but mostly the immature oocytes result from timing problems.

Lars Hamberger (Göteborg):

I would like to mention two observations on delayed polar body extrusion in the human. First, we saw a higher incidence of failure of extrusion when we decreased the osmolarity of the culture medium, by mistake, to 270 mOsm kg^{-1}. Second, we have twice followed a gradual extrusion of the second polar body. We saw 3 pronuclei when we first looked, and then we saw that gradually, over a period of time (18 h in one case and 11 h in the other case), the polar body was extruded. Both eggs cleaved normally after that. We now take those eggs, which occur at a frequency of 2–3%, and aspirate the nuclei so that we can analyse by fingerprinting if it's due to failure of polar body extrusion or polyspermy.

Edwards:

I suspect that you've got pronuclear fragmentation. You've got a pronucleus that has fragmented into several small pieces, and probably re-aggregates again at syngamy.

Spermatids as Male Gametes

Atsuo Ogura [A,C] and Ryuzu Yanagimachi [B]

[A] Department of Veterinary Science, National Institute of Health, 23-1 Toyama 1-Chome,
Shinjuku-ku, Tokyo 162, Japan.
[B] Department of Anatomy and Reproductive Biology, University of Hawaii
Medical School, Honolulu, Hawaii 96822, USA.
[C] To whom correspondence should be addressed.

Abstract. Intracytoplasmic sperm injection (ICSI) is becoming increasingly popular in human infertility clinics as an efficient method for the treatment of male infertility. It is proposed that spermatids can be used as substitutes for spermatozoa if men are unable to produce sperm in their testes. At least in the hamster and mouse, the nuclei of round spermatids were capable of participating in syngamy when incorporated into homologous mature oocytes either by microsurgical ICSI or electrofusion. Normal mouse offspring were born after electrofusion of oocytes with round spermatids. When culture *in vitro* of spermatogonia and spermatocytes is perfected, then spermatids, transforming spermatids and spermatozoa will all be able to be used as male gametes.

Extra keywords: in vitro fertilization, spermatogenic cells, ICSI, electrofusion.

Introduction

The function of spermatozoa is to fertilize mature oocytes. To achieve this goal, spermatozoa produced in the testis undergo profound structural and biochemical modifications during maturation in the epididymis and during capacitation within the female tract before they become competent to fertilize. Round spermatids, the spermatogenic cells which have just finished meiosis, are normally incapable of fertilizing, but they can if they are electrofused with mature oocytes (Ogura *et al.* 1993) or their nuclei are injected microsurgically into oocytes (Ogura and Yanagimachi 1993). This means that the nuclei of round spermatids are potentially competent to fertilize and all of the post-meiotic modifications of the male germ cell have evolved to ensure the delivery of male genomes into mature female gametes.

Recently, intracytoplasmic sperm injection (ICSI) has become increasingly popular in human IVF clinics for treating severe male factor infertility because it is more efficient than other methods of microsurgical insemination such as partial zona dissection and subzonal injection (Palermo *et al.* 1992; Van Steirteghem *et al.* 1994). Some men are infertile due to occlusion of the male reproductive tract (epididymis) or due to congenital absence of the vas deferens. If spermatozoa are present in either the epididymis or testis, they can be used for ICSI (Silber 1994a,1994b). We propose that if the testes contain round spermatids but no spermatozoa, then these spermatids can be used as substitutes for spermatozoa to fertilize oocytes.

Intracytoplasmic Injection of Isolated Spermatid Nuclei

We have chosen the golden hamster as the animal model because their oocytes tolerate microsurgical manipulation very well. Injected sperm nuclei are able to transform into pronuclei under various experimental conditions (Uehara and Yanagimachi 1976, 1977; Naish *et al.* 1987). Spermatids are relatively small cells, although the diameter of each golden hamster spermatid is about 10 μm. An injection pipette which is large enough to pick up an individual spermatid without deformation inevitably damages the oolemma during injection. Therefore, we isolated nuclei from spermatids by detergent treatment before injecting them into oocytes (Ogura and Yanagimachi 1993).

When spermatid nuclei were introduced into unfertilized oocytes without any prior stimulation, spermatid nuclei often displayed premature chromosome condensation (PCC) within the cytoplasm of unactivated or slowly activating oocytes (Ogura and Yanagimachi 1993). The best result was obtained when the oocytes were first electrically activated (1500 V cm^{-1} for 100 μs in the presence of 0·05 mM Ca^{2+} and 0·1 mM Mg^{2+}), then 10–30 min later a single spermatid nucleus was injected into each oocyte. Of the 1440 injected oocytes, 1298 (90·1%) survived the entire procedure. Injection was successful in 70–95% of the surviving oocytes, depending on the experiment. Almost all (> 95%) of the incorporated spermatid nuclei transformed into well developed male pronuclei (Fig. 1) and the ability for DNA synthesis was

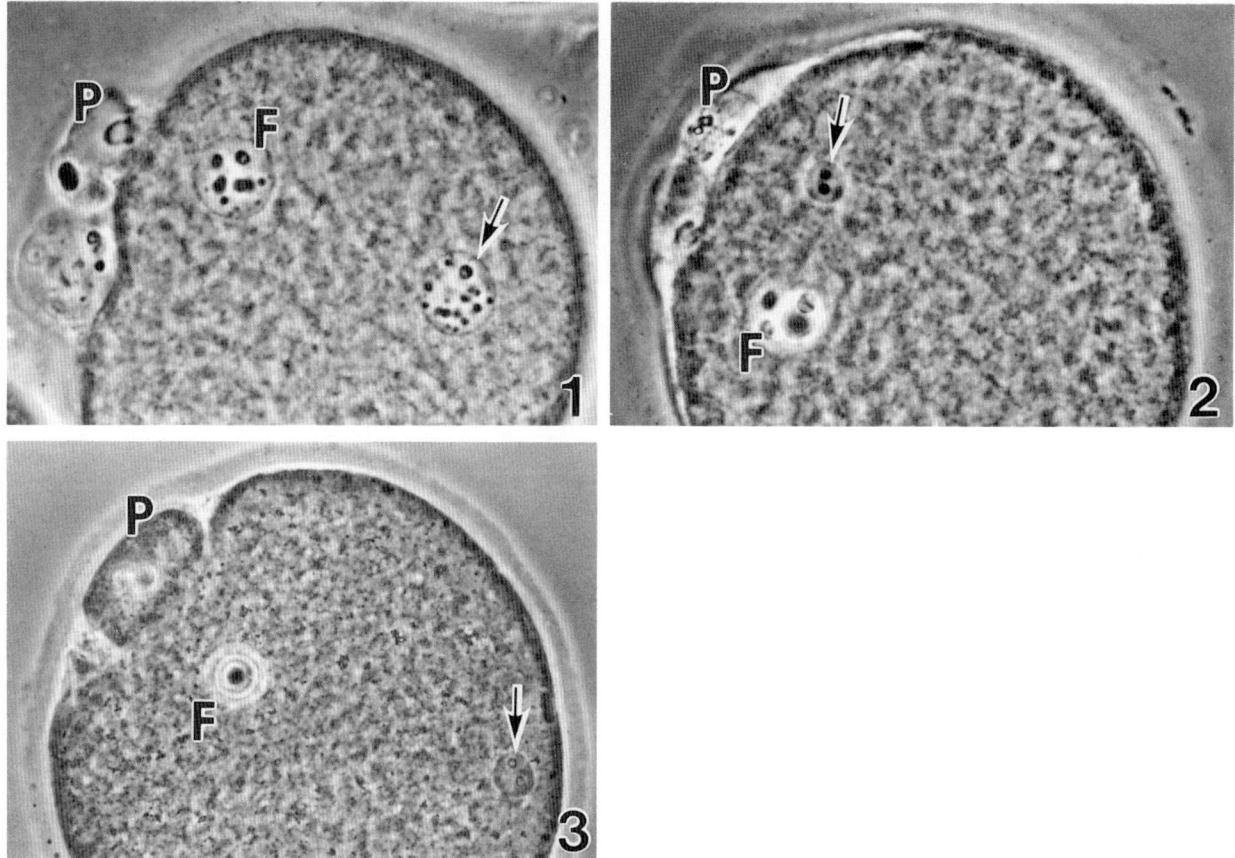

Figs. 1–3. Oocytes 3 h after microinsemination with round spermatids. (**1**) A golden hamster oocyte after intracytoplasmic injection of an isolated spermatid nucleus. A fully-grown male pronucleus is present (arrow). (**2**) A golden hamster oocyte after electrofusion with a round spermatid. It has a large female pronucleus (F) and a small spermatid-derived male pronucleus (arrow). (**3**) Mouse oocyte after electrofusion with a round spermatid. It contains a small male pronucleus (arrow). F, female pronucleus; P, second polar body.

confirmed in 89% (17/19) of these spermatid-derived male pronuclei. Of the 'fertilized' oocytes, 73% (105/143) developed to the 2-cell stage but these embryos did not develop further. We cannot expect development of hamster zygotes beyond the 2-cell stage until culture techniques *in vitro* for hamster embryos are improved (Barnett and Bavister 1992).

Oocyte–Spermatid Electrofusion

Since nuclear transfer by cell-to-cell electrofusion is considered to be less traumatic to cells than microsurgical nuclear transfer (Chang *et al.* 1992), we electrofused spermatids with oocytes (Ogura *et al.* 1993). In the golden hamster, the best result was obtained when spermatids and oocytes were treated with pronase and neuraminidase, respectively. We assume that these enzymatic treatments removed membrane-bound molecules, allowing close approximation of gametes. After these treatments, a single spermatid was inserted into the perivitelline space and a single rectangular pulse (3000 V cm^{-1}, 10 μs) was applied together with pre- and post-pulse AC field. Depending on the experiment, 20–40% of the oocyte-spermatid pairs fused (overall 26·2%, 183/699). Of all the fused oocytes, however, only 4–10% contained both large female (oocyte) and male (spermatid) pronuclei when examined 5–8 h after electrofusion. In the remaining oocytes, the spermatid pronuclei remained small (Fig. 2) even though they formed pronuclear nucleoli and synthesized DNA. About 75% of the fused oocytes developed to the 2-cell stage but did not develop further.

In the mouse, oocyte–spermatid fusion was initially very inefficient (Ogura *et al.* 1993), but became more efficient (about 30% success) in later experiments (Ogura *et al.* 1994). Unlike in the golden hamster, neuraminidase treatment of mouse oocytes had no beneficial effect on oocyte–spermatid fusion. Instead, we found that oocyte activation before electrofusion significantly increased the fusion efficiency. Since mouse oocytes could better tolerate electric pulses than hamster oocytes, they were subjected to a more intense pulse (4000 V cm^{-1}, 10 μs). As already described, about 80% of the oocytes which were electrofused with spermatids contained only one large pronucleus (Fig. 3); a small male pronucleus derived from the spermatid could not be visualized within the ooplasm of these living eggs. Since the majority of electro-stimulated mouse oocytes cleaved regardless of the success or failure of fusion, we transferred all of the 2-cell embryos to foster mothers. We have already reported the birth of six offspring following transfer of a total of 346 2-cell eggs (including unfused ones) into 8 pseudopregnant foster mothers (Ogura *et al.* 1994). Four offspring developed into fertile adults and had a normal life span (> 15 months). As of January 1995, a total of 22 offspring have been born following spermatid–oocyte fusion (Table 1). At present, we do not know whether oocytes with a small male pronucleus, those with a large male pronucleus, or those with both, developed into normal offspring.

Table 1. Mouse pups born after oocyte–spermatid fusion
Two-cell embryos, including unfused ones, were transferred to foster recipient females on Day 1 of pseudopregnancy

Total no. of embryos transferred	662
Total no. of recipient females	17
No. of recipient females which delivered pups	10
Total no. of pups born	22[A]

[A] Two pups were killed within a few days of birth. The remaining pups (12 females and 8 males) developed normally.

Future Prospects

We were able to produce normal mice by fusing spermatids with oocytes. This means that the nuclei of spermatids can provide the paternal chromosomes required for full embryonic development. It may be argued that the rather low incidence of the birth of normal offspring after spermatid–oocyte fusion could be due to the incomplete genomic imprinting of the male germ cells at the early spermatid stage. Although this might be the case, we are of the opinion that it is largely due to technical problems and we believe that the success rate will increase with the improvement of techniques for handling spermatids and oocytes.

If it is proven that spermatid nuclei are fully imprinted genomically, then spermatids could be used as substitutes for mature spermatozoa. This would be particularly useful when infertile men have no mature spermatozoa in their testes or epididymides. We do not know at present whether ICSI or electrofusion is better suited for humans. Injection of isolated spermatid nuclei into oocytes may not invoke full embryonic development because, during normal fertilization in humans, the sperm centriole seems to play an essential role in syngamy (Sathananthan *et al.* 1991) and it may be missing from spermatid nuclei. Electrofusion induces activation of oocytes at a high rate in most mammalian species, whereas injection does not do this as efficiently. Hence, if sperm cytoplasmic factors are shown to initiate activation of human oocytes (Swann *et al.* 1994), then it may be necessary to artificially induce activation of human oocytes before injection of spermatid nuclei to avoid PCC. Thus, either oocyte–spermatid electrofusion or microsurgical injection of both the nucleus and cytoplasm of the spermatid is possible, but the technical improvement of both techniques is definitely needed before they are applied to humans.

There is a group of infertile men with spermatogenic arrest at the primary spermatocyte or earlier stages (Martin du Pan and Campana 1993). Spermatogenic arrest could be due to either genetic factors or various non-genetic factors such as infections and radiotherapy. In the mouse, it is possible to culture pre-meiotic spermatogenic cells to elongated spermatids by co-culture with somatic cells, particularly Sertoli cells (Rassoulzadegan *et al.* 1993). Hence, if the causes of spermatogenic arrest in these infertile men prove to be non-genetic and the testes contain sufficient numbers of spermatogonia and/or spermatocytes, then these cells could be cultured *in vitro* until they reach the round spermatid stage.

We do not need a large number of spermatids for microinsemination. However, it is still very important to differentiate normal spermatids from abnormal ones. At present, we do not know how to differentiate genomically normal spermatids from abnormal ones without destroying the cells. At the very least, however, differentiation of live and dead cells should be performed using, for example trypan blue, to avoid injection of dead or dying spermatids into the oocytes. There may be no method with 100% accuracy, but we should look for the one with the best success rate.

Acknowledgments

These studies were supported by grants from the Japanese Ministry of Education, Science and Culture (A.O.), the Japanese Ministry of Health and Welfare (A.O.) and the US National Institute of Health (R.Y.).

References

Barnett, D.K., and Bavister, B.D. (1992). Hypotaurine requirement for in vitro development of golden hamster one-cell embryos into morulae and blastocysts, and production of term offspring from *in vitro*-fertilized ova. *Biol. Reprod.* **47**, 297–304.

Chang, D.C., Saunders, J.A., Chassy, B.M., and Sowers, A.E. (1992). Overview of electroporation and electrofusion. In 'Guide to Electroporation and Electrofusion'. (Eds D.C. Chang, B.M. Chassy, J.A. Saunders and A.E. Sowers.) pp. 1–6. (Academic Press: San Diego.)

Martin du Pan, R.C., and Campana, A. (1993). Physiopathology of spermatogenic arrest. *Fertil. Steril.* **60**, 937–46.

Naish, S.J., Perreault, S.D., and Zirkin, B.R. (1987). DNA synthesis following microinjection of heterologous sperm and somatic cell nuclei into hamster oocytes. *Gamete Res.* **18**, 109–20.

Ogura, A., and Yanagimachi, R. (1993). Round spermatid nuclei injected into hamster oocytes form pronuclei and participate in syngamy. *Biol. Reprod.* **48**, 219–25.

Ogura, A., Yanagimachi, R., and Usui, N. (1993). Behaviour of hamster and mouse round spermatid nuclei incorporated into mature oocytes by electrofusion. *Zygote* **1**, 1–8.

Ogura, A., Matsuda, J., and Yanagimachi, R. (1994). Birth of normal young after electrofusion of mouse oocytes with round spermatids. *Proc. Natl Acad. Sci. USA* **91**, 7460–2.

Palermo, G., Joris, H., Devroey, P., and Van Steirteghem, A.C. (1992). Pregnancies after intracytoplasmic injection of single spermatozoon into an oocyte. *Lancet* **340**, 17–18.

Rassoulzadegan, M., Paquis-Flucklinger, V., Bertino, B., Sage, J., Jasin, M., Miyagawa, K., van Heyningen, V., Besmer, P., and Cuzin, F. (1993). Transmeiotic differentiation of male germ cells in culture. *Cell* **75**, 997–1006.

Sathananthan, A.H., Kola, I., Osborne, J., Trounson, A., Ng, S.-C., Bongso, A., and Ratnam, S.S. (1991). Centrioles in the beginning of human development. *Proc. Natl Acad. Sci. USA* **88**, 4806–10.

Silber, S.J. (1994*a*). A modern view of male infertility. In 'The Infertile Male: Advanced Assisted Reproductive Technology'. *Reprod. Fertil. Dev.* **6**, 93–104.

Silber, S.J. (1994*b*). The use of epididymal sperm in assisted reproduction. In 'Frontiers in Endocrinology. Vol. 8. Male Factor in Human Infertility'. (Ed. J. Tesarik.) pp. 335–68. (Ares Serono Symposia: Rome.)

Swann, K., Homa, S., and Carroll, J. (1994). An inside job: the results of injecting whole sperm into eggs supports one view of signal transduction at fertilization. *Hum. Reprod. (Oxf.)* **9**, 978–80.

Uehara, T., and Yanagimachi, R. (1976). Microsurgical injection of spermatozoa into hamster eggs with subsequent transformation of sperm nuclei into male pronuclei. *Biol. Reprod.* **15**, 467–70.

Uehara, T., and Yanagimachi, R. (1977). Behaviour of nuclei of testicular, caput and cauda epididymal spermatozoa injected into hamster eggs. *Biol. Reprod.* **16**, 315–21.

Van Steirteghem, A., Liu, J., Joris, H., Nagy, Z., Staessen, C., Camus, M., Wisanto, A., Van Assche, E., and Devroey, P. (1994). Assisted fertilization by subzonal insemination and intracytoplasmic sperm injection. In 'The Infertile Male: Advanced Assisted Reproductive Technology'. *Reprod. Fertil. Dev.* **6**, 85–91.

Manuscript received 20 February 1995

Open Discussion

Ke-Hui Cui (Adelaide):

How do you extract the spermatid nucleus for injection?

Ogura:

Golden hamster spermatid nuclei were obtained after detergent treatment. A very low concentration of detergent is used for isolation of round spermatid nuclei.

Cui:

Detergent extraction of the nucleus might destroy the nuclear membrane and it therefore could have a traumatic effect on the DNA.

Ogura:

I examined the nuclear membrane and it was intact at the time of injection.

Colin Matthews (Adelaide):

What is the size of human spermatids and would we generate oocyte damage by injecting such large cells?

Sherman Silber (St Louis):

A mature elongated spermatid would be 4×6 μm. A round spermatid would be large as 10 μm and that could cause a problem.

David de Kretser (Melbourne):

The nucleus of a round spermatid would be up to 5 μm in diameter.

Bob Edwards (Cambridge):

Why didn't you use elongating spermatids?

Ogura:

We performed those experiments in the hamster using elongated spermatids and we obtained fully developed male pronuclei and normal fertilization.

Silber:

I would like to verify that we have considerable experience with injecting elongated human spermatids and they have a fertilization rate equivalent to ejaculated sperm and give rise to pregnancies. We haven't any experience with round spermatids, but we are planning to use this technique for cases of azoospermia due to maturation arrest.

Alan Trounson (Melbourne):

When we fused mouse eggs and round spermatids, the majority of the embryos stopped at the 8-cell stage after normal development to that point, and few of the transferred embryos went to term. These experiments will need to be done in the human to see if we have the same problem. Can you comment on the low capacity of the eggs to develop pronuclei and undergo embryogenesis to term?

Ogura:

There may be damage due to the electric pulse which affects development.

Trounson:

Our controls were unaffected by the pulse. My own view is that something which is needed for embryogenesis is normally acquired during mouse sperm maturation.

Ogura:

Did you examine the size of the pronuclei?

Trounson:

They were smaller and more difficult to see. The female pronuclei were normal size, but the male pronuclei were much smaller. We saw some large male pronuclei, but not many.

Ogura:

In our experiments, about 10% of the hamster oocytes had large male pronuclei, and those oocytes may have been the ones which developed into pups.

Comparative Intracytoplasmic Sperm Injection (ICSI) in Human and Domestic Species

James W. Catt[AC] and Sally L. Rhodes[B]

[A] North Shore ART, Clinic 20, Royal North Shore Hospital, St Leonards, NSW 2065, Australia.
[B] Department of Animal Science, University of Sydney, Sydney, NSW 2006, Australia.
[C] To whom correspondence should be addressed.

Abstract. The current clinical use of intracytoplasmic sperm injection (ICSI) for the alleviation of male factor infertility has prompted a re-investigation of sperm injection techniques in a number of animal species. This report examines sperm injection of *in vitro* matured oocytes in the major domestic species and compares the results with the human. Ovine, bovine and porcine oocytes can undergo fertilization and at least limited development without exogenous activation either prior to or subsequent to injection. Porcine is temperature sensitive during fertilization and the early stages of embryo development. The oocytes of all three domestic species, particularly ovine, have a tendency to activate after the injection procedure regardless of the presence or absence of sperm. The implications for early development studies and the practical use of direct sperm injection for domestic species are discussed.

Extra keywords: micromanipulation, ovine, bovine, porcine, oocyte activation, fertilization.

Introduction

There are a number of reasons for studying direct sperm injection into oocytes of animal species. These studies enable research into fundamental aspects of fertilization and early embryonic development. Historically, the use of animal models for understanding human mechanisms has proven very useful, although caution must always be used in extrapolation. There may also be application for sperm injection in animal species themselves where, for one reason or another, fertilization by *in vivo* or *in vitro* techniques is not possible.

The direct injection of sperm into the cytoplasm of the oocyte (ICSI) is not a recent innovation. Sperm injection, subsequent oocyte activation and fertilization have been used for many years as a tool in echinoderm (Hiramoto 1962) and amphibian research (Brun 1974). The first sperm injection experiments with mammals were conducted with rodent species and met with variable success. Decondensation of the sperm head into pronuclei and subsequent early cleavage has been readily achieved in the hamster (Uehara and Yanagimachi 1976). The hamster system has been the most extensively used for sperm studies because the oocytes are easy to inject without overt damage and the cytoplasm is permissive in allowing pronuclear formation with sperm from many species. Exogenous activation of hamster oocytes, either prior to or subsequent to sperm injection is not required, but has been used extensively with other species. Markert (1983) reported successful fertilization in mice but subsequent development was compromised. More recently, live births have been reported with mouse ICSI (Roknabadi *et al.* 1994) but details of the techniques used have yet to be published.

Live births resulting from ICSI were first achieved with rabbits (Hosoi *et al.* 1988), followed by cows (Goto *et al.* 1990), but there is a paucity of information on other domestic species. Clarke *et al.* (1988) showed that injection of whole ram sperm or sperm nuclei could give rise to pronuclear formation and subsequent early cleavage, and Keefer *et al.* (1990) demonstrated that bovine oocytes could be successfully injected and subsequently undergo early development. In both of these studies, however, dvelopmental competence of the embryos was not demonstrated.

All of these reports showed that injection of sperm into oocytes can cause terminal damage. The efficiency of fertilization was low and the developmental competence of the subsequent embryos was compromised. This raises the question as to why direct sperm injection in human oocytes results in high fertilization, development and pregnancy rates, equivalent to those found with embryos produced by conventional IVF (Van Steirteghem *et al.* 1993*a*, 1993*b*; Payne and Matthews 1995). Are human sperm and oocytes different from domestic species? This report re-investigates some of the basic parameters of sperm injection in domestic species using knowledge gained from human oocyte injection. Further trials are required before the methodology is proven.

The ability to use human oocytes for research is severely limited and so the development of an animal model for the human would rapidly increase our understanding of the mechanisms underlying successful sperm injection. Given the relative ease with which large numbers of oocytes suitable for injection can be obtained, domestic species ICSI would also serve as a training tool for human ICSI.

Materials and Methods

Oocyte Maturation

Oocytes were recovered from ovaries obtained from local abattoirs. The ovaries were transported to the laboratory at 30–35°C within 2 h of collection. Immature cumulus-oocyte complexes were aspirated from secondary follicles on the ovarian surface with a syringe and 19 G needle. Complexes with contiguous coronal cells were matured in 50 μL-drops of media under paraffin oil at 39°C in an atmosphere of 5% CO_2 in air. The culture medium used was M199 (Sigma, St Louis, MO, USA) supplemented with 10% foetal bovine serum (Cytosystems, Sydney, NSW), 10 mg mL^{-1} follicle stimulating hormone (FSH) (Follitropin-V; Vetrapharm, Melbourne, Australia) and 10 mg mL^{-1} luteinizing hormone (LH) (Lutropin-V; Vetrapharm). Oocytes were matured for 24 h (ovine, bovine) or for 48 h (porcine).

Sperm Preparation

Semen was collected from three rams using an artificial vagina, pooled, diluted 1:20 in HEPES-buffered synthetic oviduct medium (h-SOF) (Tervit et al. 1972) and 20 μL was underlaid beneath 0·5 mL of h-SOF. The sperm were allowed to swim-up for 30 min, before they were diluted 1:1 with 10% polyvinylpyrrolidone (PVP) (PVP-360; Sigma) before injection (Thadani 1980).

Bovine sperm, and in initial experiments porcine sperm, were prepared from frozen semen. A pellet was thawed, washed twice by centrifugation in h-SOF and diluted to 2×10^6 sperm mL^{-1}. This was then mixed with PVP as described above. In a later experiment, fresh boar semen was used, supplied as a commercial extended product. These sperm were allowed to swim-up in small droplets, and motile sperm were recovered from the surface of the droplets and diluted with 10% PVP.

Tool Manufacture

Holding pipettes were made by hand-pulling capillary glass (GC100-15; Clarke Electromedical Instruments, Reading, UK) after heating them in a microburner. The outer diameter (OD) of these pipettes was 150–200 μm and the end of the pipette was heat polished with a microforge to an inner diameter (ID) of 30–80 μm. A bend was introduced 1–2 mm back from the tip of the pipette to allow easy access to the manipulation drop.

Injection pipettes were made by drawing capillary glass (GC100T-15; Clarke Electromedical Instruments) in a P-87 pipette puller (Sutter Instrument Novato, CA, USA). The pull programme was designed to give a two-stage pull, whereby the pipette was slowly tapered to a wisp. The glass was then cut to an OD of 10 μm with a scalpel blade using a dissecting microscope. The end of the pipette was wet ground to an angle of 40–50°. The pipette was immediately washed by aspirating boiling water into it. A similar bend to the holding pipettes was introduced. After manufacture, the pipettes were dry-heat sterilized at 130°C for 12 h.

Micromanipulation

The microinjection techniques in the following series of experiments were all performed by one operator (J.W.C.) with extensive experience in human ICSI. Two Nikon inverted microscopes (Nikon Optical, Tokyo, Japan) were used for micromanipulation, both fitted with micromanipulators (Narishige Instrument, Tokyo, Japan). One was fitted with Nomarski differential interference contrast (DIC) optics and the other with Hoffman optics (Modulation Optics, Greenvale, NY, USA). When the DIC system was used, all manipulation was carried out in plastic dishes with holes cut in the centre and a glass cover slip was glued over the hole. Unmodified plastic dishes were used with Hoffman optics.

Manipulation was carried out in 10-μL droplets of HEPES-buffered M199 under paraffin oil (heavy grade; BDH, Poole, UK). One droplet contained the sperm and the other contained 5 oocytes. The oocytes were stripped of cumulus by vortexing (without aeration) for 30 s. They were placed in the middle of the droplet and moved to the edge after injection to avoid repeated manipulation.

The tools were directly connected to lengths of vinyl tubing which were, in turn, connected to 0·5-mL screw plunger syringes (Hamilton, Reno, NV, USA). The whole system was filled with Fluorinert FC40 (Sigma) and the syringe was used to completely fill the pipettes. The pipettes were lowered into a drop of medium and backfilled with 5 mm of medium. This provided very stable pressures in the pipettes which greatly simplified the injection procedure. A motile spermatozoon was trapped and then swiped, perpendicular to the tail, with the injection pipette. This immobilized the spermatozoon, which was then aspirated tail first into the pipette and held just behind the bevel. The tools were then moved to the droplet containing the oocytes, and an oocyte was aspirated onto the holding pipette. The injection pipette was then inserted into the middle of the oocyte and back pressure was exerted until the cytoplasm moved freely past the spermatozoon in the pipette. The cytoplasm and the spermatozoon were injected into the oocyte and the pipette was removed. This process was repeated until all the oocytes in the droplet had been injected. Oocytes were recovered from the micromanipulating droplet, washed twice and then placed into culture for at least another 16 h.

Sham Injections

Oocytes were sham injected using the same procedure as described above, except that sperm were omitted from the injection pipette.

No Treatment Controls

Matured oocytes were stripped of cumulus and returned to culture for a further 16 h.

In vitro Fertilization (IVF)

Ram and boar sperm were collected after swim-up; the boar sperm medium was supplemented with 5 mM caffeine and 8 mM pyruvate. Sperm (1×10^6) were added to intact cumulus–oocyte complexes (usually 5) in 50-μL droplets under oil. They were then incubated at 39°C in an atmosphere of 5% CO_2 in air.

Fertilization Assessment

After overnight incubation, the oocytes were removed from culture and fixed in acetic acid:ethanol (1:3) on slides, under Vaseline-supported coverslips. After 24 h fixation (48 h for porcine), the oocytes were cleared in absolute ethanol for 30 min and then stained with aceto–orcein (0·25% in 45% acetic acid). The oocytes were then examined using phase contrast microscopy. An oocyte was only considered to be fertilized if two pronuclei and a sperm tail could be seen inside the oocyte. If a sperm tail could not be seen, the oocyte was classified as activated but not fertilized. Penetrated but not activated oocytes were defined as those oocytes that were still at metaphase II but had a sperm within the cytoplasm. Sometimes the sperm head appeared swollen but the oocytes were still classified as

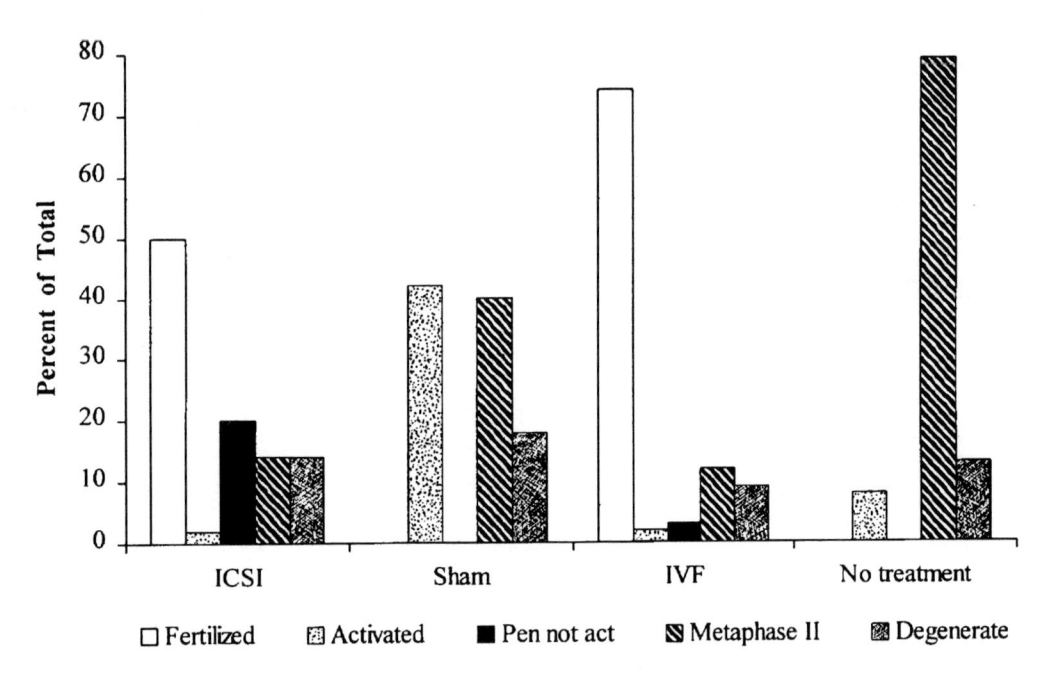

Fig. 1. Results of ovine ICSI and controls using sham injection, conventional IVF and no treatment. 'Pen not act', penetrated but not activated.

penetrated but not activated. Using this method of staining we were unable to distinguish the presence of sperm in degenerate oocytes.

In vitro Culture of Ovine Embryos

Two experiments were conducted to assess the cleavage and developmental potential of ovine oocytes from the treatment groups. Modified SOF medium which was supplemented with 10% human serum (Thompson *et al.* 1992) was used to culture the presumptive zygotes under an atmosphere of 5% O_2, 5% CO_2, 90% N_2. After a further 24 h, cleavage was assessed and embryos were fixed and stained in aceto–orcein.

In vivo Culture of Ovine Embryos

To assess *in vivo* development, both sham and sperm injected oocytes were cultured for 24 h and then transferred to ligated sheep oviducts for 6 days. The oviducts were flushed and the recovered embryos were fixed and stained for assessment.

Results

Fertilization

Ovine. The results are pooled from three replicates with a minimum of 50 oocytes in each treatment group (Fig. 1). For ICSI, there was a penetration rate of 70% (52/75), two-thirds of which (34) showed activation of the oocyte (52% of the total injected). Sham injection of ovine oocytes caused activation in 24/60 oocytes (40%) giving rise to random polar body abstriction and pronuclear formation (Fig. 2). In view of this high activation rate, the assessment of fertilization (after ICSI) was stringent and the presence of a sperm tail within the oocyte cytoplasm was a prerequisite. The activation rate in the no treatment controls was 10% (Fig. 1) indicating that the majority of the activation was a result of the injection process. The IVF control group gave a 70% fertilization rate, indicating that maturation of the oocytes was adequate for fertilization.

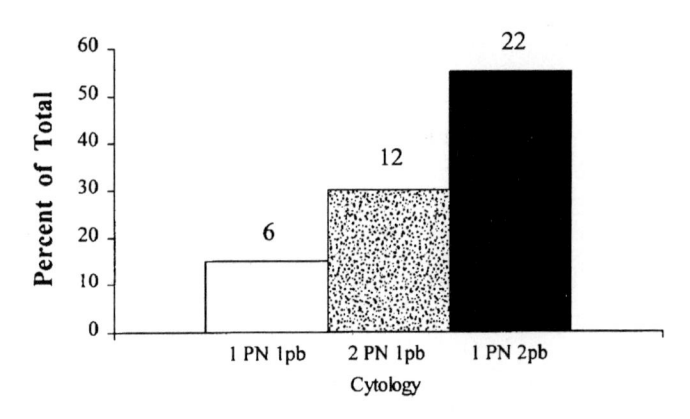

Fig. 2. Cytology of sham-injected, activated ovine oocytes. The figures above the columns are the number of oocytes examined. PN, pronuclei; pb, polar body.

Bovine. Pooled data from two replicates with a minimum of 20 oocytes in each group are presented in Fig. 3. The fertilization rate after ICSI was lower than ovine (25% *v.* 70%), probably reflecting the more technically demanding nature of injection in the bovine. The activation rate was also lower after sham injection or no treatment. In this series of experiments, bovine IVF was not performed as initial results showed that apparently normal fertilization was occurring.

Porcine. The initial results shown in Fig. 4 include three replicates with a minimum of 30 oocytes in each treatment group. Injection of these oocytes was carried out at 37°C with sperm that gave poor IVF results.

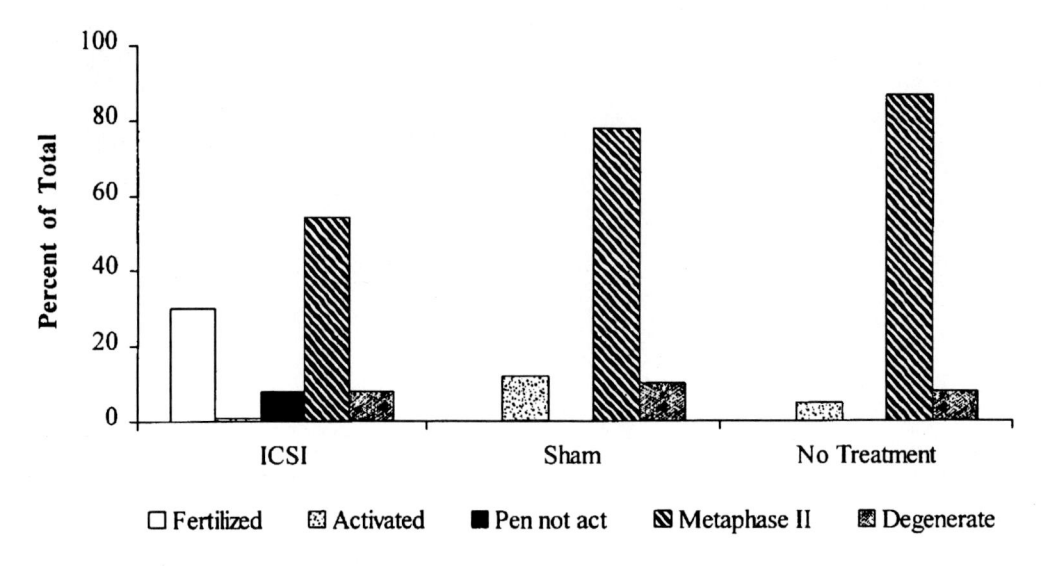

Fig. 3. Results of bovine ICSI and controls using sham injection and no treatment. 'Pen not act', penetrated but not activated.

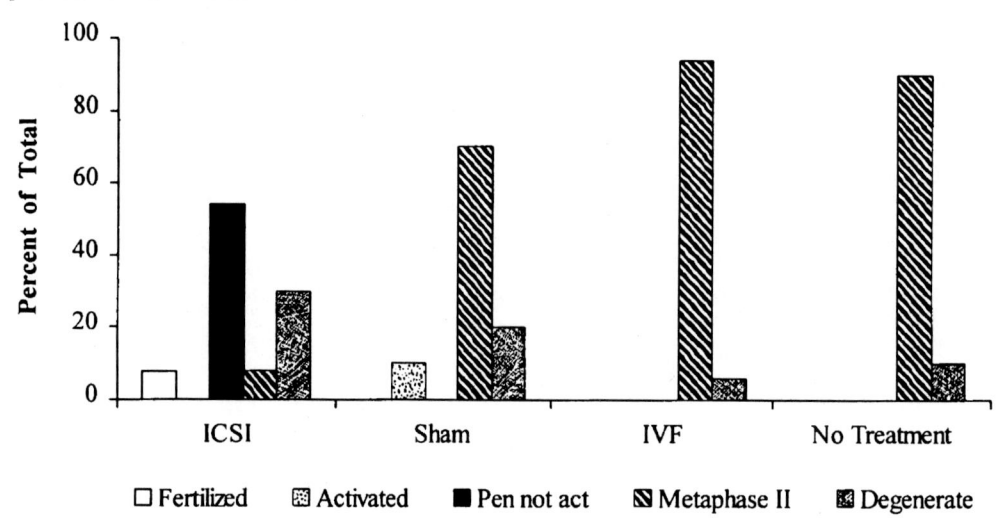

Fig. 4. Cytology of early porcine ICSI experiments, conducted at a restrictive temperature (37°C) with poor quality sperm. 'Pen not act', penetrated but not activated.

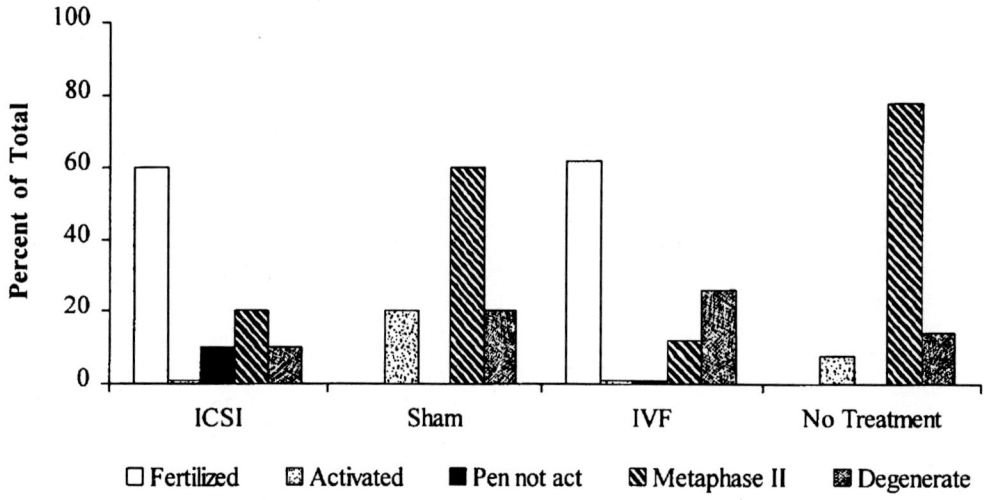

Fig. 5. Results of porcine ICSI conducted at 39°C with fresh, extended sperm. 'Pen not act', penetrated but not activated.

The results indicated that activation subsequent to sperm injection or sham injection was low (10%). Cytological analysis showed that the sperm had penetrated the oocytes but had arrested early in decondensation. The meiotic plates in these oocytes were often disrupted in a manner reminiscent of temperature-induced chromosomal abnormalities. In a further trial, therefore, the injection procedure and subsequent incubation were performed at 39°C and fresh, extended sperm were used. A total of 100 oocytes were used with 25 in each treatment group and the results are shown in Fig. 5. The fertilization rate with ICSI was 60% (15/25), similar to the ovine, but the activation rate after sham injection was similar to bovine (20%, 5/25). The IVF controls gave a fertilization rate of 70% (18/25) indicating that the oocytes were mature.

Ovine in vitro Cleavage

The ability of ovine zygotes to cleave was tested and the early cleavage stages were fixed and stained to ascertain cell and nuclei numbers (Fig. 6). The ICSI fertilization rate was 63% (17/27), and 48% (8/17) of the fertilized oocytes cleaved. The activation rate for the sham injections was 55% (12/21) of which 2 cleaved (17% of those activated). The results suggest that fertilized oocytes are more likely to divide, but more data are needed to confirm this.

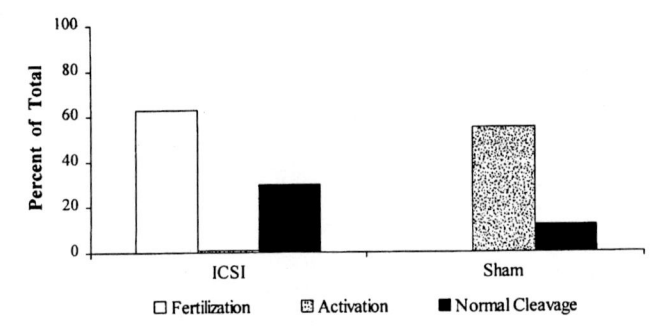

Fig. 6. Fertilization and cleavage of ICSI and sham-injected ovine oocytes *in vitro*.

Ovine in vivo Culture

One embryo transfer experiment was carried out in which 15 zygotes derived from ICSI were transferred to the ligated oviducts of a synchronized ewe recipient, and 13 of them were recovered 6 days later and fixed and stained. One blastocyst (150 cells), two morulae (70 and 27 cells) and three earlier division stages (4–8 cells with fragmentation) were recovered.

Discussion

The preliminary data presented here indicate that a re-assessment of mammalian ICSI is justified. The early work on rodents does not seem to apply to the larger domestic species, in that oocytes from domestics are permissive to microinjection of sperm and early development. There appear to be differences between species, particularly in the ability of oocytes to activate after injection. It has been suggested that in humans, it is not the injection process, but the introduction of the sperm itself that causes oocyte activation (Tesarik *et al.* 1994). This may be the case with the bovine and porcine, but not with ovine oocytes which can apparently activate as a consequence of the injection procedure. Provided that a spermatozoon is injected at the time of activation, then early development is normal. Whether these embryos are fully competent awaits further investigation.

In previous studies with domestic species, oocytes were exogenously activated by electrical or chemical stimuli either prior to or subsequent to sperm injection. Our studies show that induced activation is not a prerequisite for fertilization. This may reflect our treatment of sperm (swiping to damage the tail and induce immobilization) which might release cytoplasmic components which promote fertilization (Swann and Ozil 1994). In previous studies with domestic species, the sperm were either dead or undamaged before injection and these types of sperm give a lower incidence of normal fertilization with human ICSI (Catt *et al.* 1995).

Given that ICSI in domestic species works, then the following uses of the technique must be considered.

(1) Availability of material. The only constraint on the number of oocytes is the amount of time, expertize and money available. Since abattoir-sourced ovaries are essentially waste material, the oocytes are economical and it is ethically sound to use them.

(2) Research. The basis of how and why ICSI works is poorly understood and virtually nothing is known about what happens to the spermatozoon and oocyte in the few hours following sperm injection. Research with human material is of necessity limited, so the use of domestic species should rapidly promote research into the fundamental mechanisms of ICSI.

(3) Training. Most IVF units have found that technical competency with ICSI takes time and experience. ICSI with domestic species is technically similar to human and thus, is suitable as a training tool. Given the constraints in some units, states or countries on the use of human material for either training or producing zygotes not for transfer, then the alternative of using material from domestic species is attractive.

(4) Domestic species. The use of ICSI for domestic species and its potential use in exotic species for conservation should not be overlooked.

There are at least two areas where ICSI is already having a direct impact. One is direct propagation. For example, a premium bull might have excellent characteristics with the exception of poor quality semen. In extreme cases, the semen can be unsuitable for artificial insemination (AI) or even IVF, but ICSI can be successfully used to generate embryos. In such cases, an embryo (let alone a calf) can be worth thousands of dollars so the investment can be commercially viable.

The other current use of ICSI in domestic species is in the testing of X and Y sperm separation techniques. The ability to produce offspring of a defined sex has obvious implications for animal husbandry where exclusively male or female offspring can be advantageous. To date, the only substantiated method of separating (as opposed to enriching) male and female sperm is the use of flow cytometry. The difficulty has been to produce enough viable sperm after separation for use in AI and IVF. This has been achieved in a number of species including rabbits (Johnson et al. 1989; Morrell and Dresser 1989), pigs (Johnson 1991) and cattle (Cran et al. 1993). In our experience, ovine sperm seem to be particularly susceptible to the stresses of flow cytometry and ICSI may be a method to circumvent the problems of sperm survival. The results presented here suggest that ICSI could be used to generate embryos for testing of the methodology. The technology of sperm separation by flow cytometry has been patented and a license has recently been issued (Johnson et al. 1993) to allow its use in humans for eliminating the possibility of X-linked diseases. At present ICSI would be the method of insemination.

In conclusion, the advent of ICSI in humans has enabled us to re-assess the use of ICSI in domestic species. It can and does work, and will enable us to use the technique to further our knowledge of early fertilization events, to use it as a model and teaching aid for human ICSI, and to use it for propagating domestic species.

Acknowledgments

Justine O'Brien and Simon Robinson of the Department of Animal Sciences at Sydney University are thanked for their help and advice on ovine and porcine oocyte culture.

References

Brun, B. (1974). Studies on fertilization in *Xenopus laevis*. *Biol. Reprod.* **11**, 513–8.

Catt, J. W., Ryan, J. P., Pike, I. L, O'Neill, C., and Saunders, D. M. (1995). Clinical intracytoplasmic sperm injection (ICSI) results from Royal North Shore Hospital. In 'Intracytoplasmic Sperm Injection: the Revolution in Male Infertility'. *Reprod. Fertil. Dev.* **7**, 255–62.

Clarke, R. N., Rexroad, C. E., Powell, A. M., and Johnson, L. A. (1988). Microinjection of ram spermatozoa into homologous and heterologous oocytes. *Biol. Reprod.* **38** (Suppl. 1), 75 [Abstr.]

Cran, D. G., Johnson, L. A., Miller, N. G., Cochrane, D., and Polge, C. (1993). Production of bovine calves following separation of X- and Y-chromosome bearing sperm and *in vitro* fertilization. *Vet Rec.* **132**, 40–1.

Goto, K., Kinoshita, A., Takuma, Y., and Ogawa, K. (1990). Fertilisation of bovine oocytes by the injection of immobilised, killed spermatozoa. *Vet. Rec.* **127**, 517–20.

Hiramoto, Y. (1962). Microinjection of the live spermatozoa into sea urchin eggs. *Exp. Cell Res.* **27**, 416–26.

Hosoi, Y., Miyake, M., Utsumi, K., and Iritani, A. (1988). Development of rabbit oocytes after microinjection of spermatozoon. *Proc. 11th Int. Congr. Anim. Reprod. Artif. Insem.* **3**, 331–3.

Johnson, L. A. (1991). Sex selection in swine: altered sex ratios in offspring following surgical insemination of flow sorted X- and Y-bearing sperm. *Reprod. Dom. Animal.* **26**, 309–14.

Johnson, L. A., Flook, J. P., and Hawk, H. W. (1989). Sex preselection in rabbits: live births from X and Y sperm separated by DNA and cell sorting. *Biol. Reprod.* **41**, 199–203.

Johnson, L. A., Welch, G. R., Keyvanfar, K., Dorfmann, A., Fugger, E. F., and Schulman, J. D. (1993). Gender preselection in humans? Flow cytometric separation of X and Y spermatozoa for the prevention of X-linked diseases. *Hum. Reprod. (Oxf.)* **8**, 1733–9.

Keefer, C. L., Younis, A. I., and Brackett, B. G. (1990). Cleavage development of bovine oocytes fertilized by sperm injection. *Mol. Reprod. Dev.* **25**, 281–5.

Markert, C. L. (1983). Fertilization of mammalian eggs by sperm injection. *J. Exp. Zool.* **228**, 195–201.

Morrell, J. M., and Dresser, D. W. (1989). Offspring from inseminations with mammalian sperm stained with Hoechst 33342, either with or without flow cytometry. *Mutat. Res.* **224**, 177–83.

Payne, D., and Matthews, C. D. (1995). Intracytoplasmic sperm injection — clinical results from the Reproductive Medicine Unit, Adelaide. In 'Intracytoplasmic Sperm Injection: the Revolution in Male Infertility'. *Reprod. Fertil. Dev.* **7**, 219–27.

Roknabadi, G. A., Ng, S.-C., Liow, S. L., Bongso, A., and Ratnam S. S. (1994). Intracytoplasmic sperm injection in mouse. *Proc. 13th Ann. Meet. Fertil. Soc. Aust.*, MP116 [Abstr.]

Swann, K., and Ozil, J.-P. (1994). Dynamics of the calcium signal that triggers mammalian egg activation. *Int. Rev. Cytol.* **152**, 183–222.

Tervit, H. R., Whittingham, D. G., and Rowson, L. E. A. (1972). Successful culture, *in vitro*, of sheep and cattle ova. *J. Reprod. Fertil.* **30**, 493–7.

Tesarik, J., Sousa, M., and Testart, J. (1994). Human oocyte activation after intracytoplasmic sperm injection. *Hum. Reprod. (Oxf.)* **9**, 511–8.

Thadani, V. M. (1980). A study of hetero-specific sperm-egg interactions in the rat, mouse and deer mouse using *in vitro* fertilization and sperm injection. *J. Exp. Zool.* **212**, 435–53.

Thompson, J. G., Simpson, A. C., Pugh, P. A., and Tervit, H. R. (1992). *In vitro* development of early sheep embryos is superior in medium supplemented with human serum compared with sheep serum or human serum albumin. *Anim. Reprod. Sci.* **29**, 61–8.

Uehara, T., and Yanagamachi, R. (1976). Microsurgical injection of spermatozoa into hamster eggs with subsequent transformation of sperm nuclei into male pronuclei. *Biol. Reprod.* **15**, 467–70.

Van Steirteghem, A. C., Liu, J., Joris, H., Nagy, Z., Janssenswillen, C., Tournaye, H., Derde, M.-P., Van Assche, E., and Devroey, P. (1993*a*). Higher success rate by intracytoplasmic sperm injection than by subzonal insemination. Report of a second series of 300 consecutive treatment cycles. *Hum. Reprod. (Oxf.)* **8**, 1055–60.

Van Steirteghem, A. C., Nagy, Z., Joris, H., Liu, J., Staessen, C., Smitz, J., Wisanto, A., and Devroey, P. (1993*b*). High fertilization and implantation rates after intracytoplasmic injection. *Hum. Reprod. (Oxf.)* **8**, 1061–6.

Manuscript received 3 February 1995

Open Discussion

Alan Trounson (Melbourne):

We produce blastocysts in cattle by parthenogenetic activation and they all look as good as the blastocysts that you showed. You would have to do chromosomal studies with fluorescence *in situ* hybridization (FISH) to show that you actually have embryos that are not parthenogenetic.

Catt:

We can get early fertilization events but we haven't done embryo transfers yet so we're aren't sure of developmental competence.

Trounson:

We've produced many blastocysts from ICSI in cattle, but we're looking to make sure that they have a component of the male genome before we do any transfers.

Robert Edwards (Cambridge):

Did you use a high calcium concentration in the medium when you injected the sham operated oocytes?

Catt:

We tried high calcium, low calcium and no calcium, but we haven't seen any effect of calcium concentration in the experiments to date.

Edwards:

So the injection pipette activates the egg and gives it a calcium stimulus?

Catt:

I believe so.

Simon Fishel (Nottingham):

Do you see any differences in cleavage morphology between 2 pronuclear oocytes with one polar body and the normally fertilized ones? Could you distinguish them on that basis?

Catt:

No, in the ovine system it's very difficult. In early cleavage stage ovine embryos, it is very difficult to tell cleavage from fragmentation.

Trounson:

I think you can tell clearly *in vitro* whether you've got good embryos or not, using basically the same criteria as those for mice or humans.

Catt:

At the time of compaction and blastocyst formation the embryos look good, but not at the early stages.

Intracytoplasmic Sperm Injection (ICSI) *versus* High Insemination Concentration (HIC) for Human Conception *in vitro*

Simon Fishel [ABC], Franco Lisi [B], Leonardo Rinaldi [B], Rosella Lisi [B], Judy Timson [A], Steven Green [A], Jenny Hall [A], Steven Fleming [A], Alison Hunter [A], Ken Dowell [A] and Simon Thornton [A]

[A] NURTURE (Nottingham University Research and Treatment Unit in Reproduction), Department of Obstetrics and Gynaecology, Queen's Medical Centre, Nottingham NG7 2UH, UK.
[B] BIOGENESI, Clinica Europa, Viale Euphrate, 27, Eur, 00144 Roma 3, Italy.
[C] To whom correspondence should be addressed.

Abstract. The use of high insemination concentration (HIC) for *in vitro* fertilization (IVF) was compared with intracytoplasmic sperm injection (ICSI) in cases of male factor infertility. Sibling oocytes ($n = 252$) from 24 patients were used, 123 for HIC and 129 for ICSI. Although the incidence of fertilization was decreased with HIC (48% v. 61%), this treatment was nevertheless a viable option for many patients, especially when ICSI was not available. However, there was a higher incidence of cytoplasmic fragmentation of embryos after HIC compared with ICSI (36% v. 10%, $P = 0.003$) and the outcome was significantly affected by the severity of teratozoospermia. Using a cut-off of 5% normal forms, the incidence of fertilization with HIC for the group with < 5% normal forms was 37% compared with 72% for the group with > 5% normal forms; there was also a significant decrease in cleavage rate ($P = 0.05$) and the number of regular embryos ($P = 0.005$), and an increase in cytoplasmic fragmentation ($P = 0.006$) in patients with < 5% normal forms. No distinction was made between cases of teratozoospermia when ICSI was used. The present study confirms the value of HIC as a first line treatment for male infertility, as long as ICSI remains significantly more expensive and concerns on safety are mooted. However, the use of sibling oocytes for ICSI is recommended, especially in cases with < 5% normal sperm morphology.

Extra keywords: IVF, sperm morphology.

Introduction

Conventional *in vitro* fertilization (IVF) has been modified and refined to achieve increased rates of conception in cases of male factor infertility. Methods such as high insemination concentration (HIC), microdrop IVF (mIVF) and a combination of these two approaches are the most readily utilized techniques aside from microinjection. The first observation that IVF, either conventional IVF or HIC, was useful for treating oligozoospermia and oligoasthenozoospermia was reported by Fishel and Edwards (1982). This was followed by a series of publications indicating the value of IVF in such cases (Edwards *et al*. 1984; Cohen *et al*. 1985). Recently it has been documented that HIC, in cases of previously failed IVF, and combinations of HIC and mIVF in cases where there are too few spermatozoa for conventional IVF, can result in successful conception *in vitro* and the delivery of healthy offspring (Baker *et al*. 1993; Fishel *et al*. 1993; Tucker *et al*. 1993). However, the recent advent of micromanipulation and, in particular, the most successful of these techniques, intracytoplasmic sperm injection (ICSI), has overshadowed the use of these modified IVF insemination procedures (Palermo *et al*. 1992, 1993).

Before the introduction of ICSI, partial zona dissection (PZD) had become controversial and was subsequently abandoned by many workers (Fishel *et al*. 1993; Tucker *et al*. 1993), and subzonal insemination (SUZI) only produced relatively low fertilization rates (Fishel *et al*. 1992, 1993, 1994*a*, 1994*b*). A number of practitioners still found value in using HIC, however, this procedure was not well defined with insemination concentrations of $0.5-5 \times 10^6$ mL^{-1} being utilized. The literature is also unclear and ambiguous with regard to the impact of teratozoospermia on HIC results. Some reports indicated a significant reduction in the incidence of fertilization and implantation with very severe teratozoospermia (< 5% normal forms) (Baker *et al*. 1993; Fishel *et al*.

1994a), and the implantation rate in such cases remains a moot point. Furthermore, a recent report by Ombelet et al. (1994) demonstrated a total failure of implantation with < 5% normal forms, which is in contrast to other studies (Cohen et al. 1992; Fishel et al. 1994a).

The present study evaluated the usefulness of HIC and compared it with ICSI. The results presented in this paper have also been submitted for publication elsewhere.

Materials and Methods

Patients

For the sibling oocyte study, patients were by necessity included when there were enough motile sperm available to attempt HIC. By definition, these patients had failed conventional IVF, either on two previous occasions, or on a single occasion in which there was no binding of sperm to the zona pellucida. In all cases, however, the patients were actually referred for ICSI and HIC was offered as an option on some of the oocytes.

Ovarian Stimulation

All female partners underwent pituitary desensitization with gonadotrophin-releasing hormone analogue (Suprefact; Hoechst AG, Frankfurt, Germany) for a minimum of 4 weeks before follicular stimulation with human menopausal gonadotrophin (Pergonal; Serono, Aubonne, Switzerland or Humegon; Organon, Oss, The Netherlands) followed by 10 000 I.U. of human chorionic gonadotrophin (Profasi; Serono). Oocytes were aspirated 36 h later by transvaginal ultrasound-guided retrieval.

Preparation of Spermatozoa for ICSI

Semen samples were centrifuged initially on a discontinuous Percoll (Sigma, Poole, Dorset, UK) gradient (45%, 90%) at 500g for 10 min. The sperm pellet was carefully removed and resuspended with culture medium, and then centrifuged at 250g for 5 min. The supernatant was removed and the pellet was resuspended in ~1 mL of Earle's minimal essential medium (MEM) supplemented with 25 mM HEPES (Sigma) and 4·5% (w/v) human serum albumin (HSA). Just before ICSI, the sperm suspension was centrifuged in a microfuge at 1800g for 6 min in sterile Eppendorf microfuge tubes (Labosystems UK, Basingstoke, UK). The supernatant was removed and, depending on the concentration of spermatozoa, the pellet was resuspended in a minimum of 5 μL of MEM.

Preparation of Spermatozoa for HIC

Sperm for HIC were prepared as described above but with the following changes. After centrifugation at 250g, the sperm pellet was resuspended in approximately 1 mL of Earle's balanced salt solution containing 10% (v/v) serum (EBSS). The sperm concentration was adjusted with EBSS to ~1·0×10^6 motile sperm mL^{-1} for insemination. In some cases it was necessary to use as little as 0·2 mL to obtain the correct concentration. This medium was then gassed with 5% CO_2 in air and equilibrated at 37°C before insemination. The insemination droplet was routinely 0·2 mL, which is identical to our conventional IVF procedures.

Preparation of Oocytes and Insemination

Before ICSI, the oocyte was transferred to HEPES-buffered MEM culture medium containing 80 I.U. mL^{-1} of hyaluronidase. The oocyte-cumulus complex was maintained in the hyaluronidase for a maximum of 1 min, after which the oocyte and its attendant corona radiata cells were removed and washed through HEPES-buffered MEM before mechanical removal of the corona cells using finely-pulled, sterile Pasteur pipettes. The ICSI procedure has been described in detail elsewhere (Fishel et al. 1995).

For the HIC procedure, oocytes were maintained in their cumulus mass, and only those with an expanded cumulus and corona radiata were utilized. A maximum of two oocyte-cumulus complexes were inseminated in each 0·2-mL droplet. No differences in results have been observed that bear any relationship to either the volume of the insemination concentration or the presence of one or two cumulus masses (Fishel, unpublished data).

Once the eggs had undergone ICSI, the culture conditions were identical for the HIC and ICSI oocytes. Culturing was performed in drops under paraffin oil as described previously (Fishel and Jackson 1986; Fishel et al. 1994a). The incidence of fertilization was calculated according to the number of metaphase-II oocytes observed at the time of pronuclear scoring; this is consistent with the use of only metaphase-II oocytes for ICSI.

Statistical Analysis

Differences in the incidence of fertilization in the sibling oocyte study were evaluated using the χ^2-test for comparison between groups.

Results

Case Report

The couple JT and ST aged 31 (female) and 35 (male) were referred after four years of primary infertility. Thorough examination of the female revealed little. In contrast, the male had a follicle-stimulating hormone (FSH) concentration of 12·0 I.U. L^{-1} with a first semen assessment demonstrating a volume of 3·5 mL, a sperm concentration of 1×10^6 sperm mL^{-1} and 50% sperm motility; a repeat ejaculate at a later date showed azoospermia. The couple were referred for IVF using donor sperm and/or ICSI — they had previously completed four cycles of donor insemination (DI).

Thirteen metaphase-II oocytes were obtained by transvaginal ultrasound-guided retrieval. On the day of oocyte collection, the husband's semen sample contained a total count of 1·8×10^6 motile sperm. The sperm were prepared by Percoll gradient centrifugation and, after further centrifugation, were finally resuspended at the insemination concentration in 0·4 mL. Nine of the oocytes underwent ICSI and four underwent HIC at a concentration of 1·0×10^6 sperm mL^{-1}. The four oocyte-cumulus complexes were inseminated in two 0·2-mL droplets. Five of the ICSI oocytes underwent fertilization (56%), whereas all 4 of the HIC oocytes fertilized (100%). On the following day, at embryo transfer, there were 6 Grade-1 embryos (no cytoplasmic fragments, smooth blastomere membranes), 4 from HIC and 2 from ICSI. Three Grade-1 HIC embryos were transferred at the 4-cell stage, and 3 supernumerary embryos (2 from ICSI and 1 from HIC) were cryopreserved at the 4-cell stage. The remaining embryos were not suitable for freezing after a further 24 h in culture. According to our routine policy, this patient was maintained on a daily dose of

50 mg Gestone administered intramuscularly, and at the time of writing had an ongoing singleton pregnancy at 29 weeks.

Many such anecdotal cases exist and a number of uncontrolled studies have reported the value of HIC (Table 1). Controlled, sibling oocyte studies comparing HIC and ICSI are difficult to perform for clinical reasons—we have attempted to study the efficacy of HIC versus ICSI in 24 patients in whom the trial was clinically reasonable and acceptable to the patients.

Table 1. High insemination concentration (HIC) versus intracytoplasmic sperm injection (ICSI)
From Tucker et al. (1993). ET, embryo transfer

	HIC	ICSI
No. of oocytes	356	251
No. of fertilized oocytes	177	47
Fertilization rate	52%	19%
No. of ETs	23	15
Viable pregnancies	12	3
Viable pregnancy rate per ET	52%	20%

Table 2. High insemination concentration (HIC) versus intracytoplasmic sperm injection (ICSI) sibling oocyte study (24 patients)
M II, metaphase II

	HIC	ICSI
No. of cycles with fertilization	17 (71%)	22 (92%)
No. of M II oocytes	123	129
No. of fertilized oocytes (fertilization rate)[A]	59 (48%)	79 (61%)
No. of cleaved embryos[B]	45 (76%)	70 (89%)
No. of regular embryos[C,D]	22 (49%)	59 (84%)
No. of Grade 2/3 embryos[D]	16 (36%)[E]	7 (10%)[E]

[A] No three-pronuclear oocytes were produced in this study.
[B] Values in parentheses are percentages of the fertilized oocytes.
[C] Regular blastomeres with < 25% perivitelline fragments.
[D] Values in parentheses are percentages of the cleaved embryos.
[E] χ^2-test, HIC versus ICSI, $P = 0.003$.

HIC versus ICSI—Sibling Oocyte Study

In these patients, the HIC insemination concentration was maintained at $\sim 1.0 \times 10^6$ motile sperm mL^{-1} even in cases of extreme teratozoospermia. Overall, 17 of the 24 patients (71%) achieved fertilization with HIC whereas 22 (92%) achieved fertilization with ICSI. In all of the 17 patients who achieved fertilization with HIC, at least one oocyte was fertilized after ICSI.

Table 2 demonstrates the fertilization and cleavage rates as well as the cleavage morphology in those oocytes undergoing HIC compared with those undergoing ICSI. No three-pronuclear zygotes were observed in this study, hence all the fertilized oocytes had only two pronuclei. The fertilization rate was calculated as the number of fertilized oocytes divided by the number of metaphase-II oocytes. Degenerate oocytes ($n = 19$) and one-pronuclear oocytes ($n = 5$) were counted as failed fertilization. The data demonstrate a trend towards a higher fertilization rate and cleavage rate with ICSI, and a significantly higher incidence of cytoplasmic fragmentation in those embryos inseminated with HIC compared with ICSI ($P = 0.003$).

It is difficult to make an overall observation on pregnancy outcome in this study because, of the 22 patients undergoing embryo transfer, 16 had a mixture of HIC and ICSI embryos transferred. In addition, 3 patients had only HIC embryos transferred and a further 3 had only ICSI embryos transferred. Two of the 3 who had HIC embryos transferred have ongoing pregnancies, whereas 1 of the 3 patients who had only ICSI embryos transferred now has an ongoing pregnancy. Overall, there were 9 ongoing pregnancies (41%).

Effect of Teratozoospermia on HIC and ICSI

The data from the sibling oocyte trial were further subdivided into two groups, those with < 5% normal forms and those with > 5% normal forms (according to Kruger strict criteria; Hall et al. 1993). Table 3 demonstrates the tendency towards a reduced HIC fertilization rate (37%) in patients with < 5% normal forms compared

Table 3. High insemination concentration (HIC) versus intracytoplasmic sperm injection (ICSI)—effect of sperm morphology

	< 5% normal forms		> 5% normal forms	
	HIC	ICSI	HIC	ICSI
No. of oocytes	84	86	39	43
No. of fertilized oocytes	31 (37%)	50 (58%)	28 (72%)	29 (67%)
No. of cleaved embryos[A]	20 (65%)[B]	45 (90%)	25 (89%)[B]	25 (86%0
No. of regular embryos[C,D]	6 (30%)[E]	38 (84%)	19 (76%)[E]	21 (84%)
No. of Grade 2/3 embryos[D]	12 (60%)[F]	5 (11%)	4 (16%)[F]	2 (8%)

[A] Values in parentheses are percentages of the fertilized oocytes.
[B] χ^2-test; HIC, < 5% normal forms versus > 5% normal forms, $P = 0.05$.
[C] Regular blastomeres with < 25% perivitelline fragments.
[D] Values in parentheses are percentages of the cleaved embryos.
[E] χ^2-test; HIC, < 5% normal forms versus > 5% normal forms, $P = 0.005$.
[F] χ^2-test; HIC, < 5% normal forms versus > 5% normal forms, $P = 0.006$.

with those with > 5% normal forms (72%). There was no difference in the incidence of fertilization between the two groups when ICSI was used (58% v. 67%).

Patients with < 5% normal forms had a significantly reduced incidence of cleavage and compromised cleavage morphology following HIC (Table 3), which was not observed in the ICSI oocytes. Because of the mixed transfer of HIC and ICSI embryos, it was not possible to distinguish between the effect of the two morphology groups on implantation and pregnancy rates with HIC and ICSI.

Discussion

This study confirms the value of HIC for treating cases of compromised semen quality. However, we did not evaluate different high sperm insemination concentrations (from 1×10^6 to 5×10^6 sperm mL^{-1}).

In a recent report, Tucker et al. (1993) compared HIC, SUZI and ICSI in cases with previous fertilization failure or severe male factor infertility. Their data showed a 52% fertilization rate per oocyte with HIC compared with only 17% and 19% with SUZI and ICSI respectively. The viable pregnancy rates per cycle were 36%, 12·5% and 20% for HIC, SUZI and ICSI respectively (see Table 1). They commented that HIC 'can be used in many instances very successfully as a front line treatment for potential fertilization failure'.

Ord et al. (1993) utilized HIC in patients who had a total motile sperm count of $< 5 \times 10^6$ in the pre-treatment sample. Eighty percent of the patients achieved fertilization and the overall fertilization rate was 38%. Twenty-three clinical pregnancies were achieved at a pregnancy rate of 43% per embryo transfer. They divided the patients into two groups depending on the pre-treatment concentration of sperm; Group I had a total motile sperm count of $1 \cdot 5 - 5 \times 10^6$, whereas Group II had a total motile sperm count of $< 1 \cdot 5 \times 10^6$. The fertilization rates per oocyte were 54% and 25% for Groups I and II, respectively, and the take-home baby rates were 35% and 19% respectively. Their study also included 28 patients who had experienced previous failure of fertilization in one or more IVF cycles. Overall, 89% of these patients achieved fertilization and 36% (8) achieved a clinical pregnancy. Unfortunately, the reports by Ord et al. (1993), Tucker et al. (1993) and Wiker et al. (1993) did not comment on the effect of sperm morphology on HIC outcome.

A study by Ombelet et al. (1994) examined the effect of teratozoospermia on in vitro fertilization. Sperm morphology was scored according to very strict criteria (Kruger et al. 1987; Menkveld et al. 1990). The authors quoted an unpublished study which indicated a clear threshold for fertilization at 9% normal forms when using $0 \cdot 1 \times 10^6$ sperm mL^{-1} per oocyte for insemination. Their data indicated that a 'normal' fertilization rate was restored in cases with 'moderate teratozoospermia' (5–8% normal forms) using an insemination concentration of $0 \cdot 5 \times 10^6$ sperm mL^{-1} per oocyte, but this increased number of sperm did not restore the fertilization rate if the sperm morphology was < 5% normal forms. This approach had been previously suggested by Oehninger et al. (1988) who restored fertilization and pregnancy rates in patients with severe sperm morphology abnormalities.

The study by Ombelet et al. (1994) demonstrated fertilization rates per oocyte of 37·9%, 78·6% and 79·4% for < 5%, 5–8% and > 8% normal forms respectively; hence, there was a significant reduction at the 5% cut-off. However, the pregnancy rates per cycle were 0% ($n = 12$), 15·8% ($n = 38$) and 42% ($n = 50$) for < 5%, 5–8% and > 8% normal forms, respectively, with take-home baby rates of 0%, 13·0% and 38·9% respectively. They concluded that a relationship existed between embryo quality and the degree of morphological 'normality' of the sperm in the semen. Although there was no physiological explanation for this, they suggested that there may be an influence of the paternal genome on the proliferation of extra-embryonic tissue (Hilscher 1991).

Baker et al. (1993) stated that their fertilization rate for patients with < 20% normal forms 'approximately doubled' by using HIC at concentrations of $0 \cdot 2 - 1 \cdot 0 \times 10^6$ sperm mL^{-1}. They also reported that, in contrast to the study of Oehninger et al. (1988), they could find no evidence for an increase in adverse pregnancy outcome, with a viable pregnancy rate of 14%. However, many researchers would not accept < 20% normal forms as a significant cut-off. A clearer indication seems to be < 14% with Kruger strict criteria or even < 9% (Ombelet et al. 1994). Baker et al. (1993) reported that in those patients with < 5% normal forms (or a sperm concentration of $< 5 \times 10^5$ mL^{-1}), 'on average about 40% of the treatments had low (< 20%) or zero fertilization rates'. However, it is difficult to interpret such claims without clear randomized controlled studies and adequately defined criteria.

There is inconsistency between the observed pregnancy rate after embryo transfer in patients exhibiting < 5% normal morphology when HIC is utilized (Ombelet et al. 1994) compared with micro-assisted fertilization (Cohen et al. 1992; Fishel et al. 1993, 1994b). The latter studies showed viable pregnancy rates in patients with extremely severe teratozoospermia (0–5% normal forms) and this phenomenon is being observed more frequently now with ICSI (Palermo et al. 1995; Payne and Matthews 1995; Tournaye et al. 1995). The interesting observation by Cohen et al. (1992) that implantation was only compromised in cases of severe teratozoospermia when PZD was utilized, but not SUZI, indicates an iatrogenic effect. We observed a similar effect in our unit. We propose that the defects observed in embryo quality in the present study might be due to the high concentration of motile sperm, immotile sperm and other seminal debris present in the insemination medium, rather than the genetic composition of the fertilizing spermatozoon *per se*. This is also a more likely explanation for the findings of Ombelet *et al.* (1994).

Our policy is consistent with that of Tucker *et al.* (1993) and Baker *et al.* (1993) in that 'the main aim should always be to use the simplest and least expensive procedures.....with the greatest long-term chance of healthy children.' Tucker *et al.* (1993) advocated the use of ICSI in preference to HIC only when the latter has failed or the number of available sperm was limited or when prior significant fertilization failure has occurred. Baker *et al.* (1993) go further and caution the use of ICSI since we are ignorant of the underlying cause of the impairment in spermatogenesis, and 'male infertility may be associated with germ-cell mutations, (and) DNA mutations in sperm may transmit heritable characteristics — including susceptibility to infertility — expressed in future generations.'

Conclusions

From this study, as well as data gleaned from other published studies, it is clear that HIC can produce viable pregnancies for couples with severely compromised semen characteristics and/or significant previous IVF failure, even in cases of < 5% normal forms. However, in men with < 5% normal sperm morphology, decreased fertilization and embryo viability may result and this, in turn, would be consistent with a lower incidence of pregnancy. In such cases, ICSI would be a better option overall, taking into consideration expense and safety. When concerns about the safety of ICSI are fully allayed and its cost can be brought in line with conventional IVF, then ICSI is likely to become the first line option. Despite concerns that 'ICSI may beget ICSI', it might actually be the method of choice for all cases of IVF in the future.

Currently, however, we recommend that in cases of < 5% normal sperm morphology, ICSI should be used initially unless enough eggs are harvested to attempt a combination of ICSI and HIC. In cases with > 5% normal sperm, HIC is a viable treatment option if the cohort of oocytes is too small to split. In those patients who achieve fertilization with HIC, ICSI becomes unnecessary in subsequent cycles.

Acknowledgments

We fully acknowledge the support of our other colleagues in this study, Drs Atillia Floccari, George Ndukwe, A. Solomonsz, Saad Al-Hassan and M. Aloum. We also gratefully acknowledge the technical support of Helen McDermott and the excellent assistance of Rosie Metcalf in putting the manuscript together.

References

Baker, H.W.G., Liu, D.Y., Bourne, H., and Lopata, A. (1993). Diagnosis of sperm defects in selecting patients for assisted fertilization. *Hum. Reprod. (Oxf.)* **8**, 1779–80.

Cohen, J., Edwards, R.G., Fehilly, C., Fishel, S., Hewitt, J., Purdy, J., Rowland, G., Steptoe, P., and Webster, J. (1985). In vitro fertilization: a treatment for male infertility. *Fertil. Steril.* **43**, 422–32.

Cohen, J., Alikani, M., Adler, A., Berkeley, A., Davis, O., Ferrara, T., Graf, M., Grifo, J., Liu, H.C., Malter, H.E., Reing, A., Suzman, M., Talansky, B.E., and Rosenwaks, Z. (1992). Microsurgical fertilization procedures: the absence of stringent criteria for patient selection. *J. Assist. Reprod. Genet.* **9**, 197–206.

Edwards, R.G., Fishel, S.B., Cohen, J., Fehilly, C.B., Purdy, J.M., Slater, J.M., Steptoe, P.C., and Webster, J.M. (1984). Factors influencing the success of *in vitro* fertilization for alleviating human infertility. *J. In Vitro Fertil. Emb. Transfer* **1**, 3–23.

Fishel, S.B., and Edwards, R.G. (1982). Essentials of fertilisation. In 'Human Conception *in vitro*'. (Eds R.G. Edwards and J.M. Purdy.) pp. 193–5. (Academic Press: London.)

Fishel, S., and Jackson, P. (1986). Preparation for human *in vitro* fertilisation in the laboratory. In '*In vitro* Fertilisation, Past, Present and Future'. (Eds S.B. Fishel, and E.M. Symonds.) pp. 77–87. (IRL Press: Oxford.)

Fishel, S., Timson, J., Lisi, F., and Rinaldi, L. (1992). Evaluation of 225 patients undergoing subzonal insemination for the procurement of fertilization *in vitro*. *Fertil. Steril.* **57**, 840–9.

Fishel, S., Dowell, K., Timson, J., Green, S., Hall, J., and Klentzeris, L. (1993). Micro-assisted fertilization with human gametes. *Hum. Reprod. (Oxf.)* **8**, 1780–4.

Fishel, S., Timson, J., Lisi, F., Jacobsen, M., Rinaldi, L., and Globetz, L. (1994a). Micro-assisted fertilization in patients who have failed subzonal insemination. *Hum. Reprod. (Oxf.)* **9**, 501–5.

Fishel, S., Dowell, K., Lisi, F., and Rinaldi, L. (1994b). Subzonal insemination and zona breaching techniques for assisting conception *in vitro*. *Baillière's Clin. Obstet. Gynaecol.* **8**, 65–84.

Fishel, S., Lisi, F., Rinaldi, L., Green, S., Hunter, A., Dowell, K., and Thornton, S. (1995). Systematic examination of immobilising spermatozoa before intracytoplasmic sperm injection in the human. *Hum. Reprod. (Oxf.)* **10**. (In press.)

Hall, J.A., Fishel, S.B., and Timson, J. (1993). Evaluation of human sperm morphology in relation to conventional *in-vitro* fertilization (IVF) and micro-assisted fertilization (MAF). *Hum. Reprod. (Oxf.)* **8** (Suppl. 1), 90. [Abstr.]

Hilscher, W. (1991). The genetic control and germ cell kinetics of the female and male germ line in mammals including man. *Hum. Reprod. (Oxf.)* **6**, 1416–25.

Kruger, T.F., Acosta, A.A., Simmons, K.F., Swanson, R.J., Matta, J.F., Veeck, L.L., Morshedi, M., and Brugo, S. (1987). New method of evaluating sperm morphology with predictive value for human *in vitro* fertilization. *Urology* **30**, 248–51.

Menkveld, R., Stander, F.S.H., Kotze, T.J.W., Kruger, T.F., and van Zyl, J.A. (1990). The evaluation of morphological characteristics of human spermatozoa according to stricter criteria. *Hum. Reprod. (Oxf.)* **5**, 586–92.

Oehninger, S., Acosta, A.A., Morshedi, M., Veeck, L., Swanson, R.J., Simmons, K., and Rosenwaks, Z. (1988). Corrective measures and pregnancy outcome in *in vitro* fertilization in patients with severe sperm morphology abnormalities. *Fertil. Steril.* **50**, 283–7.

Ombelet, W., Fourie, F. le R., Vandeput, H., Bosmans, E., Cox, A., Janssen, M., and Kruger, T. (1994). Teratozoospermia and *in vitro* fertilization; a randomized prospective study. *Hum. Reprod. (Oxf.)* **9**, 1479–84.

Ord, T., Patrizio, P., Balmaceda, J.P., and Asch, R.H. (1993). Can severe male factor infertility be treated without micromanipulation? *Fertil. Steril.* **60**, 110–15.

Palermo, G., Joris, H., Devroey, P., and Van Steirteghem, A.C. (1992). Pregnancies after intracytoplasmic injection of single spermatozoon into an oocyte. *Lancet* **340**, 17–18.

Palermo, G., Joris, H., Derde, M.-P., Camus, M., Devroey, P., and Van Steirteghem, A. (1993). Sperm characteristics and outcome of human assisted fertilization by subzonal insemination and intracytoplasmic sperm injection. *Fertil. Steril.* **59**, 826–35.

Palermo, G. D., Cohen, J., Alikani, M., Adler, A., and Rosenwaks, Z. (1995). Development and implementation of intracytoplasmic sperm injection (ICSI). In 'Intracytoplasmic Sperm Injection: the Revolution in Male Infertility'. *Reprod. Fertil. Dev.* **7**, 211–18.

Payne, D., and Matthews, C. D. (1995). Intracytoplasmic sperm injection—clinical results from the Reproductive Medicine Unit, Adelaide. In 'Intracytoplasmic Sperm Injection: the Revolution in Male Infertility'. *Reprod. Fertil. Dev.* **7**, 219–27.

Tournaye, H., Liu, J., Nagy, Z., Joris, H., Wisanto, A., Bonduelle, M., Van der Elst, J., Staessen, C., Smitz, J., Silber, S., Devroey, P., Liebaers, I., and Van Steirteghem, A. (1995). Intracytoplasmic sperm injection: the Brussels experience. In 'Intracytoplasmic Sperm Injection: the Revolution in Male Infertility'. *Reprod. Fertil. Dev.* **7**, 269–79.

Tucker, M., Wiker, S., and Massey, J. (1993). Rational approach to assisted fertilization. *Hum. Reprod. (Oxf.)* **8**, 1778.

Wiker, S.R., Tucker, M.J., Wright, G., Malter, H.E., Kort, H.I., and Massey, J.B. (1993). Repeated sperm injection under the zona following initial fertilization failure. *Hum. Reprod. (Oxf.)* **8**, 467–9.

Manuscript received 10 April 1995

Open Discussion

Colin Matthews (Adelaide):

I think you have raised some important points about the number of sperm inseminated. It is very interesting that, although pregnancies were generated, there seems to be reduced embryo quality when excess sperm were used. Do you think that in routine IVF we might be producing poorer embryos given the number of sperm used for inseminating oocytes?

Fishel:

I think that is a very important point, because the concentration of sperm that we use in conventional IVF is non-physiological. We are probably getting as high if not a higher quality of embryo from ICSI.

Sherman Silber (St Louis):

When you see a whole field of morphologically abnormal sperm, do you select the best sperm or do you think that if we inject exclusively sperm with the poorest morphology, we will get the same results?

Fishel:

When you're sitting at the microscope and you have a choice, you always go for the 'best looking' sperm. However, I am not convinced that it makes any difference at all, and what really matters at the end of the day is technique. Nevertheless, we still have to learn whether there are sperm which are lacking components which makes them non-viable.

Lou Warnes (Adelaide):

Do you adjust the total number of sperm for insemination based on the sperm morphology?

Fishel:

We never use high numbers (5×10^6 motile) if the morphology is in the normal range, the maximum we go to is 1×10^6 motile in those cases. We only go to the higher concentrations if samples have poor morphology. There is insufficient data to establish a statistically significant regression or hierarchical cut-off as to what would be the best concentration. The point is that if you have a sample with poor morphology, the number of sperm that are able to fertilize is lower and therefore you need to increase the concentration. Up to 1×10^6 sperm with < 5% normal forms does increase the fertilization rate but we find that it does compromise embryo quality. You put abnormal sperm like that into the egg by ICSI or even SUZI and you get better embryos.

Michael Tucker (Atlanta):

I would like to confirm that good semen preparation and clean sperm samples is the key to success with HIC, otherwise you generate embryos with poor morphology.

I am still a conservative proponent of ICSI but I think it's certainly a valid technique. I also think that what we need to establish is what's best for the patient. If a clinic can provide ICSI at a cost which is comparable with conventional IVF, then I'm in favour of it, and that is exactly what we have done in Atlanta. We have taken the financial question out of the equation concerning whether or not ICSI should be applied, so that all our patients pay the same fee whether they get ICSI or not. Consequently we are left with a clinical decision rather than a financial one.

Harold Bourne (Melbourne):

Concerning the immotile sperm that you injected, did you stroke their tails before injection, or did you just inject them without damaging the tail?

Fishel:

Both. The data is not distinct because we used to just inject them without immobilizing them because they were already immotile. Now we routinely damage the sperm tail even if they are immotile.

David de Kretser (Melbourne):

When you immobilize sperm by stroking their tail, do you choose where you immobilize them, on the midpiece or the principal piece?

Fishel:

We try and immobilize them just a little further down than the neck, sometimes in the midpiece. We do one of three things. First, we suck up to about 50% of the sperm into the injection pipette and then move the pipette vigorously while the sperm is half in it. Second, at the interface between the oil and PVP layer, we just come across at 180° to the sperm and that also works. Finally, we find it very difficult to immobilize sperm when they are in the centre of the droplet because you've got to get the angle of the pipettes just right.

Alan Trounson (Melbourne):

Our own results showed a 75% fertilization rate for both immobilized and motile sperm. We saw sperm swimming weakly in the ooplasm after injection.

Fishel:

In our studies, injecting immobilized sperm made a dramatic difference, and whenever we could see sperm moving inside the ooplasm, the fertilization rate was less than half what we achieved when we immobilized the sperm. We have seen this time and again.

Sperm Preparation for Intracytoplasmic Injection: Methods and Relationship to Fertilization Results

Harold Bourne [AF], Nadine Richings [B], De Yi Liu [C], Gary N. Clarke [D], Offer Harari [ABE] and H. W. Gordon Baker [C]

[A] Reproductive Biology Unit, Royal Women's Hospital, 132 Grattan Street, Carlton, Vic. 3053, Australia.
[B] Melbourne IVF, 320 Victoria Parade, East Melbourne, Vic. 3002, Australia.
[C] Department of Obstetrics and Gynaecology, University of Melbourne, Royal Women's Hospital, Carlton, Vic. 3053, Australia.
[D] Department of Pathology, Royal Women's Hospital, Carlton, Vic. 3053, Australia.
[E] Current address: Bnai Zion Medical Center, Department of Obstetrics and Gynecology, Faculty of Medicine, Technion, PO Box 4940, Haifa 31048, Israel.
[F] To whom correspondence should be addressed.

Abstract. Sperm preparation for intracytoplasmic sperm injection (ICSI) is described and the effect of high speed centrifugation during preparation on fertilization rate is evaluated. No significant differences were found in the 2-pronuclear or abnormal fertilization rates between sibling oocytes injected with sperm prepared by swim-up or mini-Percoll combined with high speed centrifugation. The high fertilization rate obtained with both methods indicates that high speed centrifugation is not necessary to prepare sperm for ICSI. Fertilization rates were also compared for sperm obtained from ejaculates, fresh and frozen epididymal aspirates, and testicular biopsies. High fertilization rates were obtained from all groups but they were significantly higher in those oocytes injected with epididymal sperm (78% per oocyte surviving injection). The high fertilization rate with epididymal sperm may reflect sperm quality or may result from the method of sperm preparation for injection. Fertilization after the injection of sperm from which the tail was dislodged during immobilization was compared with that obtained using intact sperm. A significantly lower rate of 2-pronuclear fertilization was found in those oocytes injected with sperm heads only (55%) compared with intact sperm (68%), although cleavage rates between the two groups were similar. The use of hypo-osmotic medium to select potentially live sperm from an immotile sample is also described and fertilization was obtained after the injection of sperm with a structural defect which were selected using this technique. These results indicate that high fertilization rates can be obtained with ejaculated, epididymal and testicular sperm without special treatment. Fertilization can also be achieved using ICSI with immotile sperm selected by hypo-osmotic swelling and from the injection of sperm heads. However, the injection of sperm heads only may not be appropriate because of the risk of mosaicism from defective or absent sperm centrosomes.

Extra keywords: ICSI micromanipulation, epididymal sperm, testicular sperm, sperm centrosome.

Introduction

The development of intracytoplasmic sperm injection (ICSI) by Palermo *et al.* (1992) has enabled the treatment of male infertility due to severe oligozoospermia and cases in which fertilization *in vitro* was not possible because of other sperm defects (Van Steirteghem *et al.* 1993*a*, 1993*b*). In addition, ICSI has markedly improved the outcome in patients with less severe sperm problems and has produced consistent fertilization rates and pregnancies using both epididymal and testicular sperm from patients with genital tract obstructions (Schoysman *et al.* 1993; Silber *et al.* 1994; Tournaye *et al.* 1994).

The original methods described for preparing sperm for injection involved the use of high speed centrifugation. Whether this is necessary to enable the sperm to decondense and form pronuclei (PN) after injection is unknown and a comparison of standard methods with this protocol is therefore warranted.

The requirement for such a small number of sperm for ICSI makes it feasible to freeze poor quality samples for subsequent microinjection where previously it was thought impractical to do so because of the loss of viable sperm after cryopreservation. This would be of particular use in patients from whom sperm are collected surgically or by biopsy, or in cases in which sperm are stored before chemotherapy or for other medical indications. In these cases, poor quality samples are common and the use of freezing with a view to using ICSI for insemination would maximize the use of the limited sperm numbers and reduce the need for further intervention.

Although fertilization and pregnancies have been achieved using epididymal and testicular sperm (Schoysman et al. 1993; Silber et al. 1994), it has not yet been demonstrated whether sperm from these sites are able to fertilize as reliably after intracytoplasmic injection as ejaculated sperm. In this context, a comparison of the fertilization rates using sperm isolated from ejaculates, epididymal aspirates and testicular biopsies is indicated.

In this report, we describe the methods we have used to prepare sperm for ICSI and fertilization rates are compared for sperm obtained from ejaculates, fresh and frozen epididymal aspirates, and testicular biopsies. The effect of high speed centrifugation on the fertilization rate has been examined and fertilization after the injection of sperm heads only is reported and is compared to the rate obtained with intact sperm. We also describe a method for selecting potentially live sperm for injection from samples in which only immotile sperm are present.

Materials and Methods

Patients

Couples with infertility due to severe oligozoospermia ($<2\times10^6$ sperm mL^{-1}), previous failure of standard *in vitro* fertilization (IVF), male genital tract obstruction, high abnormal sperm morphology (>85%), poor motility (<25% progressive or <40% total) or other severe sperm defects were treated by ICSI and IVF. Data were analyzed from 164 cycles undertaken at the Royal Women's Hospital between July 1993 and May 1994. A further 12 cycles up to September 1994 were included for patients with specific indications (male genital tract obstruction and completely immotile sperm).

Ovarian stimulation was achieved by a short protocol of gonadotrophin releasing hormone analogue (Lucrin; Abbott Australasia, Kurnell, NSW, Australia) and human menopausal gonadotrophin (hMG) (Humegon; Organon, Lane Cove, NSW or Pergonal; Serono, Frenchs Forest, NSW). Oocytes were collected by transvaginal ultrasound-guided follicular aspiration 36 h after injection of human chorionic gonadotrophin (hCG) (Pregnyl; Organon) and were cultured in human tubal fluid (HTF) medium (Irvine Scientific, Irvine, CA, USA) containing 10% patient's serum (PS). Luteal phase support was given for 12 days after oocyte retrieval in the form of progesterone pessaries (100 mg day^{-1}) or injections of hCG (1000 I.U. every 3 days).

Oocyte Preparation

Oocytes were denuded of cumulus by brief exposure (< 1 min) to HEPES-buffered HTF–PS containing 100 I.U. mL^{-1} of hyaluronidase (Bovine Type IV; Sigma, St Louis, MO, USA or Hyalase; Fisons, Castle Hill, NSW). Adherent coronal cells were dislodged by aspiration of oocytes through a fine bore glass pipette in fresh HEPES–buffered HTF–PS. Following cumulus removal, oocytes were washed through two further changes of HEPES-buffered HTF–PS before returning to fresh HTF–PS for culture. Most injections were performed on mature oocytes on the day of collection, although in a small number of cases, additional *in vitro* matured oocytes were injected the day after collection.

Sperm Collection and Preparation Methods

Sperm were isolated from ejaculated, epididymal and testicular samples and were prepared for injection as described below. Samples were prepared and used on the day of oocyte collection or after overnight incubation at room temperature in the case of *in vitro* matured oocytes. On the day of preparation, the final suspension was kept at 37°C after processing.

The methods used to prepare ejaculated and epididymal sperm were as follows:

Standard mini-Percoll (MP). Isotonic Percoll and 50%, 70% and 95% dilutions were made as described by Ord et al. (1990). Discontinuous gradients were prepared by placing 0·3 mL or 0·5 mL of 95% isotonic Percoll in the bottom of a conical centrifuge tube (Falcon 2099; Becton Dickinson, Lincoln Park, NJ, USA) followed by layering similar aliquots of 70% and 50% isotonic Percoll. Semen was mixed 1:1 with HEPES- or bicarbonate-buffered HTF–PS and centrifuged for 10 min at 300g. The pellet was resuspended in a small volume of medium (< 1 mL) and 0·3-mL or 0·5-mL aliquots were overlaid on one or two discontinuous MP gradients before centrifugation for 20–40 min at 300g. In some cases, 0·3–0·5 mL of raw semen was placed directly onto multiple gradients. After centrifugation, the 95% layer and pellet were transferred to a clean tube, diluted with 1 mL of medium and washed once or twice (300g for 5–10 min) before resuspension in <1 mL of HEPES-buffered HTF–PF for use.

Mini-Percoll and high speed centrifugation (MP–high speed). Samples were diluted with an equal volume of HEPES- or bicarbonate-buffered HTF–PS and centrifuged at 1800g for 5 min. The pellet was resuspended in a small volume ($\leq 0\cdot5$ mL) of HEPES-buffered HTF–PS, placed onto a 95%/70%/50% MP gradient (0·3 mL or 0·5 mL layers) as described above and centrifuged for 20–40 min at 300g. Following centrifugation, the 95% layer and pellet were removed and mixed with 1 mL of fresh medium and the Percoll was removed by one or two washes (1800g, 5 min). The final sperm pellet was resuspended in a small volume ($\leq 0\cdot5$ mL) of HEPES-buffered HTF–PS for use.

Swim-up. Raw semen (~0·5 mL) was placed in a 5 mL tube (Falcon 2003; Becton Dickinson), overlaid with 1–2 mL of HTF–PS and incubated, loosely capped, for at least 1 h at 37°C in an atmosphere of 5% CO_2. Following incubation, the top layer containing motile sperm was harvested and transferred to a clean tube, diluted with an approximately equal volume of medium and centrifuged for 5 min at 300–400g. The resulting pellet was resuspended in HEPES-buffered HTF–PS and diluted to a concentration of <300 000 sperm mL^{-1} for injection.

Resuspension. Samples were mixed with an equal volume of HEPES- or bicarbonate-buffered HTF–PS and centrifuged for 5–10 min at 1800g. The pellet was resuspended in $\leq 0\cdot5$ mL of HEPES-buffered HTF–PF for use.

Ejaculated sperm. Sperm from ejaculates were isolated from fresh samples produced on the day of oocyte collection or from previously stored frozen samples. In most cases, samples were prepared using a MP–high speed protocol. If there were sufficient sperm with good forward progression in the sample ($>5\cdot0\times10^6$ mL^{-1}), then a swim-up suspension was prepared. In some cases in which very few sperm were present (<10 sperm in the whole chamber of a Neubauer haemocytometer), a simple resuspension only was done.

For the frozen samples, semen was mixed 3:1 with glycerol–egg yolk–citrate medium, sealed in 0·5 mL plastic straws and cooled at $-1\cdot5$°C min^{-1} from 20°C to -6°C followed by -6°C min^{-1} down to −100°C before storing in liquid nitrogen. The cryoprotective medium was based on Clarke *et al.* 1988, but lacked Kanamycin. The final mixture contained approximately 30% glycerol, 1·5% glucose, 1·0% sodium citrate, 1·3% glycine and 17% egg yolk. The diluent (~400 mOsm kg^{-1} excluding glycerol, pH 7·0) was added to the semen in 5 aliquots over 10 min at room temperature. The final percentage of glycerol in the diluted sample was 7·0–7·5%. Prior to use, straws were air thawed and the samples were prepared using either standard MP gradients or the MP–high speed protocol.

Epididymal sperm. In patients with a genital tract obstruction, epididymal sperm were collected by microsurgical epididymal sperm aspiration (MESA) or percutaneous cyst aspiration. In most cases, fresh epididymal sperm were prepared using standard MP gradients, however, in a few cycles, the MP–high speed protocol was used. If there was only minimal blood contamination in the fresh aspirate, then the resuspension only method was employed. The resultant final suspensions were used either fresh or after cryopreservation.

Excess sperm were usually available for cryopreservation in a glucose–citrate–glycine (GCG) buffer with glycerol as cryoprotectant. The GCG–glycerol medium was modified slightly from that used for ejaculated semen. The main difference was the exclusion of egg yolk which produced a microscopic precipitate when the sperm were mixed with HTF–PS. This made microscopy difficult, but there was no evidence that post-thaw recovery was compromised. The cryoprotectant contained 1·0% glucose, 0·9% sodium citrate, 1·0% glycine and 23% glycerol and had an osmolarity excluding glycerol of ~370 mOsm kg^{-1} and a pH of 7·5. Samples were mixed with an approximately equal volume of patient's serum, diluted with GCG–glycerol medium (1:2), loaded into 0·5-mL straws and cooled using the same programme as for ejaculated semen. The percentage of glycerol in the final sample was approximately 7·6%. In one case in which access to the standard protocol was not available, sperm were frozen in 0·25-mL straws using a 1, 2-propanediol–sucrose protocol as described by Lassalle *et al.* (1985) for embryos. For use, straws were thawed in air and the sperm were separated from the cryoprotectant using MP–high speed, standard MP gradients or the resuspension method.

Testicular sperm. Testicular tissue (~0·5 cm in diameter) was obtained by open biopsy when no motile sperm were collected by MESA. In patients with an intratesticular blockage, testicular tissue was obtained by fine needle biopsy under local anaesthesia using a modified 20 G Menghini needle as described by Mallidis and Baker (1994). The pieces of tissue were placed into a small Petri dish (Falcon 3001; Becton Dickinson) containing 1–2 mL of HEPES-buffered HTF–PS and dissected using fine scissors and/or 25 G needles. After dissection, the medium and tissue debris were transferred to a clean 5 mL tube (Falcon 2003) and pipetted vigorously to disperse the sperm. The resulting coarse suspension was left for a short time (<5 min) to allow the large tissue clumps and debris to settle. In one instance, this suspension was used without further processing. In the remaining cases, the top layer of the suspension was either separated on a three step Percoll gradient (0·3–1·0 mL layers) with the final wash done at 500*g*, or it was prepared by centrifugation for 10 min at 500*g* and resuspension in approximately 0·3 mL of HEPES-buffered HTF–PS.

Microinjection Procedure

Prior to use, a small drop (~30 μL) of the final sperm suspension was spread onto a Petri dish (Falcon 1006; Becton Dickinson) along with small drops (~10 μL) of fresh HEPES-buffered HTF–PS for holding the oocytes. These were covered with 6 mL of temperature equilibrated paraffin oil (BDH, Poole, UK) or mineral oil (Sigma) and the dish was placed on the heated stage of a Diaphot TMD inverted microscope (Nikon, Tokyo, Japan) for injection. For testicular samples, the Petri dish for injection was made soon after the sperm had been prepared and the dish was left on a hotplate at 37°C until needed.

Microinjection was based on the protocol described by Palermo *et al.* (1992) but without the use of polyvinylpyrrolidone (PVP). Briefly, motile sperm were aspirated from the sperm suspension into a fine pipette (outer diameter 6–10 μm), transferred to fresh HEPES-buffered HTF–PS containing an oocyte and immobilized by crushing the tail against the bottom of the dish with the injection pipette. The immobilized spermatozoon was re-aspirated and injected into the cytoplasm of a mature oocyte after pushing the pipette through the zona pellucida and piercing the oolemma. Following injection, oocytes were placed into fresh HTF–PS for culture.

Preparation and Use of Hypo-osmotic Medium

One patient with completely immotile sperm due to a sperm structural defect had two cycles of treatment in which the sperm were selected for injection by observing tail coiling in hypo-osmotic medium. Hypo-osmotic medium of ~100 mOsm kg^{-1} was prepared by adding 0·5 mL of HEPES-buffered HTF–PS to 1·0 mL of Nanopure water (Sybron/Barnstead, Boston, Massachusetts, USA) followed by filtration through a 0·2 μm filter. This method of preparing hypo-osmotic medium was used because of its simplicity and also to avoid exposing sperm to the additional factors found in conventional hypo-osmotic media. A small drop of this solution was plated onto the Petri dish for injection along with the sperm suspension and fresh drops of HEPES-buffered HTF–PS. Immotile sperm were aspirated from the sperm suspension and transferred to the hypo-osmotic solution. Immediately after contacting the hypo-osmotic medium, the tail of some sperm began to coil and these sperm were transferred to the iso-osmotic HEPES-buffered HTF–PS drop for injection. After flushing the sperm out, the injection pipette was repeatedly washed by aspiration with fresh medium to ensure removal of the solution carried over from the hypo-osmotic droplet.

Oocyte Survival and Assessment of Fertilization

Oocytes were classified as surviving the procedure if they remained intact and did not display any signs of lysis or degeneration over the 2 days following injection. Fertilization was assessed by the observation of pronuclei 15–20 h after injection using an inverted microscope at 200× magnification.

Controlled Trials and Comparisons of Fertilization Results

Mini-percoll–high speed centrifugation v. swim-up. In 26 cycles of ICSI, fertilization rates were compared for oocytes injected with sperm isolated from fresh ejaculates and prepared by either the MP–high speed or swim-up protocols. For each patient, half the oocytes were injected with intact sperm processed using the MP–high speed method and the remaining sibling oocytes were injected with sperm prepared by swim-up.

Ejaculated v. epididymal v. testicular sperm. Fertilization rates were compared between cycles using sperm obtained from fresh ejaculates, fresh and frozen epididymal aspirates, and fresh testicular biopsies. In all categories, only cycles in which all oocytes were injected with freshly immobilized and intact sperm were analysed.

Intact sperm v. sperm heads only. In 36 cycles, some of the oocytes were injected with sperm heads and the remaining sibling oocytes were injected with intact sperm. This was not a controlled trial since injection of heads was only undertaken if the tail was accidentally dislodged during immobilization. Sperm were isolated from fresh ejaculates and prepared using MP–high speed or standard MP protocols, except in four cases in which a simple resuspension was used.

Statistical Analysis

The comparisons between frequencies of fertilization in the various groups were done using a χ^2-test for significance.

Results

The results from the 176 cycles are summarized in Table 1. A survival rate of 93% was obtained with 68% of these oocytes fertilizing and displaying 2 PN. A comparison of fertilization rates for oocytes injected with sperm prepared by MP–high speed or swim-up are shown in Table 2. There were no significant differences in either the 2 PN or polyploid fertilization rates, nor in the rate of oocytes developing 1 PN between the two groups.

Table 1. Overall results from intracytoplasmic sperm injection, irrespective of sperm preparation method or the source of sperm

PN, pronuclei

No. of cycles	176
No. of oocytes injected	1659
No. of oocytes which survived injection	1545 (93%)
No. of fertilized oocytes	
2 PN	1057 (68%)[A]
> 2 PN	71 (4·6%)[A]
1 PN	78 (5·0%)[A]

[A] Values in parentheses represent percentages of the oocytes surviving injection.

Table 2. Fertilization after intracytoplasmic injection of sibling oocytes with sperm prepared by mini-Percoll–high speed centrifugation (MP–high speed) or swim-up (26 cycles)

PN, pronuclei

	MP–high speed	Swim-up
No. oocytes injected and survived	113	113
No. of fertilized oocytes[A]		
2 PN	80 (71%)	76 (67%)
> 2 PN	5 (4·4%)	3 (2·7%)
1 PN	6 (5·3%)	7 (6·2%)

[A] 3×2 χ^2, $P = 0.755$; not significant.

The fertilization rates for ejaculated, epididymal and testicular sperm are shown in Table 3. An analysis comparing the 2 PN and abnormal (1 PN plus >2 PN) fertilization rates between ejaculated, epididymal and testicular sperm showed non-uniformity due to the high 2 PN fertilization rate obtained with epididymal sperm. There were no other significant differences between the groups. It is worth noting that the fertilization rates from frozen and fresh epididymal sperm were similar.

The results from cycles in which oocytes were injected with intact sperm or sperm heads only showed a significantly lower 2 PN fertilization rate in those oocytes injected with isolated heads (Table 4). However, the percentage of fertilized oocytes which cleaved and were transferred or frozen was similar for intact sperm (82%) or sperm heads only (85%). There were no other significant differences in this analysis.

In the 2 cycles in which sperm were selected using hypo-osmotic medium, fertilization was achieved in 2 of the 4 oocytes which survived the procedure.

Discussion

The overall rates for 2 PN, 1 PN and polyploid fertilization in this study were similar to those reported by Van Steirteghem *et al.* (1993*b*). The first reports of sperm preparation for ICSI involved high speed centrifugation to concentrate the sample before separation on a Percoll gradient and also during the final washing steps after Percoll (Palermo *et al.* 1993; Van Steirteghem *et al.* 1993*a*, 1993*b*). Whether this was necessary to produce sperm capable of decondensing and forming a PN after injection was unknown. It may have been that high speed centrifugation was needed to disrupt the sperm membrane and allow enzymes in the oocyte cytoplasm access to the sperm nucleus. However, a comparison of fertilization rates using sperm prepared by MP–high speed and swim-up showed no significant differences in normal or abnormal fertilization rates between the two methods, and the high fertilization rate obtained with sperm prepared by swim-up indicates that high speed centrifugation is not necessary to prepare sperm for intracytoplasmic injection. However, its use may be of benefit in maximizing the yield from samples in which only a few sperm are present.

Table 3. Comparison of intracytoplasmic sperm injection fertilization rates using sperm from ejaculates, epididymal aspirates or testicular biopsies

PN, pronuclei

	Ejaculated sperm	Epididymal sperm fresh	Epididymal sperm frozen	Testicular sperm
No. of cycles	95	20	8	6
No. oocytes injected and survived	761	176	51	68
No. of fertilized oocytes[A]				
2 PN	525 (69%)	137 (78%)	41 (80%)	44 (65%)
> 2 PN	31 (4·1%)	6 (3·4%)	3 (5·9%)	4 (5·9%)
1 PN	40 (5·2%)	12 (6·8%)	2 (3·9%)	6 (8·8%)

[A] Results of 6×2 χ^2-test for 2 PN *v.* abnormal (1 PN plus > 2 PN) fertilization with ejaculated, epididymal and testicular sperm shows non-uniformity due to the high fertilization rate with epididymal sperm. $\chi^2 = 14.0$, $P < 0.03$.

Although it has been shown that high speed centrifugation is not needed to prepare sperm for ICSI, it is also apparent that it is not detrimental. This is in contrast to the effect of centrifugation on sperm function in standard IVF. The generation of reactive oxygen species (ROS) from defective sperm during centrifugation impairs the function of normal sperm in the same suspension if unfractionated samples are centrifuged (Aitken and Clarkson 1988). In those cases in which oocytes were injected with sperm prepared by MP–high speed and swim-up, sufficient sperm were present for the generation of ROS during MP–high speed preparation, but no differences in the fertilization rate were observed. As the effect of ROS generation during centrifugation reduces sperm function associated with motility, oolemma binding and fusion, it is not surprising that fertilization after ICSI was not affected since these steps are essentially bypassed. At present, it is unknown whether the peroxidation that can occur from centrifugation extends its deleterious effect to events occurring after fertilization. To study this would require quantifying the production of ROS during the sperm preparation methods we have used and determining if there were any relationship with the outcome of ICSI embryos.

Table 4. Results from the injection of intact sperm and sperm heads only (tail was dislodged during immobilization). Data are from 36 cycles

PN, pronuclei

	Intact sperm	Sperm heads
No. oocytes injected and survived	292	118
No. of fertilized oocytes		
2 PN	198 (68%)[A]	65 (55%)[A]
> 2 PN	16 (5·5%)	2 (1·7%)
1 PN	16 (5·5%)	2 (1·7%)

[A] $\chi^2 = 20\cdot 4$, $P < 0\cdot 001$.

The capacity of sperm to fertilize at the same rate after swim-up or MP–high speed separation suggests that sperm morphology may not be related to fertilization after ICSI. Swim-up has been shown to produce a higher yield of normal forms from poor quality samples (Ng *et al.* 1992) and normal morphology is strongly correlated with the fertilization rate in standard IVF (Liu *et al.* 1988). If morphology were strongly correlated with fertilization after ICSI, then a higher fertilization rate would be expected in those oocytes injected with sperm prepared by swim-up. This was clearly not the case in our experiments. However, confirmation of this requires an analysis of the sperm characteristics in the samples used for injection.

The 2 PN fertilization rate using epididymal sperm was higher than the rate for both ejaculated and testicular sperm and may reflect an inherent better quality of the epididymal sperm. This is plausible since the infertility in these patients is due to a genital tract obstruction, and spermatogenesis in most cases is essentially normal. However, the contribution of female factors to this high fertilization rate cannot be discounted.

The good results achieved with epididymal sperm and ICSI contrasts strongly with the poor results obtained using epididymal sperm and standard IVF (Silber *et al.* 1994), partial zona dissection (PZD) or sub-zonal insemination (SUZI) (Garrisi *et al.* 1993). The low fertilization rate obtained with epididymal sperm using standard IVF may be related to sperm maturity (Silber *et al.* 1994). However, the consistently high fertilization rate obtained in this study using epididymal and testicular sperm indicates that sperm maturity may be irrelevant with ICSI. The need for sperm to acrosome react prior to oolemma binding (Liu and Baker 1994) may be the reason for the low fertilization rate with epididymal sperm using PZD or SUZI. Epididymal sperm obtained from patients with a genital tract obstruction are predominantly of normal morphology with good quality acrosomes (Liu, unpublished observations). A high percentage of sperm with intact acrosomes would mean there are fewer sperm able to bind to the oolemma and the chance of fertilization would be decreased.

The fertilization rates for epididymal and testicular sperm in this study were higher than those reported previously with ICSI (Silber 1994; Tournaye *et al.* 1994; Van Steirteghem *et al.* 1994). The method of immobilizing the sperm for injection in this study differs from previous methods in that PVP was not used to retard sperm motility. Movement is frequently seen after crushing the sperm tail and the procedure is often repeated until the sperm is completely immotile. The small amount of movement that is initially observed after crushing the sperm tail is not likely to be seen if PVP is present, and it may be that this extensive immobilization step in our procedure is advantageous in preparing epididymal and testicular sperm for ICSI. Evidence against this possibility was presented by Lacham-Kaplan and Trounson (1994) who obtained similar fertilization rates after injection of motile and immobilized sperm into human oocytes although it is assumed that this was with ejaculated and not epididymal or testicular sperm. Alternatively, PVP might interfere with the intracytoplasmic processing of these sperm after injection. Epididymal and testicular sperm have surfaces of different composition and charge to ejaculated sperm and PVP may preferentially coat these sperm and hinder the sequence of events that would normally occur after injection. The effect of female factors such as patient age or oocyte factors might also contribute to the differences in fertilization rate seen in these studies. Further investigation is required to evaluate the effect of PVP on the fertilizing capacity of epididymal and testicular sperm after ICSI.

Results from the injection of sperm after the tail was dislodged during immobilization show that fertilization can occur with sperm heads, but at a lower rate than for intact sperm. The lower fertilization rate may result from damage incurred during decapitation, resulting in a reduced ability to form PN. The results presented here were not part of a controlled trial bacause sperm heads were injected if they were accidentally removed during immobilization. It is possible that the sperm in which the tail was lost were more susceptible to damage and were therefore inherently less likely to fertilize even if they were injected intact.

The zygotes obtained after fertilization with sperm heads cleaved at a similar rate to those resulting from intact sperm, so the role of the centrosome in these embryos is interesting. The centrosome is a specialised organelle which is involved in the organization of spindle fibres that function during cell division. After decapitation, it is possible that the centrosome is left behind in the midpiece. The point where the head attaches to the tail at the implantation fossa appears to be a likely point for separation. Recent evidence suggests that the centrosome in humans is inherited via the sperm (Sathananthan et al. 1991; Palermo et al. 1994) as it is in many other species. The ability of zygotes fertilized with sperm heads only to cleave, suggests that the centrosome or at least sufficient remnants of it, is injected with the sperm head, although spindle formation by a maternal microtubule organizing centre in the absence of a sperm centrosome cannot be discounted. Electron microscopic studies are needed to determine the level of damage and to what extent the centrosome is retained in sperm head preparations produced by decapitation.

The results from the use of hypo-osmotic selection of immotile sperm are inconclusive. The swelling of sperm in hypo-osmotic medium is related to the presence of a functional membrane (Jeyendran et al. 1984) and so the sperm which show tail coiling are more likely to be viable. Although fertilization was achieved with sperm selected by this method, the number of oocytes injected was too small to draw any conclusions. Motile or weakly motile sperm were found in all the cases treated except the patient with a structural defect. In the testicular samples, it was noted that the sperm observed during dissection and immediately after preparation were often immotile. However, motile sperm were found after the sample had been incubated for a few hours, although in many cases the number of motile sperm was few and an extensive search of the sperm suspension was required to locate them. The likelihood of not finding motile sperm from patients without a sperm structural defect is low and so the need for selecting sperm by hypo-osmotic swelling may be limited. Further evaluation of this technique is required to determine its usefulness.

In summary, sperm preparation using high speed centrifugation is not required to obtain a high fertilization rate after ICSI. The choice of method probably need only be based on ease, availability of sperm and the degree of contamination with debris or blood cells. High fertilization rates can be obtained with epididymal and testicular sperm without any special treatment of the sperm. Excess sperm from microsurgical aspirations or biopsies, or semen from patients with specific medical problems should be frozen for later use even if the quality is poor. However, the injection of sperm heads may not be appropriate unless there is no other choice due to the risk of mosaicism and cleavage anomalies from defective or absent centrosomes.

Acknowledgments

We thank the medical, nursing and laboratory staff of the Reproductive Biology Unit for their assistance in the management of these patients. In particular, we wish to acknowledge Michele McDonald, Felix Nieto and Anne Vassiliadis for their role in performing ICSI and Jessica Costa for the manufacture of pipettes. We also thank Peter Elliot and Henry Oh from the Andrology laboratory at Royal Women's Hospital for the cryopreservation of sperm samples.

References

Aitken, R.J., and Clarkson, J.S. (1988). Significance of reactive oxygen species and antioxidants in defining the efficacy of sperm preparation techniques. *J. Androl.* **9**, 367–76.

Clarke, G.N., Hyne, R.V., Du Plessis, Y., and Johnston, W.I.H. (1988). Sperm antibodies in human *in vitro* fertilization. *Fertil. Steril.* **49**, 1018–25.

Garrisi, J.G., Chin, A.J., Dolan, P.M., Nagler, H.M., Vasquez-Levin, M., Navot, D., and Gordon, J.W. (1993). Analysis of factors contributing to success in a program of micromanipulation-assisted fertilization. *Fertil. Steril.* **59**, 366–74.

Jeyendran, R.S., Van der Ven, H.H., Perez-Pelaez, M., Crabo, B.G., and Zaneveld, L.J.D. (1984). Development of an assay to assess the functional integrity of the human sperm membrane and its relationship to other semen characteristics. *J. Reprod. Fertil.* **70**, 219–28.

Lacham-Kaplan, O., and Trounson, A. (1994). Micromanipulation assisted fertilization: comparison of different techniques. In 'Frontiers in Endocrinology. Vol. 8. Male Factor in Human Infertility'. (Ed. J. Tesarik.) pp. 287–304. (Ares-Serono Symposia: Rome.)

Lassalle, B., Testart, T., and Renard, J.-P. (1985). Human embryo features that influence the success of cryopreservation with the use of 1,2-propanediol. *Fertil. Steril.* **44**, 645–51.

Liu, D.Y., Du Plessis, Y.P., Nayudu, P.L., Johnston, W.I.H., and Baker, H.W.G. (1988). The use of *in vitro* fertilization to evaluate putative tests of human sperm function. *Fertil. Steril.* **49**, 272–7.

Liu, D.Y., and Baker, H.W.G. (1994). Acrosome status and morphology of human spermatozoa bound to the zona pellucida and oolemma determined using oocytes that failed to fertilize *in vitro*. *Hum. Reprod. (Oxf.)* **9**, 673–9.

Mallidis, C., and Baker, H.W.G. (1994). Fine needle tissue aspiration biopsy of the testis. *Fertil. Steril.* **61**, 367–75.

Ng, F.L.H., Liu, D.Y., and Baker, H.W.G. (1992). Comparison of Percoll, mini-Percoll and swim-up methods for sperm preparation from abnormal semen samples. *Hum. Reprod. (Oxf.)* **7**, 261–6.

Ord, T., Patrizio, P., Marello, E., Balmaceda, J.P., and Asch, R.H. (1990). Mini-Percoll: a new method of semen preparation for IVF in severe male factor infertility. *Hum. Reprod. (Oxf.)* **5**, 987–9.

Palermo, G., Joris, H., Devroey, P., and Van Steirteghem, A.C. (1992). Pregnancies after intracytoplasmic injection of single spermatozoon into an oocyte. *Lancet* **340**, 17–8.

Palermo, G., Joris, H., Derde, M-P., Camus, M., Devroey, P., and Van Steirteghem, A.C. (1993). Sperm characteristics and outcome of human assisted fertilization by subzonal insemination and intracytoplasmic sperm injection. *Fertil. Steril.* **59**, 826–35.

Palermo, G., Munne, S., and Cohen, J. (1994). The human zygote inherits its mitotic potential from the male gamete. *Hum. Reprod. (Oxf.)* **9**, 1220–5.

Sathananthan, A.H., Kola, I., Osborne, J., Trounson, A., Ng, S.-C., Bongso, A., and Ratnam, S.S. (1991). Centrioles in the beginning of human development. *Proc. Natl Acad. Sci. USA* **88**, 4806–10.

Schoysman, R., Vanderzwalmen, P., Nijs, M., Segal, L., Segal-Bertin, G., Geerts, L., van Roosendaal, E., and Schoysman, D. (1993). Pregnancy after fertilisation with human testicular spermatozoa. *Lancet* **342**, 1237.

Silber, S.J. (1994). The use of epididymal sperm in assisted reproduction. In 'Frontiers in Endocrinology. Vol. 8. Male Factor in Human Infertility'. (Ed. J. Tesarik.) pp. 335–68. (Ares-Serono Symposia: Rome.)

Silber, S.J., Nagy, Z.P., Liu, J., Godoy, H., Devroey, P., and Van Steirteghem, A.C. (1994). Conventional *in-vitro* fertilization versus intracytoplasmic sperm injection for patients requiring microsurgical sperm aspiration. *Hum. Reprod. (Oxf.)* **9**, 1705–9.

Tournaye, H., Devroey, P., Liu, J., Nagy, Z., Lissens, W., and Van Steirteghem, A. (1994). Microsurgical epididymal sperm aspiration and intracytoplasmic sperm injection: a new effective approach to infertility as a result of congenital bilateral absence of vas deferens. *Fertil. Steril.* **61**, 1045–51.

Van Steirteghem, A.C., Liu, J., Joris, H., Nagy, Z., Janssenswillen, C., Tournaye, H., Derde, M.-P., Van Assche, E., and Devroey, P. (1993*a*). Higher success rate by intracytoplasmic sperm injection than by subzonal insemination. Report of a second series of 300 consecutive treatment cycles. *Hum. Reprod. (Oxf.)* **8**, 1055–60.

Van Steirteghem, A.C., Nagy, Z., Joris, H., Liu, J., Staessen, C., Smitz, J., Wisanto, A., and Devroey, P. (1993*b*). High fertilization and implantation rates after intracytoplasmic sperm injection. *Hum. Reprod. (Oxf.)* **8**, 1061–6.

Van Steirteghem, A., Devroey, P., Joris, H., Nagy, P., Liu, J., Camus, M., Wisanto, A., Staessen, C., Silber, S., and Liebaers, I. (1994). Criteria of patient selection for micromanipulation assisted conception. In 'Frontiers in Endocrinology. Vol. 8. Male Factor in Human Infertility'. (Ed. J. Tesarik.) pp. 325–34. (Ares-Serono Symposia: Rome.)

Manuscript received 25 January 1995

Open Discussion

Robert McLachlan (Melbourne):

What cryoprotectant do you use for the epididymal sperm? Do you ever cryopreserve testicular sperm from biopsies or do you biopsy in each cycle, which is what we've been doing?

Bourne:

Normally you only get a small number of sperm in the fine needle testicular biopsies, but in one case we retrieved a large number of testicular sperm, more than I've seen with some of our MESA cases, and we froze them. However, they haven't been used yet because the patient was pregnant after a fresh embryo transfer.

Sherman Silber (St Louis):

When you do the HOS test for selecting live, immotile sperm, how long do you leave them in the 100 mOsm solution before you put them back in HEPES-buffered medium?

Bourne:

Only a few seconds. The tail starts to coil up immediately the spermatozoon is ejected into the hypo-osmotic solution, so you pick it up almost straight away.

Intracytoplasmic Sperm Injection: Instrumentation and Injection Technique

Dianna Payne

Reproductive Medicine Laboratories, Department of Obstetrics and Gynecology, The University of Adelaide, The Queen Elizabeth Hospital, Woodville, SA 5011, Australia.

Extra keywords: ICSI, injection pipette, holding pipette, fertilization, oocyte activation.

Introduction

A technique which is successful in one laboratory sometimes cannot be successfully applied in other laboratories, and this can be a particular problem if the technique is complex and has 'tricks' associated with it. The technique might not be fully and exhaustively detailed in a publication due to limited space in the Materials and Methods section, and yet it is often the small and seemingly unimportant points which hold the key to success. Furthermore, a specific technique might be equally successful in two laboratories which use profoundly different methodology because the same important points are applied in both and may have been arrived at independently. The trick in the application of any technique is to identify the essential components and be aware that some aspects of the technique, often enshrined in gold by a particular laboratory, may be idiosyncratic and not necessarily pivotal to its successful application.

In this paper, I present a detailed description of the preparation of glass instruments for intracytoplasmic sperm injection (ICSI) and the injection technique that we use. I must stress that this is the way that ICSI has been performed successfully in our laboratory (see Payne and Matthews 1995 for clinical results) and there are subtle differences in the procedures used in other laboratories which have also successfully applied ICSI. Where possible, I outline some of these variations.

Preparation of Holding and Injection Pipettes

General Design of Instruments

The manufacture and use of precision glass instruments is critical for success with ICSI. Although there are several important design considerations, other features can be varied to suit the microscope or micromanipulators that are used, or the personal preferences of the operator. The pipettes can be straight for almost horizontal side entry into drops of medium on depression well slides, or they can have one or more bends in them so that they can be brought in from above a Petri dish. We routinely use Z shaped pipettes which enter at a shallow angle relative to the horizontal, but still clear the lip of a glass Petri dish lid. The important point is that the tips of the holding and injection pipettes must be horizontal so that the minimum amount of pressure needs to be exerted on the oocyte during injection.

We routinely use holding pipettes with an outside diameter (OD) of ~120 μm, but other operators prefer to use narrower pipettes with an OD of 60 μm (Palermo et al. 1992). We have tried narrower holding pipettes but we believe that those which we describe below are easier to use, especially during the initial learning curve. There is no difference in efficacy, however, providing that ICSI can be performed using the chosen holding pipette.

There are two features of the injection pipettes which are important for ICSI. First, they must be bevelled and sharp. Second, they should have an OD at the tip of 6–8 μm — if narrower than 6 μm there may be difficulty moving sperm in and out of the pipettes, and if wider than 8 μm there is too much disruption of the oocyte cytoplasm during injection. Providing that these criteria are met, the bevel angle can vary from 28–30° (Hamberger et al. 1995; Palermo et al. 1995a) to about 45–50° (Van Steirteghem et al. 1993a), and the pipettes can either be fitted with a sharp spike or they can be used without a spike (Catt et al. 1995).

Glassware Preparation

Thick- and thin-walled borosilicate glass capillaries (Clarke Electromedical Instruments, Reading, UK) are soaked overnight in 1N hydrochloric acid (HCl) and then rinsed extensively in running water until the effluent has a neutral pH. The capillaries are soaked overnight twice in 18 Ω Milli Q water (Millipore Corporation, Bedford, Massachusetts, USA) and after each soaking they are rinsed extensively in fresh Milli Q water. The capillaries are then dried at 120°C and subsequently stored in clean, covered glass containers before the manufacture of instruments.

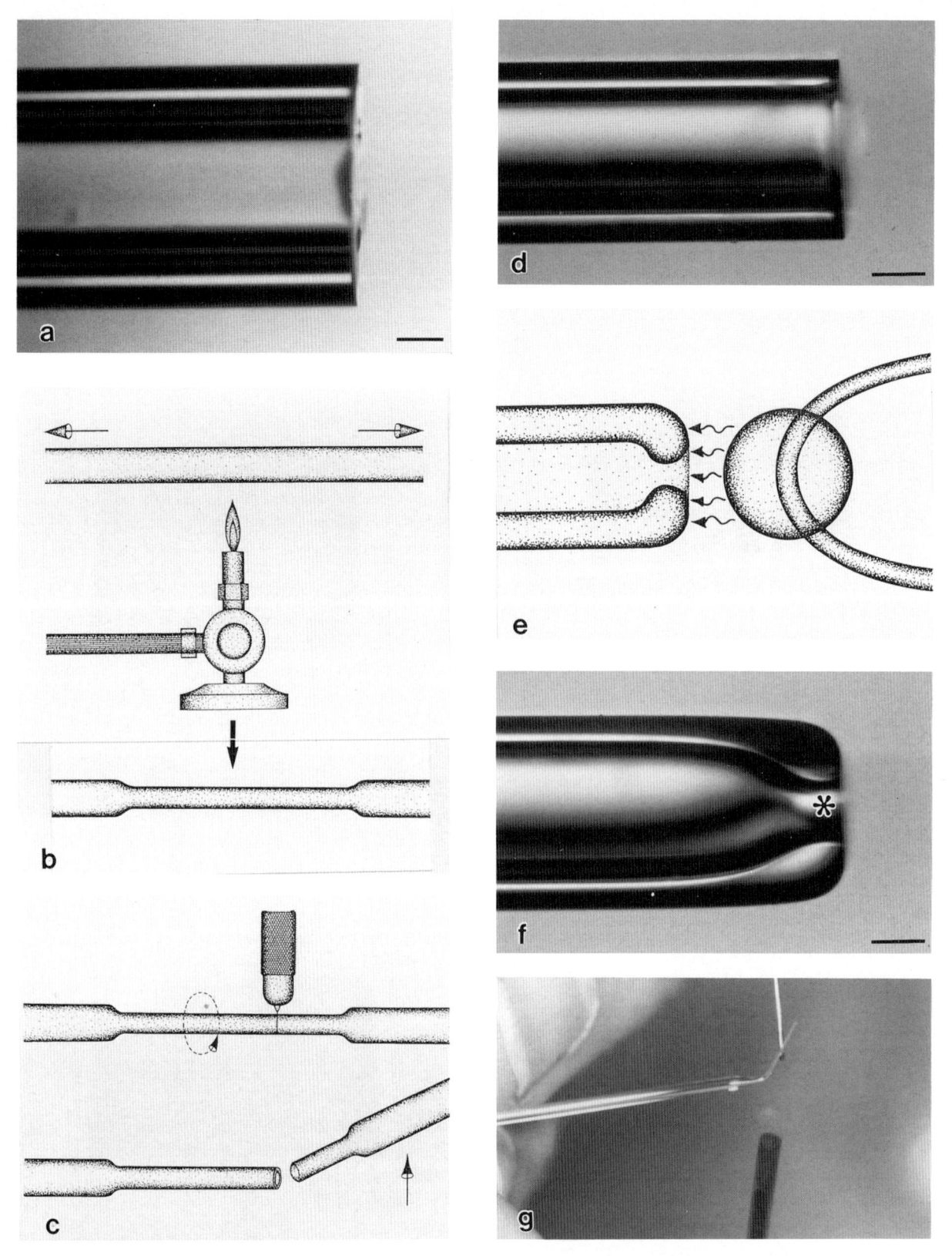

Fig. 1. The manufacture of a holding pipette. (*a*) A glass capillary after washing—note the thick walls. (*b*) The glass capillary is pulled by hand over a microflame to a diameter of approximately 120 μm. (*c*) The glass is scored with a diamond-encrusted dental burr and broken along the score line. (*d*) The resultant holding pipette—note that the break is flat and clean. (*e*) The pipette tip is heat-polished with the radiant heat (arrows) from a small glass bead which is fused onto the filament of the microforge. (*f*) A polished holding pipette—the opening (*) is 30–40 μm in diameter. (*g*) The holding pipette is bent to the appropriate angle using a microflame and a 26 G needle with its end bent over to form a hook. Bars *a*, 200 μm; *d* and *f*, 50 μm.

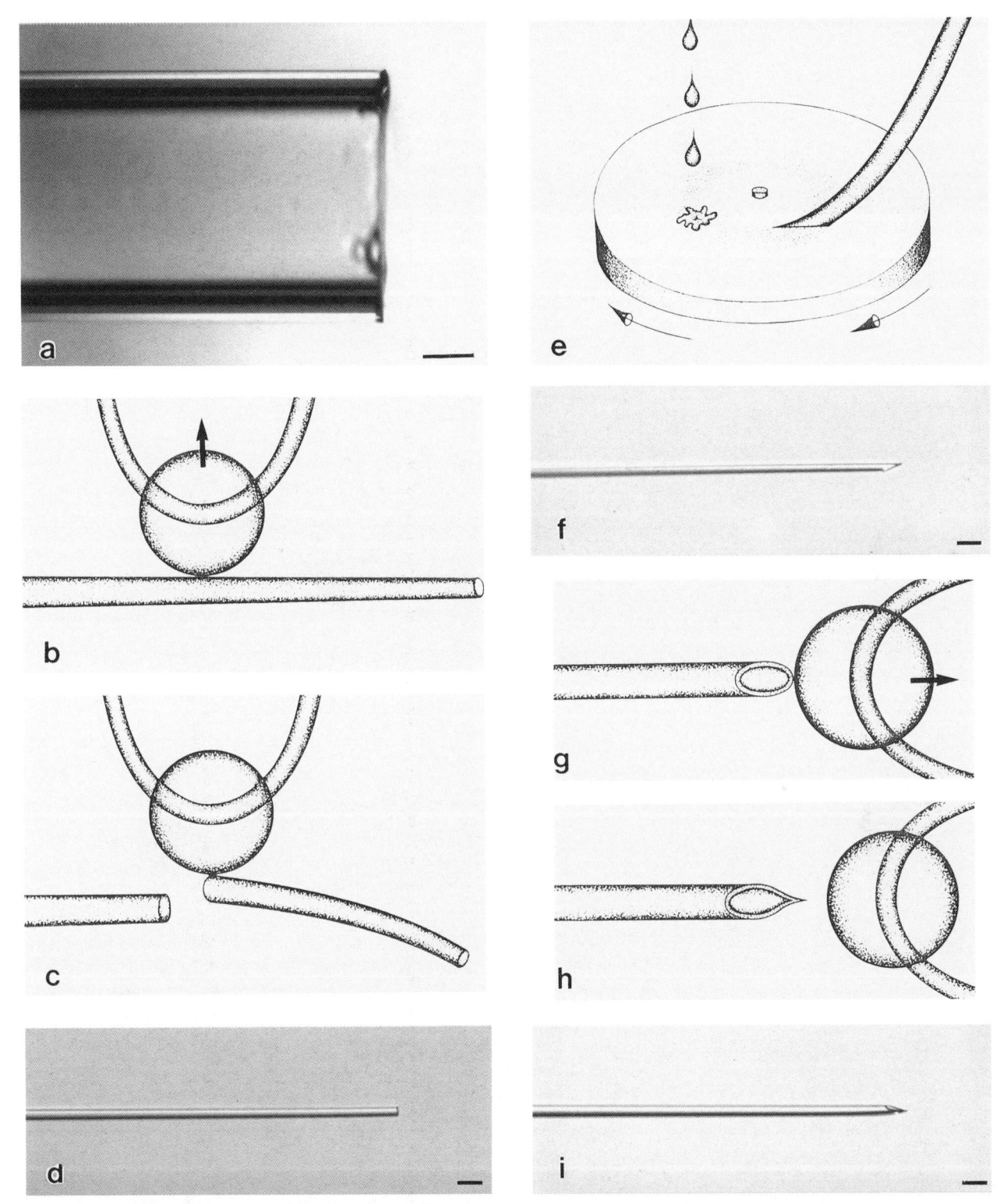

Fig. 2. The manufacture of an injection pipette. *(a)* A glass capillary after washing—note the thin walls. *(b and c)* The capillary is drawn out on a pipette puller and the glass taper is broken where its outer diameter is approximately 6 µm using the microforge. The glass bead is heated to a dull red, and the taper is placed against it at the desired thickness as shown in *(b)*. The current to the filament is then turned off, and the filament retracts as it cools, breaking the glass taper as shown in *(c)*. *(d)* The glass taper after breaking—note that the break is clean and flat. *(e)* A 40–45° bevel is ground onto the tip of the taper using a capillary tip grinder—note that water drops onto the grinding path. *(f)* The injection pipette after grinding. *(g and h)* A spike is created on the tip of the bevelled injection pipette by lightly pushing the end of the bevel against a very deep red glass bead attached to the microforge filament *(g)*, then the glass bead is drawn sharply away to produce a sharp spike *(h)*. *(i)* A finished injection pipette with a spike. Bars: *a*, 200 µm; *d, f* and *i*, 20 µm.

Manufacture of Holding Pipettes

The capillaries we use to manufacture the holding pipettes have an OD of 1 mm and an inner diameter (ID) of 0·58 mm (Fig. 1a). We originally pulled the holding pipettes by hand over a microflame (Model B; Microflame, Minneapolis, Minnesota, USA) to an O.D. of ~120–150 μm (Fig. 1b). However, holding pipettes are now pulled on a model P-87 Flaming/Brown micropipette puller (Sutter Instrument, Novato, California, USA) to an OD of ~120 μm with a taper of 1 μm every 400 μm over a length of approximately 5 mm. We have found that although the puller was not designed to pull capillaries to this dimension, a U-shaped platinum–iridium filament of 5·5-mm width produces consistent results. The programme settings we use are heat 580, pull 60, velocity 50, time 250 and pressure 430.

Once the capillary has been pulled, the glass is scored with a diamond-encrusted dental burr at the point where the OD is ~120 μm, and the capillary is then broken (Fig. 1c). The face of this break must be vertical and flat (Fig. 1d) and pipettes with uneven or oblique breaks should be discarded. The holding pipette is heat polished using the radiant heat from a small glass bead (~100 μm in diameter) which has been fused onto the platinum–iridium filament of a microforge (Bachofer GmbH, Reutlingen, Germany) (Fig. 1e). The ID of the polished portion of the holding pipette is ~30–40 μm (Fig. 1f) which allows the oocyte to be held securely with minimal distortion. The holding pipette is then bent over the microflame to the appropriate angles, using a 26 G needle with a small hook in its tip to control the position of the glass as it bends (Fig. 1g).

Manufacture of Injection Pipettes

Thin-walled borosilicate capillaries which have an OD of 1·0 mm and an ID of 0·78 mm (Fig. 2a) are pulled to an OD of ~7 μm with a taper of 1 mm every 400 mm over a length of 5 mm. It is important that the sides of the pipette are approximately parallel as uneven sides can make it difficult to control fluid in the pipette. A box-shaped, platinum–iridium filament of 2-mm width is used in the pipette puller. The programme settings we use are heat 590, pull 50, velocity 40, time 30 and pressure 500.

The pulled capillary is broken where its OD is ~6–7 μm using the microforge (Figs 2b and 2c). The small glass bead on the microforge filament is heated until it is just tacky, and the glass capillary is touched against the glass bead (Fig. 2b). When the current to the filament is turned off, the filament cools and retracts, and the glass sticking to the bead is broken as the filament pulls away (Fig. 2c), giving a clean break at that point (Fig. 2d).

The tip of the pipette is then ground to an angle of 40–45° using a capillary tip microgrinder (Bachofer GmbH, Reutlingen, Germany). Correct pressure must be applied to the glass capillary — too little pressure will result in an incompletely ground tip, and too much pressure will produce an elongated ground surface. The grinding wheel is irrigated with 18 Ω Milli Q water at a rate of 1 drop every 4 s which keeps the capillary free of glass dust during grinding (Fig. 2e). The pipette is then rinsed 5 times with absolute alcohol and 5 times with 18 Ω Milli Q water. The ground surface is inspected at 500× magnification on an inverted microscope to ensure that the bevel is satisfactory (Fig. 2f).

A sharp spike is created on the tip of the pipette by touching the point of the bevel against the glass bead of the microforge and then quickly pulling the bead away (Figs 2g and 2h). The glass bead must be sticky, but it should also be slightly hotter than when it is used to break injection pipettes. The bead should faintly glow a very deep red. Spikes which are too long cause lysis of the oocyte, so long spikes should be broken off against the thick edge of the holding pipette before injection or the pipette should be discarded. An example of a good spike is shown in Fig. 2i.

The pipette can be bent to the appropriate angle(s) with the aid of a hooked 26 G needle. Because injection pipettes are very fine, it is easier to bend them using the microforge than a microflame.

Heat Sterilization of Pipettes

The finished holding and injection pipettes are stored in clean, dust-free glass or plastic containers. They are heat sterilized at 150°C for 2 h before use.

Problems Encountered During Pipette Manufacture

The capillaries scorch during manufacture. This can be a problem, particularly when holding pipettes are heat-polished. It occurs when the glassware has not been adequately cleaned before the manufacture of instruments.

The glass bead on the forge becomes less tacky even though the same amount of current is applied. This can be overcome by gradually increasing the filament current so that the bead glows to yellow–white hot, followed by reducing the current to the normal working level.

The injection pipette is difficult to break OR *the spike on the tip of the injection pipette is very difficult to make.* It is important in all steps of instrument manufacture to ensure that the top of the glass bead and the glass filament are in sharp focus at the same time so that they can be oriented with respect to each other.

The spike on the injection pipette is too long OR *the hole at the tip of the injection pipette is very elongate after the spike has been made.* In both cases the bead temperature is too hot. Reduce the temperature, focus on the top of the bead and the point of the bevel very clearly, then touch the bead against the bevel, press it

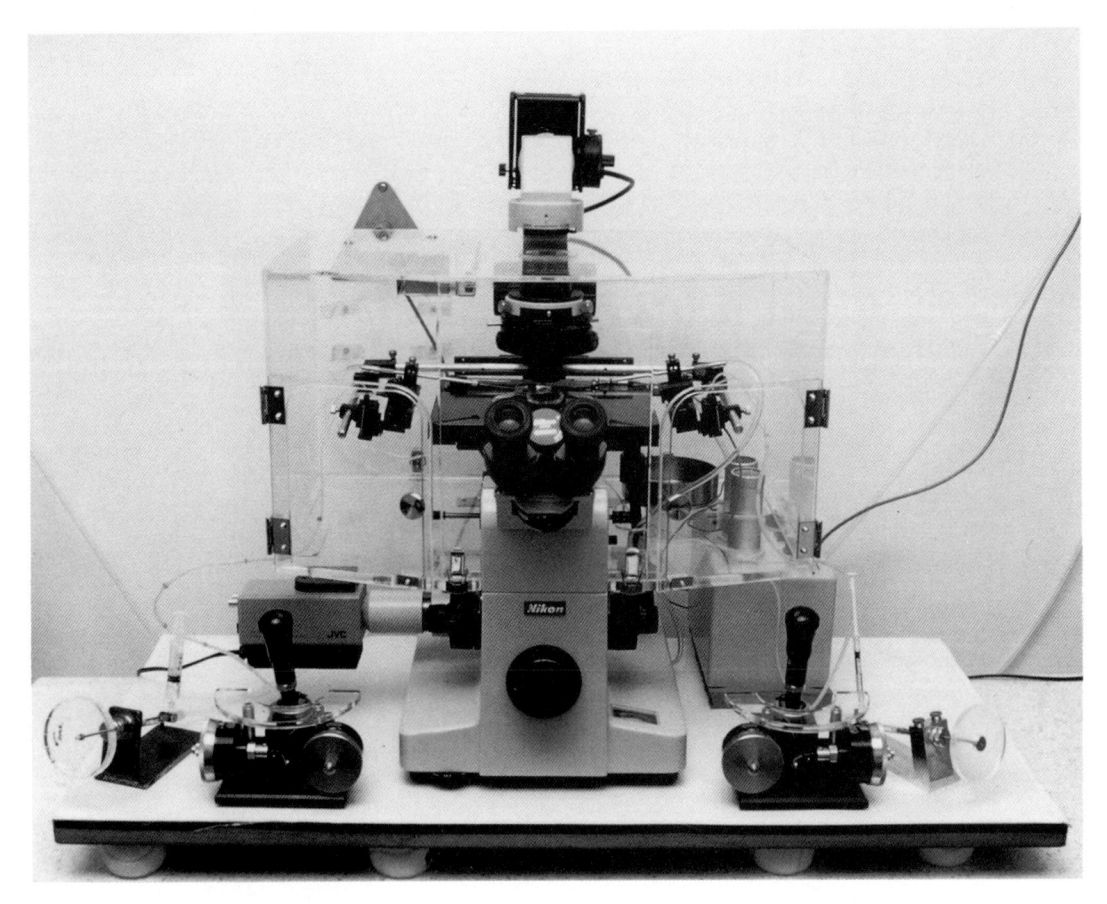

Fig. 3. The micromanipulator set-up includes an inverted microscope fitted with Nomarski DIC optics, 2 joystick manipulators, and an environmental chamber equipped with a heater and a CO_2 controller. The set-up sits on a heavy slate base which is cushioned by 2 pneumatic wheelbarrow tyres and 8 half court tennis balls to reduce vibration.

against the point of the pipette slightly—the shaft of the pipette will bend a little, and then quickly pull the bead away.

Injection pipettes clog up with glass filings during grinding. The water must drip onto the path of the injection pipette so that there is a column of water in the injection pipette which rises and falls as the water drops onto the grinding wheel. This will ensure that the pipette is kept free of glass particles during grinding by carrying away the particles as they form.

Pipettes are inconsistent in diameter. It is important to check the outer diameter of each manufactured pipette, especially injection pipettes, against a calibrated graticule at high magnification (500×). We have also found it useful to use a graticule in the stereo microscope on the microforge to check the diameter of pipettes—high quality optics are required.

Commercially Available Pipettes

The manufacture of glass instruments is time consuming and has a considerable learning curve. Furthermore, the pipette puller, microforge and grinder are expensive, and unless a unit intends doing a significant number of ICSI procedures each week, it may be difficult to recoup the initial financial outlay. Several companies now offer high quality ICSI pipettes for sale, and if suitable glass instruments can be obtained in this way, then it might be advantageous to explore this avenue before committing the laboratory to the expense and time involved in making pipettes.

Injection Technique

General Micromanipulator Set up

We use two micromanipulation set-ups (Fig. 3) which each consist of a Diaphot inverted microscope equipped with Nomarski differential interference contrast (DIC) optics, a perspex environmental chamber and heater (Nikon, Tokyo, Japan), and a CO_2 controller (Forma Scientific, Marietta, OH, USA). The chamber is maintained at 37°C and a constant, humidified atmosphere of 5% CO_2 in air. Prior to and after microinjection, oocytes are handled in converted premature infant incubators which are similarly gassed with 5% CO_2 in air, humidified and heated to 37°C. The advantage of this system is that we can maintain oocytes in bicarbonate-buffered culture medium at all times without having to change to HEPES-buffered medium for the micromanipulation procedures. Nevertheless, many units achieve excellent results using heated microscope stages and HEPES-buffered media for injection (Van Steirteghem et al. 1993a, 1993b).

For the suction and injection systems, we use semi-rigid, fine bore teflon tubing filled with low viscosity silicon oil (200 fluid/50 CS; Dow Corning, Blacktown, NSW, Australia). Metal instrument holders (Leica, Wetzlar, Germany) are used to mount and hold the glass holding and injection pipettes on the micromanipulators. Suction for the holding pipette is generated using a 0·5 mL screw plunger glass syringe (Hamilton, Reno, Nevada, USA) and care is taken to ensure that there are no air bubbles in the lines. We control the degree of suction in the injection pipette using a 1 mL disposable tuberculin syringe (Becton Dickinson, Singapore), and the judicious use of air spaces in the syringe and injection pipette permits very fine control of the injection pressure. Two upright joystick type manipulators with Z control (Type MO 202; Narishige, Tokyo, Japan) complete each set-up (Fig. 3).

Since the microscopes are fitted with Nomarski DIC optics, we use glass Petri dish lids (Glaswerk, Wertheim, Germany) for micromanipulation and they provide an excellent image. Many other units use Hoffman modulation contrast optics (Catt et al. 1995) which permits the use of plastic Petri dishes, but in our experience, the quality and clarity of the image is inferior to that which can be obtained using Nomarski DIC optics and glass dishes.

Preparation of Polyvinylpyrrolidone

A 10% solution of polyvinylpyrrolidone (PVP) (PVP-360; Sigma, St Louis, MO, USA) in Milli Q water is dialysed for 36 h at 4°C against 14 changes of 18 Ω Milli Q water using dialysis membranes with a molecular weight cut-off of 14 kDa (Union Carbide, Chicago, IL, USA). The membranes are boiled for 2 h in 0·2 M sodium bicarbonate (BDH, Poole, Dorset, UK) and 1 mM EDTA (Sigma), then rinsed extensively in 18 Ω Milli Q water before use. The resulting dialysate is freeze-dried and stored in capped culture tubes at room temperature. A 10% solution of PVP is prepared in bicarbonate-buffered human tubal fluid (HTF) medium (Quinn et al. 1985) as required. It is filter sterilized through a 0·8 μm filter and then stored at 4°C for up to 4 weeks. Although some operators obtain good fertilization rates without using PVP (Bourne et al. 1995), we believe that the use of PVP has been an important factor in the success of our ICSI programme. The viscosity of a 10% solution dramatically slows even fast moving sperm, and improves the control of fluid movement in and out of the injection pipette. In turn, precise control means that sperm can be manipulated with great accuracy and that very little injection vehicle is introduced into the oocyte during injection.

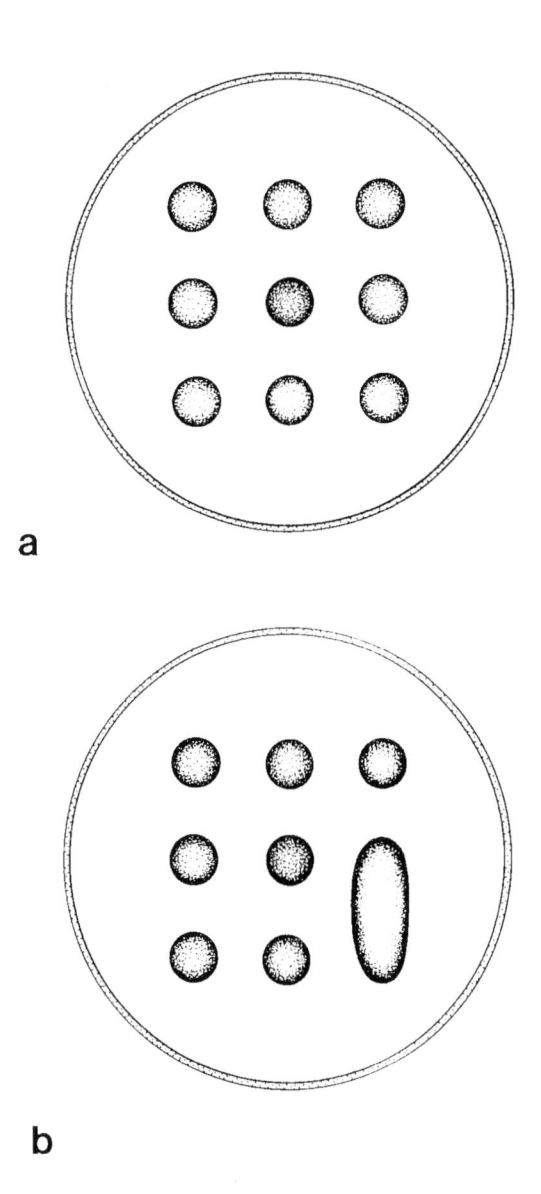

Fig. 4. Arrangement of culture medium drops in the injection dishes. (a) Eight 5-μL drops of medium containing the oocytes surround a central 5-μL drop of 10% PVP; (b) when only occasional motile sperm are recovered from the ejaculate or the procedure uses testicular or epididymal sperm, a long drop of medium (15 μL) replaces two of the 5-μL drops. The sperm suspension is added to the long drop and sperm are selected one at a time, and transported to the central drop of PVP where they are immobilized.

Preparation of Culture Media and Dishes

Eight drops (5 μL each) of bicarbonate-buffered HTF medium are placed around a single 5-μL drop of the 10% PVP solution in a glass Petri dish lid (Fig. 4). The drops are quickly and carefully covered with 3 mL of culture grade mineral (paraffin) oil (Sigma) and equilibrated at 37°C at 5% CO_2 for several hours before injection. It is important that each dish is prepared separately so that the 5-μL drops of medium do not evaporate significantly before they are covered with oil.

Preparation of Oocytes and Sperm for Injection

Cumulus–oocyte complexes are exposed to 1 mg mL^{-1} (690 I.U. mL^{-1}) hyaluronidase (ovine, Type III; Sigma) for about 30s and then rinsed through 4 changes of HTF medium before mechanically denuding the coronal cells with a fine bore, hand-pulled pipette. Rough pipetting will rupture the zona pellucida and cause lysis of the oocyte. Unless the coronal cells are very loosely attached, it is advisable to use a large bore pipette to remove some of the cells before progressing to a narrower bore pipette to strip the residual cells. Cumulus-free oocytes are cultured for at least 30 min before injection.

Immediately before injection, oocytes are placed singly in the 5-μL drops of HTF medium under oil and approximately 1 μL of sperm suspension is added to the 5-μL drop of 10% PVP (Fig. 4a). When only an occasional motile sperm is recovered from the ejaculate, the sperm suspension is placed in an elongated drop (Fig. 4b) and motile sperm are picked out of the debris with the injection pipette and transferred to the central drop containing PVP. Severely oligozoospermic semen samples often contain high numbers of non-sperm cells and significant amounts of debris, which can both clog injection pipettes. Even sperm which are essentially immotile or merely twitching are transferred to PVP before injection. If a man is known to have completely immotile sperm, it is worthwhile performing a dye exclusion test for sperm viability before the treatment cycle. Alternatively, the hypo-osmotic swelling test can be used to select viable sperm for ICSI (Desmet *et al.* 1994; Bourne *et al.* 1995).

Injection Procedure

Many aspects of the procedure described below were originally developed in Brussels (Palermo *et al.* 1992; Van Steirteghem *et al.* 1993a).

Immobilizing the spermatozoon. The orientation of the injection pipette, holding pipette and the drops of medium is shown in Fig. 5. We examine the sperm in the PVP drop at a magnification of 200×, and select morphologically 'acceptable' sperm which are swimming slowly along the base of the Petri dish lid. In some cases the sperm only twitch. In severe teratozoospermic samples, few if any of the sperm are morphologically 'normal' so we select those sperm which most closely approximate a normal morphology. When a spermatozoon has been selected, the injection pipette is raised and positioned over the midpiece of the sperm tail (Fig. 6a), and while the spermatozoon is still moving slowly, the injection pipette is brought down onto the midpiece.

If the pipette is in contact with the tail and the tail is on the bottom of the dish, the spermatozoon will stop moving forward (Fig. 6b). The injection pipette is then drawn sharply across the tail (Fig. 6c) which immediately immobilizes the spermatozoon. If it retains any motility at all, even a slight flexing of the tail, the procedure is repeated until complete immobilization occurs. This procedure is also carried out on immotile or twitching sperm. The immobilized spermatozoon is then aspirated into the injection pipette tail first (Fig. 6d) and is positioned close to the pipette opening (Fig. 6e). The injection pipette is transferred to a 5-μL drop containing an oocyte.

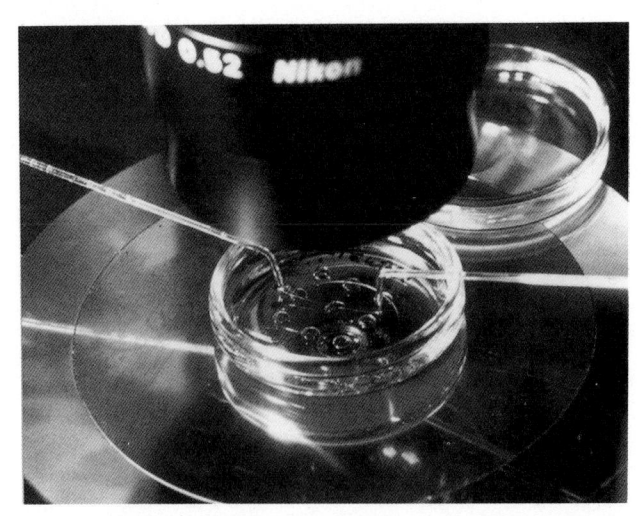

Fig. 5. Z-shaped pipettes and glass Petri dish lids are used for micromanipulation.

Intracytoplasmic sperm injection. The oocyte is held flat against the holding pipette using gentle suction. We ensure that the oocyte is in contact with the bottom of the dish — this provides an extra axis of support during injection. The injection pipette is positioned so that the oocyte plasma membrane and the tip of the injection pipette are both in sharp focus — this ensures injection through the middle of the oocyte. The polar body is oriented at 12 o'clock and the bevel of the injection pipette faces 6 o'clock (Fig. 7a). Practitioners have found that on some occasions, the injected sperm become involved in the metaphase chromosomes of the oocyte (Dozortsev *et al.* 1994a; Flaherty *et al.* 1995), so we always orient the injection pipette with the bevel facing 6 o'clock in an attempt to reduce the incidence of this abnormal outcome. Since this practice has not completely prevented the presence of sperm among the metaphase chromosomes of the oocyte, it seems that the polar body is not always a reliable indicator of the site of germinal vesicle breakdown (Palermo *et al.* 1995b).

The spermatozoon is positioned near the pipette opening. The injection pipette is then pushed steadily

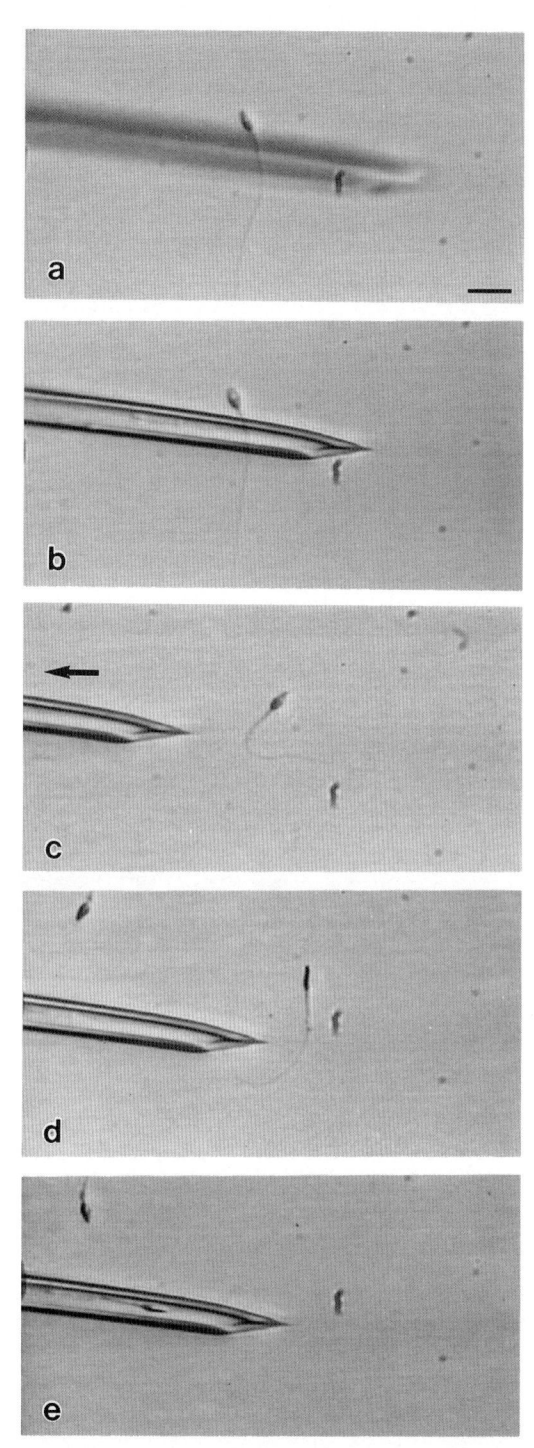

Fig. 6. Sperm immobilization before injection. *(a)* A motile spermatozoon which is moving slowly along the bottom of the dish (in viscous PVP) is located, the tail is arranged perpendicular to the injection pipette and the pipette is raised above the midpiece; *(b)* the pipette is brought down into contact with the tail—forward progression ceases; *(c)* the pipette is drawn across the tail very quickly in the direction of the arrow. This procedure should immobilize the spermatozoon immediately, but if it still retains some motility, then the procedure is repeated; *(d)* the spermatozoon is aspirated into the pipette tail first; *(e)* the sperm head is positioned close to the opening of the pipette. Bar, 10 μm.

against the zona pellucida (ZP) (Fig. 7*a*) until it pierces the ZP and is situated well within the oocyte, surrounded by a shallow furrow (Fig. 7*b*). In our experience the oocyte plasma membrane does not usually rupture at this time, although Palermo *et al.* (1995*b*) reported that it does. To ensure that the oolemma does rupture, the oocyte cytoplasm is aspirated back into the injection pipette (Fig. 7*c*) until there is a sudden increase in the speed of cytoplasm movement in the pipette, which indicates that the membrane has ruptured. The cytoplasm is gently pushed back into the oocyte along with the spermatozoon and a minimal volume of PVP solution (Fig. 7*d*), and the injection pipette is then withdrawn from the oocyte, leaving the spermatozoon in the oocyte (Fig. 7*e*). There should be relatively little disturbance of the oocyte cytoplasm during injection. A large amount of cytoplasmic disturbance indicates that the diameter of the injection pipette might be too large (>8 μm) or that the replacement of the cytoplasm was too hurried. The actual injection of the spermatozoon into the oocyte usually takes no longer than 5 s, however, Palermo *et al.* (1995*b*) describe a more complex methology which takes around 1 min to accomplish.

The oocyte plasma membrane slowly (1–5 min) assumes its original conformation (Fig. 7*f*). Once all of the oocytes in a particular dish have been injected, each oocyte is checked again to ensure that the spermatozoon is indeed located within the cytoplasm—this indicates that the procedure has been successful. Oocytes that have been unsuccessfully injected and contain a spermatozoon in the perivitelline space (PVS) are re-injected with a fresh spermatozoon.

The oocytes are washed through a change of HTF medium and they are then cultured overnight in 10-μL drops of HTF under mineral oil. To avoid the effects of embryo toxicity, the mineral oil is tested weekly in an *in vitro* sperm viability assay which is similar to the one described by Critchlow *et al.* (1989). Mineral oil can quickly develop embryo toxicity during short-term or long-term storage (Payne *et al.* 1994), even in unopened bottles, so it is essential that it is tested regularly.

Oocytes are examined at 200× approximately 17 h post-injection for evidence of fertilization (2 pronuclei, 2 polar bodies), and zygotes are then cultured for a further 48 h in fresh drops of HTF under mineral oil. Up to 3 good quality embryos are transferred to the uterus, and any suitable supernumerary embryos are cryopreserved.

Problems Encountered during Injection

Failed injection. If the oocyte plasma membrane is not ruptured, the spermatozoon will not be deposited in the cytoplasm when the needle is withdrawn, even though it may look as though it is (Fig. 8*a*). During the next 5 min, the spermatozoon will be drawn back with

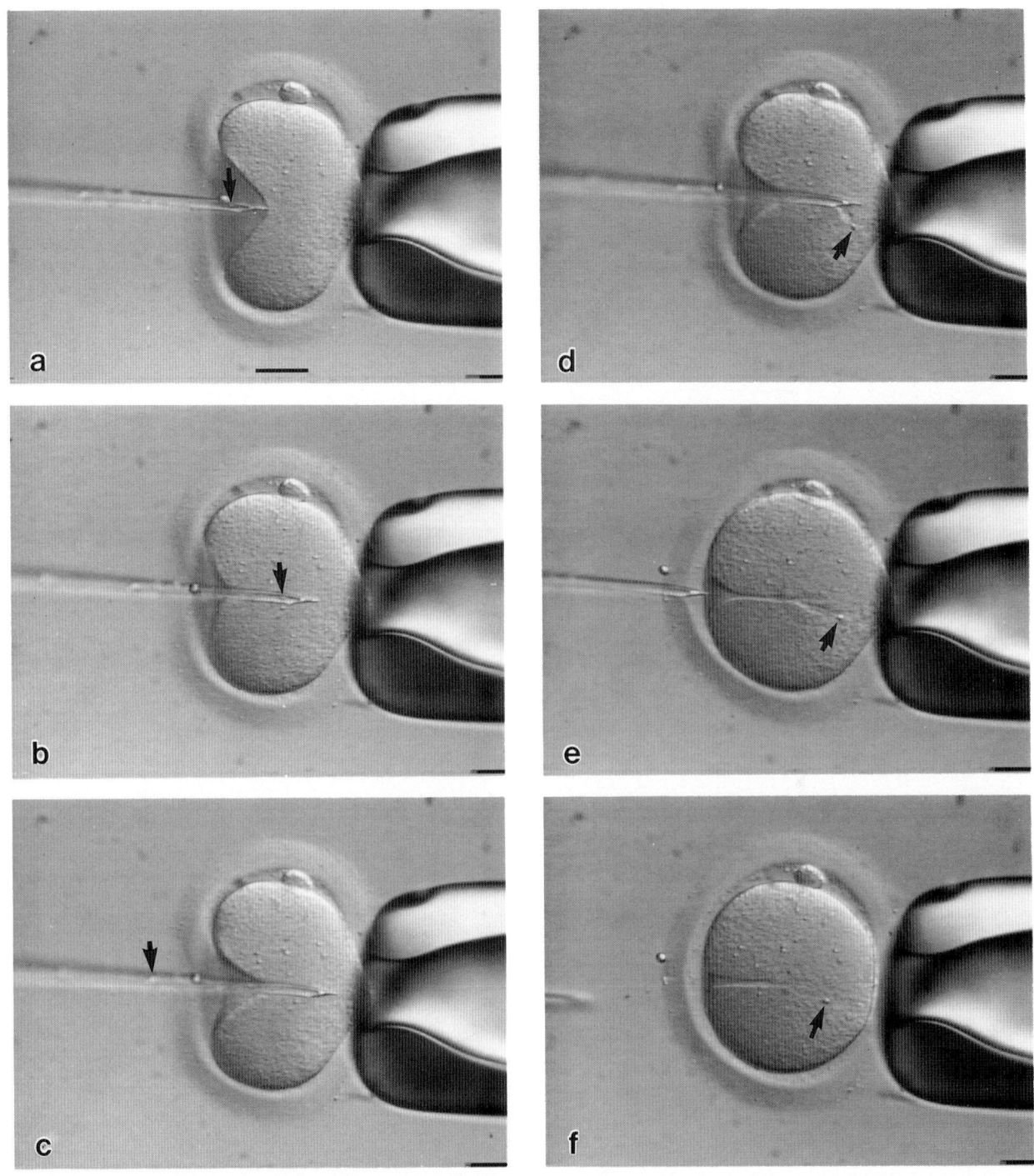

Fig. 7. Intracytoplasmic sperm injection. In each micrograph, the sperm head is indicated by an arrow. *(a)* The oocyte is held snugly against the holding pipette, with the polar body at 12 o'clock, and the injection pipette is pushed against the zona pellucida which distorts the oocyte. *(b)* As the injection pipette penetrates the zona pellucida it lies deep within the oocyte, but the oocyte plasma membrane has not yet ruptured—the spermatozoon is still near the end of the injection pipette (arrow). *(c)* The cytoplasm of the oocyte is drawn back into the injection pipette, increasing the tension on the plasma membrane. The spermatozoon also moves backwards into the body of the injection pipette (arrow). There is a sudden rush of cytoplasm into the pipette as the oocyte plasma membrane ruptures. *(d)* The cytoplasm and the spermatozoon are pushed back into the oocyte so that the spermatozoon lies within the oocyte (arrow). *(e)* The injection pipette is gently withdrawn from the oocyte—the spermatozoon remains in the cytoplasm (arrow). *(f)* The oocyte plasma membrane heals rapidly and the oocyte resumes its original shape within 5 min. The spermatozoon remains stationary within the oocyte during this process (arrow). Bar, 30 μm.

the membrane as the oocyte resumes its original shape (Figs 8b and 8c) and it will eventually be ejected into the PVS (Fig. 8d).

Oocyte lysis during injection. An injection pipette with a long, sharp spike can cause immediate rupture of the oolemma and lysis of the oocyte. These pipettes can be successfully modified at the time of injection by driving the spike against the holding pipette several times. This breaks the end of the spike but still leaves the pipette sharp enough to penetrate the ZP with minimal distortion. These 'modified' pipettes do not cause lysis.

If the plasma membrane at the equator of the oocyte and the injection pipette are both in sharp focus during injection, then the minimum area of plasma membrane will be pulled back into the injection pipette as the membrane is broken. If, however, injection is attempted with the injection pipette above or below the equator of the oocyte (tip of the pipette not in the same plane of focus as the oocyte membrane), then an oblique entry into the oocyte will ensue and a larger area of plasma membrane will be pulled back into the injection pipette. When the membrane eventually ruptures, a large tear results which can induce irreparable damage to the membrane and lysis of the oocyte.

When the surface of the holding pipette is not flat, or the holding pipette is too narrow, the force of the injection pipette against the ZP can cause the oocyte to roll off the holding pipette, resulting in considerable distortion of the oocyte. Similarly, if the injection pipette is too blunt, the oocyte can be badly distorted before the pipette penetrates the ZP or the oolemma. When the holding pipette is too close to the bottom of the dish, the oocyte cannot be held securely and this results in it rolling off the holding pipette with considerable distortion during injection. The risk of lysis increases markedly when the oocyte is grossly distorted.

Conclusions

The following are essential for the success of any micromanipulation programme:

(1) There must be a good routine IVF programme already in place before trying to introduce demanding micromanipulation techniques.

(2) All aspects of micromanipulation must be carried out with the same rigid attention to cleanliness and sterility as used in routine IVF.

(3) There must be alert and vigilant consideration of any factors which might reduce sperm and oocyte survival, such as over-exposure of oocytes to hyaluronidase (Fishel *et al.* 1992; Van Steirteghem *et al.* 1993b), rough handling of oocytes during denuding, temperature and pH fluctuations, and undue distortion of the egg during injection (Payne 1994).

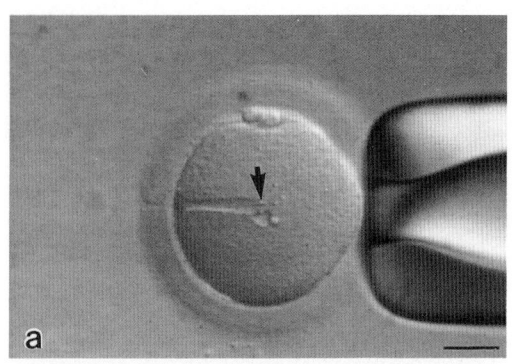

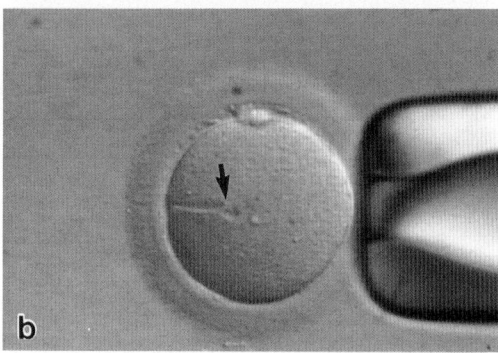

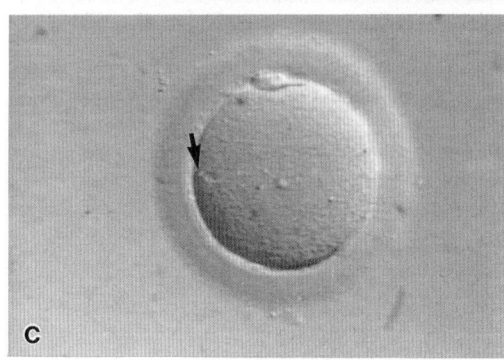

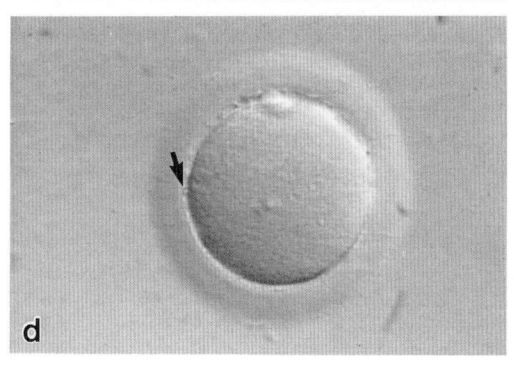

Fig. 8. This sequence of micrographs illustrates a failed injection attempt in which the oocyte plasma membrane was drawn back into the injection pipette, but not far enough to rupture it. Consequently, the spermatozoon was never deposited into the cytoplasm. *(a)* The spermatozoon (arrow) appears to be located within the cytoplasm of the oocyte; *(b* and *c)* the spermatozoon (arrow) moves peripherally with the membrane as the oocyte resumes its original shape; *(d)* the spermatozoon (arrow) is eventually ejected into the perivitelline space. Bar, 30 μm.

(4) High quality glass instruments are essential. It is axiomatic for those skilled in micromanipulative procedures that good quality instruments are responsible for much of the success of these techniques.

In our experience, two technical actions are crucial to the success of ICSI: sperm immobilization and rupture of the oocyte plasma membrane. Sperm must be completely immobilized before injection. The spermatozoon will quickly regain motility in the reduced viscosity of the oocyte cytoplasm if it has not been fully immobilized and this should be avoided. Moreover, sperm immobilization has important consequences for fertilization. When the injection pipette is drawn sharply across the sperm tail, the plasma membrane is ruptured (Dozortsev *et al.* 1994*b*) and this may allow cytoplasmic factors in the oocyte which induce sperm head decondensation to enter the spermatozoon (Flaherty *et al.* 1995; Payne 1995). There is also evidence that sperm cytosolic factors are responsible for activation of the oocyte after ICSI (Dozortsev *et al.* 1995), and in a recent study in which sperm were not routinely immobilized before ICSI, the fertilization rate was reduced due to failure of oocyte activation. Furthermore, the majority of these unfertilized oocytes formed 2 pronuclei when activated by exposure to calcium ionophore (Tesarik *et al.* 1995). Rupture of the sperm plasma membrane, which is achieved and indicated by immobilization, is essential for obtaining good fertilization rates after ICSI. Incomplete or tentative immobilization leads to reduced fertilization rates and this can be easily corrected if immobilization is performed more enthusiastically (Catt *et al.* 1995; Palermo *et al.* 1995*b*).

The oocyte plasma membrane must be ruptured or else the spermatozoon will not be deposited into the oocyte and it will merely be left in an invagination of the oolemma. This is equivalent to single sperm sub-zonal injection (SUZI) which generally yields poor fertilization rates (15–20%). Sperm which are left in such an invagination will be ejected into the PVS (Catt *et al.* 1995). McLachlan *et al.* (1995) reported that their fertilization rate improved significantly when greater care was taken to rupture the oocyte plasma membrane.

Successful application of the ICSI technique requires a considerable learning curve, particularly for those new to micromanipulation. Setting up the glass instruments, developing a conceptual understanding of up and down in a two-dimensional microscope field of view, maintaining clean, useable instruments during the course of the procedure, and coping with the million and one perturbations that always seem to occur, requires experience and many hours of practice. It is unrealistic to expect immediate competence with any micromanipulative technique just because a video makes it look easy. There are also many time consuming activities behind the scenes which are just as essential for success but which are not immediately obvious to the casual observer. These must also be given due consideration when establishing the technique in the laboratory.

ICSI has been a major breakthrough in the treatment of male factor infertility and any IVF unit wishing to offer a comprehensive service must consider ICSI as an essential component.

Acknowledgments

I thank Nick Swann for his excellent diagrams, Matt Makinson for assistance with photography, and Sean Flaherty for assistance with preparation of the manuscript.

References

Bourne, H., Richings, N., Harari, O., Watkins, W., Speirs, A. L., Johnston, W. I. H., and Baker, H. W. G. (1995). The use of intracytoplasmic sperm injection for the treatment of severe and extreme male factor infertility. In 'Intracytoplasmic Sperm Injection: the Revolution in Male Infertility'. *Reprod. Fertil. Dev.* **7**, 237–45.

Catt, J. W., Ryan, J. P., Pike, I. L., O'Neill, C., and Saunders, D. M. (1995). Clinical intracytoplasmic sperm injection results from Royal North Shore Hospital. In 'Intracytoplasmic Sperm Injection: the Revolution in Male Infertility'. *Reprod. Fertil. Dev.* **7**, 255–62.

Critchlow, J. D., Matson, P. L., Newman, M. C., Horne, G., Troup, S. A., and Lieberman, B. A. (1989). Quality control in an *in-vitro* fertilization laboratory: use of human sperm survival studies. *Hum. Reprod. (Oxf.)* **4**, 545–9.

Desmet, B., Joris, H., Nagy, Z., Liu, J., Bocken, G., Vankelecom, A., Van Ranst, H., Devroey, P., and Van Steirteghem, A. C. (1994). Selection of vital immotile spermatozoa for intracytoplasmic sperm injection by the hypo-osmotic swelling test. *Hum. Reprod. (Oxf.)* **9** (Suppl. 4), 24. [Abstr.]

Dozortsev, D., De Sutter, P., and Dhont, M. (1994*a*). Behaviour of spermatozoa in human oocytes displaying no or one pronucleus after intracytoplasmic sperm injection. *Hum. Reprod. (Oxf.)* **9**, 2139–44.

Dozortsev, D., De Sutter, P., and Dhont, M. (1994*b*). Damage to the sperm plasma membrane by touching the sperm tail with a needle prior to intracytoplasmic injection. *Hum. Reprod. (Oxf.)* **9** (Suppl. 4), 40. [Abstr.]

Dorzortsev, D., Rybouchkin, A., De Sutter, P., Qiam, C., and Dhont, M. (1995). Human oocyte activation following intracytoplasmic injection: the role of the sperm cell. *Hum. Reprod. (Oxf.)* **10**, 403–7.

Fishel, S., Timson, J., Lisi, F., and Rinaldi, L. (1992). Evaluation of 225 patients undergoing subzonal insemination for the procurement of fertilization *in vitro*. *Fertil. Steril.* **57**, 840–9.

Flaherty, S. P., Payne, D., Swann, N. J., and Matthews, C. D. (1995). Assessment of abnormal fertilization and fertilization failure after intracytoplasmic sperm injection (ICSI). In 'Intracytoplasmic Sperm Injection: the Revolution in Male Infertility'. *Reprod. Fertil. Dev.* **7**, 197–210.

Hamberger, L., Sjögren, A., Lundin, K., Söderlund, B., Nilsson, L., Bergh, C., Wennerholm, U.-B., Wikland, M., Svalander, P., Jakobsson, A. H., and Forsberg, A.-S. (1995). Microfertilization techniques: the Swedish experience. In 'Intracytoplasmic Sperm Injection: the Revolution in Male Infertility'. *Reprod Fertil. Dev.* **7**, 263–8.

McLachlan, R. I., Fuscaldo, G., Rho, H., Poulos, C., Dalrymple, J., Jackson P., and Holden, C. A. (1995). Clinical results from intracytoplasmic sperm injection at Monash IVF. In 'Intracytoplasmic Sperm Injection: the Revolution in Male Infertility'. *Reprod. Fertil. Dev.* **7**, 247–53.

Palermo, G., Joris, H., Devroey, P., and Van Steirteghem, A. C. (1992). Pregnancies after intracytoplasmic injection of single spermatozoon into an oocyte. *Lancet* **340**, 17–18.

Palermo, G., Cohen, J., Alikani, M., Adler, A., and Rosenwaks, Z. (1995a). Development and implementation of intracytoplasmic sperm injection (ICSI). In 'Intracytoplasmic Sperm Injection: the Revolution in Male Infertility'. *Reprod Fertil. Dev.* **7**, 211–18.

Palermo, G. D., Cohen, J., Alikani, M., Adler, A., and Rosenwaks, Z. (1995b). Intracytoplasmic sperm injection: a novel treatment for all forms of male factor infertility. *Fertil. Steril.* (In press.)

Payne, D. (1994). Embryo viability associated with microassisted fertilization. *Baillière's Clin. Obstet. Gynaecol.* **8**, 157–75.

Payne, D. (1995). Micro-assisted fertilization. *Reprod Fertil. Dev.* **7**. (In press.)

Payne, D., and Matthews, C. D. (1995). Intracytoplasmic sperm injection—clinical results from the Reproductive Medicine Unit, Adelaide. In 'Intracytoplasmic Sperm Injection: the Revolution in Male Infertility'. *Reprod Fertil. Dev.* **7**, 219–27.

Payne, D., Flaherty, S. P., Jeffrey. R., Warnes, G. M., and Matthews, C. D. (1994). Successful treatment of severe factor infertility in 100 consecutive cycles using intracytoplasmic sperm injection. *Hum. Reprod. (Oxf.)* **9**, 2051–7.

Quinn, P., Kerin, J. F., and Warnes, G. M. (1985). Improved pregnancy rate in human *in vitro* fertilization with the use of a medium based on the composition of human tubal fluid. *Fertil. Steril.* **44**, 493–8.

Tesarik, J., and Sousa, M. (1995). More than 90% fertilization rates after intracytoplasmic sperm injection and artificial induction of oocyte activation with calcium ionophore. *Fertil. Steril.* **63**, 343–9.

Van Steirteghem, A. C., Joris, H., Liu, J., Nagy, Z., Bocken, G., Vankelecom, A., Desmet, B., and Van Ranst, H. (1993a). Protocol intracytoplasmic sperm injection (ICSI). In 'First International Course on Assisted Fertilization by Intracytoplasmic Sperm Injection'. pp. 1–10. (ESHRE Campus Workshop: Brussels.)

Van Steirteghem, A. C., Liu, J., Joris, H., Nagy, Z., Janssenswillen, C., Tournaye, H., Derde, M.-P., Van Assche, E., and Devroey, P. (1993b). Higher success rate by intracytoplasmic sperm injection than by subzonal insemination. Report of a second series of 300 consecutive treatment cycles. *Hum. Reprod. (Oxf.)* **8**, 1055–60.

Manuscript received 4 April 1995

Open Discussion

Lars Hamberger (Göteborg):

I think we have come to the point where we really need to compare details. First, we do not use spikes and we use a 28° bevel on our injection pipettes—they penetrate the egg very well. Second, we never insert the sperm unless we have applied a negative pressure so that we can see that the cytoplasm comes up into the injection pipette. In this way, we have no problems penetrating the oolemma, although as you pointed out, you have to have a very good regulation. Finally, we have recently gone down to 5–6 μm diameter pipettes, just wide enough so that we can get the head of the spermatozoon into the pipette. This has significantly increased our fertilization rate, so in our experience at least, 8-μm diameter pipettes are slightly too thick.

Payne:

We initially used injection pipettes of about 5–6-μm diameter, but we found it quite difficult to aspirate sperm into them. This was possibly because, in putting the spike on the pipette, we altered the conformation of the hole at the end of the pipette. So we went to slightly larger injection pipettes to overcome the problem. Our fertilization rate is routinely 69%, with 65% normal fertilization, so the diameter of the pipettes is not compromising our fertilization rate. As you saw in the video, very little injection vehicle goes into the oocyte and there is very little disruption of the oocyte cytoplasm. But I take your point, it's better to have narrower injection pipettes than thicker ones.

Simon Fishel (Nottingham):

I think we'll learn a lot in this meeting that the sperm itself is less important than the procedure.

Assessment of Fertilization Failure and Abnormal Fertilization after Intracytoplasmic Sperm Injection (ICSI)

Sean P. Flaherty[A], Dianna Payne,
Nicholas J. Swann and Colin D. Matthews

*Reproductive Medicine Laboratories, Department of Obstetrics and Gynaecology,
The University of Adelaide, The Queen Elizabeth Hospital, Woodville, SA 5011, Australia.*
[A] *To whom correspondence should be addressed.*

Abstract. The assessment of fertilization is an important part of intracytoplasmic sperm injection (ICSI) and oocytes are routinely examined about 17 h after injection using Nomarski differential interference contrast optics. However, it is not possible to conclusively determine the aetiology of fertilization anomalies in this manner, so cytological studies were undertaken to determine the causes of failed and abnormal fertilization after ICSI. Oocytes which exhibited no evidence of fertilization, one pronucleus (PN) or 3 PN were fixed in glutaraldehyde, stained with Hoechst 33342 and examined by fluorescence microscopy to identify PN, metaphase chromosomes, sperm heads and polar bodies. A total of 428 unfertilized oocytes were examined from 170 ICSI cycles. Overall, 82% of these unfertilized oocytes were still at metaphase II (non-activated) while the remaining 18% were activated and had 1 PN and two polar bodies. The majority (71%) of the metaphase II oocytes contained a swollen sperm head, which indicates that the spermatozoon was correctly injected but the oocyte did not activate and complete its second meiotic division. The swollen sperm head was located among the metaphase chromosomes in 4·3% of these oocytes, while in some cases (6·6%), the sperm chromosomes had undergone premature chromosome condensation (PCC). Other aetiologies of failed fertilization in these metaphase oocytes were ejection of the spermatozoon from the oocyte (19%) and complete failure of sperm head decondensation (10%). A similar pattern of anomalies was found in 1 PN oocytes, although the ratios were different (swollen sperm head, 51%; ejection of the spermatozoon, 19%; undecondensed sperm head, 30%). Seventy abnormally fertilized oocytes were also examined, of which 63 had 3 PN and a single polar body, indicating that the unextruded second polar body developed into the third PN. In conclusion, the present study demonstrates that the principal cause of fertilization failure after ICSI is failure of oocyte activation and not ejection of the spermatozoon from the oocyte. It is also apparent that further studies are needed to elucidate the mechanisms that control oocyte activation and sperm head decondensation in injected oocytes.

Extra keywords: DNA, sperm head decondensation, oocyte activation, pronuclei, calcium, premature chromosome condensation.

Introduction

Since its introduction by Palermo *et al.* (1992), intracytoplasmic sperm injection (ICSI) has become the most efficient treatment modality for all forms of male factor infertility. ICSI overcomes the relatively low fertilization rates (10–40%) and high polyspermy rates (up to 40%) of subzonal injection (SUZI) and is a more efficacious treatment (Fishel *et al.* 1992; Palermo *et al.* 1993; Van Steirteghem *et al.* 1993a, 1993b; Payne *et al.* 1994a, 1994b). ICSI is also more efficient than routine IVF for treating cases of severe teratozoospermia (Payne *et al.* 1994b) and it can be used successfully with epididymal and testicular sperm (Silber *et al.* 1995). Furthermore, there appears to be no increase in the rate of fetal abnormalities after ICSI (Bonduelle *et al.* 1994; Tournaye *et al.* 1995).

ICSI fertilization rates of 60–70% are obtained once the injection procedure has been optimized (Palermo *et al.* 1993; Van Steirteghem *et al.* 1993a; Payne *et al.* 1994b), and it is easy to become complacent about the outstanding results that can be obtained with this technique. However, there are several important points that should be made about ICSI fertilization rates. First, the fertilization rate is only 60–70%, which indicates that a significant proportion (30–40%) of the oocytes are potentially wasted. Second, poor fertilization rates (0–50%) sometimes occur, despite successful injection of sperm into each oocyte (Payne *et al.* 1994b). The reasons for fertilization failure after ICSI are largely unknown. Third, some oocytes develop 1 pronucleus (1 PN) or 3 PN after ICSI. Palermo *et al.* (1993) speculated that 3 PN form because the oocyte retains the second polar body, but there is little experimental evidence to substantiate this contention. These three factors limit the efficacy of ICSI, and predicate that, although ICSI is successful for many couples with male factor infertility, some will still have a poor chance of conception because of low fertilization rates.

In the present paper, we describe procedures for the assessment of fertilization and the determination of the causes of failed and abnormal fertilization. Our specific aims were to determine what happened after injection in: *(1)* oocytes that showed no evidence of fertilization at all; *(2)* 1 PN oocytes; and *(3)* 3 PN oocytes. Some of the results have been published in Flaherty *et al.* (1995).

Materials and Methods

Patient Selection

For the studies on failed and abnormal fertilization, oocytes were examined from 170 (161 couples) of 282 consecutive ICSI cycles between January and August 1994. The project was approved by the Ethics of Human Research Committee at The Queen Elizabeth Hospital and informed written consent was obtained from each participating couple.

The mean±s.d. female age at treatment was $33 \cdot 7 \pm 4 \cdot 7$ years (range 24 to 48) and the mean±s.d. duration of infertility was $5 \cdot 9 \pm 3 \cdot 6$ years (range $1 \cdot 5$–22). Couples were offered ICSI for one of the following reasons: *(1)* severe oligozoospermia with only occasional motile sperm in the semen ($n = 41$); *(2)* semen that was too poor for routine IVF (<200 000 motile sperm recovered on Percoll gradients; ($n = 93$); *(3)* previous failed or poor (<25%) fertilization in routine IVF ($n = 9$); *(4)* epididymal sperm aspiration ($n = 9$); and *(5)* first cycle of IVF with <20% normal sperm morphology ($n = 9$). ICSI offers patients in group 5 a much better chance of fertilization than routine IVF (Payne *et al.* 1994*b*; Payne and Matthews 1995).

Preparation of Spermatozoa

Semen samples were produced by masturbation, collected into sterile containers and analysed according to the standards of the World Health Organization (1987). Ejaculated sperm were separated from seminal plasma using discontinuous Percoll gradients (Payne *et al.* 1991) or mini-Percoll gradients (Ord *et al.* 1990). When only occasional motile sperm were present in the ejaculate, they were concentrated by three cycles of centrifugation at 300–500g and resuspension in human tubal fluid (HTF) medium (Quinn *et al.* 1985; Payne *et al.* 1994*b*). Epididymal sperm were aspirated from dissected proximal epididymal tubules using a plastic micropipette and collected in HEPES-buffered HTF. They were maintained at 35°C and prepared for ICSI by three cycles of centrifugation (100g, 5 min) and resuspension in HTF. The final sperm suspensions were stored at 37°C in an atmosphere of 5% CO_2.

Ovarian Stimulation, Oocyte Preparation and ICSI

The procedures for stimulation of follicular growth, collection of oocytes and preparation of oocytes for injection have been described elsewhere (Payne *et al.* 1991, 1994*a*, 1994*b*) and detailed descriptions of the manufacture of injection and holding pipettes, sperm immobilization and the injection procedure are given by Payne (1995). Injection pipettes had an external diameter of 7–8 μm and a 45° bevelled tip, and they were fitted with a spike. Care was taken to ensure that each spermatozoon was completely immobilized and that the oolemma was ruptured before the spermatozoon was injected into the oocyte. All procedures were carried out in 5-μL drops of HTF covered with light paraffin oil (BDH, Poole, Dorset, UK) using a Nikon Diaphot inverted microscope equipped with an environmental chamber that was maintained at 37°C and 5% CO_2. Each oocyte was carefully checked after injection to ensure that the spermatozoon was in the oocyte and had not been dragged out into the perivitelline space (PVS). Oocytes were washed in HTF and cultured overnight in a 10-μL drop of HTF under oil at 37°C in an atmosphere of 5% CO_2.

Assessment of Fertilization

Oocytes were examined about 17 h after injection using Nomarski differential interference contrast (DIC) optics. We routinely used a Nikon Diaphot inverted microscope equipped with an environmental chamber (37°C, 5% CO_2) to ensure that oocyte and zygote viability was not compromised. Each oocyte was carefully examined for the presence and location of PN, polar bodies and the spermatozoon, and the PVS of each unfertilized oocyte was examined to determine if the spermatozoon had been ejected from the oocyte.

Embryo Transfer and Pregnancy Testing

Fertilized oocytes were transferred to fresh 10-μL drops of HTF under oil and cultured at 37°C in an atmosphere of 5% CO_2 to the 6–8-cell stage (68 h after injection). Up to three embryos were then transferred to the uterus and any supernumerary embryos were frozen. A quantitative β-hCG of >25 I.U. on Days 15 and 22 after embryo transfer was considered a positive pregnancy test. Clinical pregnancies were confirmed by ultrasound.

Preparation of Oocytes for Fluorescence Microscopy

Oocytes which showed no evidence of activation or fertilization and those which had 1 PN or 3 PN were fixed in $0 \cdot 1$–$0 \cdot 5$% glutaraldehyde in $0 \cdot 1$ M cacodylate buffer at 4°C for 2–3 h. They were sometimes fixed in glutaraldehyde for up to three days, but this produced an unacceptably high level of background fluorescence after Hoechst 33342 staining. After fixation, oocytes were rinsed thoroughly in four changes of phosphate-buffered saline containing $0 \cdot 05$% sodium azide (PBS) and were then stained with 20 μg mL^{-1} Hoechst 33342 (Sigma, St Louis, MO, USA) for 30–60 min in the dark. Stained oocytes were then rinsed in four changes of PBS and mounted individually on slides and slightly compressed under 22×22 mm coverslips supported on all sides by petroleum jelly. Each slide was coded and then stored at 4°C in a black box.

The slides were all scored by one observer (S.P.F.) who did not know the origin of the oocyte or the fertilization rate for that cycle. Oocytes were carefully examined using phase contrast and fluorescence microscopy (UV excitation). The presence and location of polar bodies, sperm heads (swollen or undecondensed) and PN were recorded for each oocyte. If the location of an undecondensed sperm head was unclear, the oocyte was rotated under the coverslip to determine if it was inside the oocyte or in the PVS.

The various categories were defined as follows. Normally fertilized oocytes contained two distinct PN and two polar bodies. Abnormally fertilized oocytes contained 3 PN and one polar body. Unfertilized oocytes either exhibited 1 PN and two polar bodies or were still at metaphase II and possessed a single polar body. Metaphase II oocytes which contained an undecondensed or swollen sperm head were classified as unfertilized.

Results and Discussion

Assessment of Fertilization

Pronuclei start to form about 5 h after ICSI (Nagy *et al.* 1994; Payne, unpublished observations), so routine fertilization checks at 17 h after injection will show fertilized oocytes at a time when their PN are fully formed and expanded. The male and female PN cannot be easily distinguished, but the two PN should be of comparable size, located centrally in the oocyte, and they should contain prominent nucleoli. Glassy membranous vacuoles are sometimes found in oocytes at retrieval or after fertilization, and they are distinguished from PN by the absence of nucleoli. After fertilization, the organelles contract centrally, leaving a translucent cortical zone beneath the oolemma. A fertilized oocyte should contain 2 polar bodies in close proximity to one another in the PVS, although it is not uncommon for the first polar body to have moved or fragmented (Fig. 1).

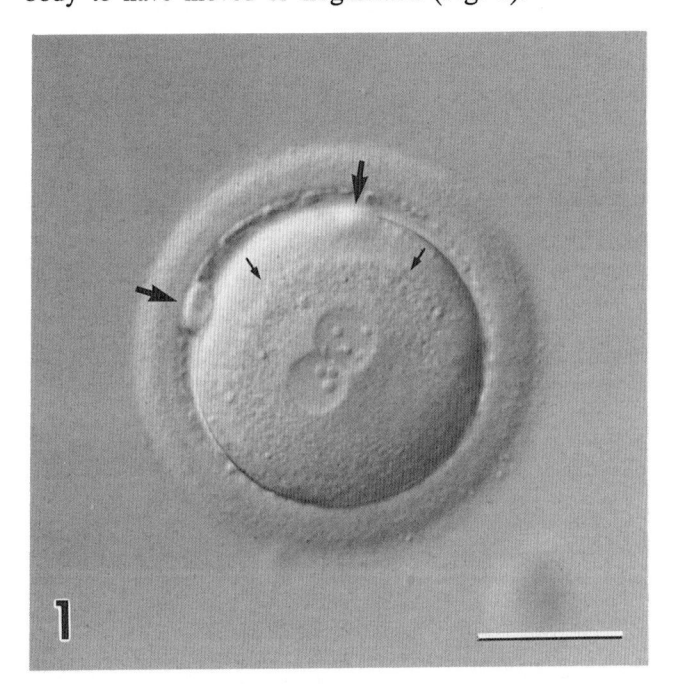

Fig. 1. A fertilized oocyte about 17 h after ICSI. Note the two uniform pronuclei with nucleoli, the two polar bodies (large arrows) and the organelle-free cortical region (small arrows). Nomarski DIC optics. Bar, 50 μm.

We carefully examine all unfertilized oocytes to determine if the spermatozoon was ejected from the oocyte into the PVS. Unusual or abnormal PN in fertilized oocytes are also noted, and these comprise PN of variant sizes (one large, one small), and instances where there are two normal-sized PN and a micro-PN.

Assessment of Oocytes using Hoechst Dyes

Hoechst 33342 and 33258 have been used to assess the cytological characteristics of unfertilized and fertilized human oocytes after routine IVF and SUZI (O'Rand et al. 1986; Gwatkin et al. 1989; Urner et al. 1993). In this study, we used Hoechst 33342 to determine why oocytes were unfertilized or showed abnormal fertilization after ICSI. Oocytes were fixed in glutaraldehyde to optimally preserve their morphology. They can be stored in this fixative for several days or even weeks before staining, but we found that this leads to an accumulation of Hoechst background fluorescence in the ooplasm which obscures PN and weakly staining sperm heads. Hence, we routinely only fix oocytes for a few hours and then store them at 4°C in PBS containing a preservative (sodium azide) until they are stained and mounted. The staining method we describe is simple, flexible and reliable, and the fluorescence emission from Hoechst 33342 is relatively stable, so the observer can examine each oocyte very carefully without worrying about the fluorescence fading quickly. It has the added advantage that the stained oocytes can be stored for many weeks in the dark at 4°C either before or after they have been mounted on slides. We mount oocytes individually on slides under 22×22-mm coverslips supported on all sides by petroleum jelly, which not only prevents evaporation during storage but also permits the coverslip to be gently compressed to flatten the oocyte or to be rotated slightly. It is not advisable to seal the coverslip edges with mountants because they compress and distort the oocyte as they dry.

Overall Fertilization Rates

The overall clinical results from our ICSI programme are presented elsewhere (Payne and Matthews 1995) and will not be covered here in detail. During the course of the present study, we examined unfertilized and abnormally fertilized oocytes from 170 of 282 consecutive ICSI cycles. In these 282 cycles, a total of 2460 oocytes were injected, of which 1742 (70·8%) were normally fertilized and 110 (4·5%) were abnormally fertilized. These fertilization rates are comparable to other published reports (Palermo et al. 1993; Van Steirteghem et al. 1993a; Payne et al. 1994b). Fig. 2 shows that acceptable fertilization rates (50–100%) were obtained in 84% of the cycles, whereas poor fertilization rates (0–50%) occurred in 16% of the cycles. Complete fertilization failure occurred in 6 cycles, and in each of these cases, only 1 oocyte (2 cycles) or 2 oocytes (4 cycles) were injected.

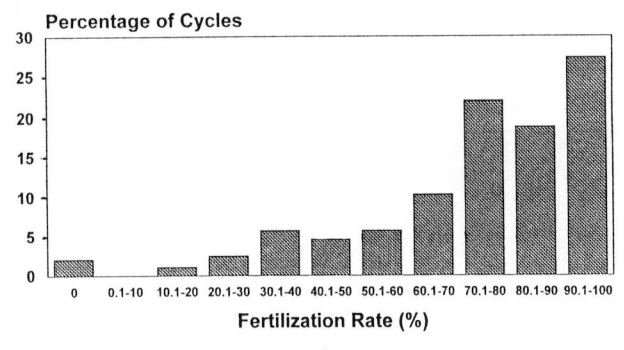

Fig. 2. Frequency distribution of fertilization rates during the study.

Table 1. Cytological observations on unfertilized oocytes

Non-activated oocytes (metaphase, one polar body) and activated oocytes (1 PN, two polar bodies) were fixed 17 h after injection. Values in parentheses are percentages of the number of oocytes examined. n, number of oocytes examined. PN, pronuclei

	Non-activated oocytes $n = 350$	Activated oocytes[A] $n = 75$
Swollen sperm head	247 (71%)	38 (51%)
Sperm ejected	66 (19%)	14 (19%)
Undecondensed sperm head	37 (10%)	23 (30%)

[A] Three oocytes which had 2 PN but only one polar body were excluded.

A total of 428 unfertilized oocytes were examined after Hoechst 33342 staining (Table 1). Overall, 350 (82%) of these oocytes were still at metaphase II and only contained a first polar body. Of the other 78 (18%) unfertilized oocytes, 75 were activated and had ejected a second polar body and possessed a female PN. The remaining 3 oocytes were activated and had 2 PN, a swollen sperm head and one polar body, which suggests that they failed to extrude the second polar body after activation and both sets of egg chromosomes developed into PN.

Unfertilized, Metaphase II Oocytes

About 71% of the unfertilized, metaphase II oocytes (19% of the injected oocytes) contained a swollen sperm head, indicating that the sperm had been correctly injected into the ooplasm but the oocyte did not activate and complete its second meiotic division (Table 1; Figs 3 and 4). Swollen sperm heads at different stages of decondensation were observed, from very early stages in which swelling was restricted to the posterior margin of the nucleus to later stages in which the nuclei were enlarged and clumps of chromatin were visible (Fig. 5). In 7% of these oocytes, the sperm head had decondensed completely into individual clumps of chromatin and long thin strands (Figs 6 and 7), which is indicative of premature chromosome condensation (PCC). In addition, a small proportion (5%) of these metaphase oocytes had abnormal or disarrayed metaphase chromosomes (Fig. 8).

Dozortsev *et al.* (1994*a*) recently reported similar findings to ours in a study of unfertilized ICSI oocytes. They found about 50% of the oocytes contained a swollen sperm head, and the same percentage of sperm heads (7%) underwent PCC. Numerous studies have also demonstrated the presence of sperm in unfertilized metaphase oocytes after routine IVF and SUZI (Pieters *et al.* 1989; Schmiady and Kentenich 1989; Balakier and Casper 1991; Selva *et al.* 1991; Plachot and Crozet 1992; Tejada *et al.* 1992; Urner *et al.* 1993). However, there appear to be two main differences between the results for unfertilized IVF and ICSI oocytes. First, the incidence of metaphase oocytes containing swollen sperm heads is much lower in unfertilized IVF oocytes (2·5–30% v. 50–70%), and this suggests that the high proportion of oocytes containing swollen sperm heads after ICSI relates in some way to microinjection. Second, most of the sperm in unfertilized IVF oocytes exhibit PCC, whereas this only occurs in about 7% of the unfertilized ICSI oocytes (Dozortsev *et al.* 1994*a*; the present study). In PCC, the sperm chromosomes prematurely condense into elongated chromatids in response to chromosome condensing factors in the ooplasm, and this is thought to be indicative of oocyte immaturity (Schmiady *et al.* 1986; Angell *et al.* 1991; Calafell *et al.* 1991).

An additional finding in 4% of the unfertilized, metaphase II oocytes was that the swollen sperm head was located among the metaphase chromosomes (Fig. 9). In some of these oocytes, the sperm head was in the spindle region near the metaphase plate, whereas in others it was completely enmeshed in the chromosomes. Dozortsev *et al.* (1994*a*) also reported this occurrence in unfertilized ICSI oocytes. In this laboratory, we always take great care to align the first polar body at 12 o'clock before injecting the oocyte at 3 or 9 o'clock so as to avoid the metaphase spindle (Palermo *et al.* 1993). This result suggests that the polar body must have moved from the spindle region at the time of injection, giving a false impression of the spindle's location. This probably also happens in a small proportion of fertilized oocytes.

In approximately 19% of the metaphase oocytes, the spermatozoon was ejected from the oocyte, and in 76% of these cases it was found in the PVS (Table 1; Fig. 10). In the remaining oocytes, it was attached to the outer surface of the zona pellucida near or in the hole through which the injection pipette had passed, or it was not seen at all and must have been ejected from the PVS into the surrounding culture medium. This result was unexpected because we originally hypothesized that ejection of the spermatozoon into the PVS would be a common finding in unfertilized oocytes. Indeed, this is the case in some ICSI programmes (Catt *et al.* 1994), whereas in others it appears to be even less common than in our study (Dozortsev *et al.* 1994*a*). These data suggest that technique may be an important component of this

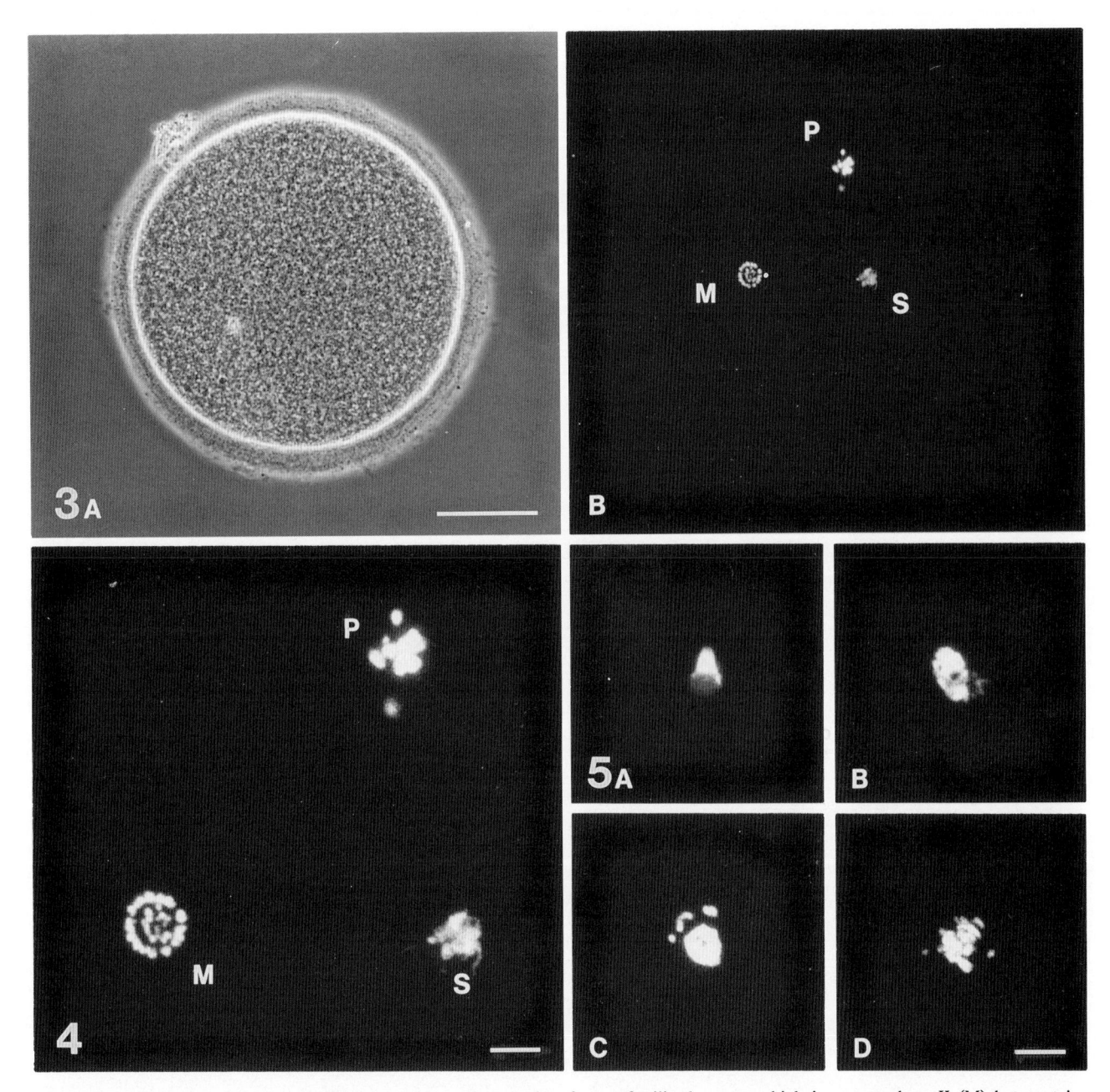

Figs 3–5. (**3A**) Phase contrast and (**3B**) fluorescence micrographs of an unfertilized oocyte which is at metaphase II (M) but contains a swollen sperm head (S). P, polar body. Bar, 50 μm. (**4**) Higher magnification of 3A showing the metaphase chromosomes (M), the swollen sperm head (S) and the first polar body (P). Bar, 10 μm. (**5**) High magnification fluorescence micrographs of swollen sperm heads in unfertilized oocytes. Various stages of sperm head decondensation are shown, from early stages (**5A**) to late stages (**5D**). Sperm nuclei often exhibited one or more DNA spots (5C). Bar, 10 μm.

aetiology. All the oocytes in the present study were carefully checked about 5–20 min after injection, when the injection furrow had completely healed, to ensure that the spermatozoon was within the ooplasm. Hence, we assume that ejection of the spermatozoon into the PVS must have occurred during culture and was not the immediate result of an unsuccessful injection attempt.

Complete failure of sperm head decondensation despite successful injection occurred in about 11% of the unfertilized, metaphase oocytes (Table 1; Fig. 11). Dozortsev *et al.* (1994a) reported a much higher percentage (38%) of this aetiology in their study. We currently do not know if this represents a gamete defect or a technical problem, but as suggested by Dozortsev *et al.* (1994a), we believe that it is due to incomplete sperm immobilization. Immobilization of the spermatozoon with the injection pipette damages the sperm membrane (Dozortsev *et al.* 1994b), and this probably enables the

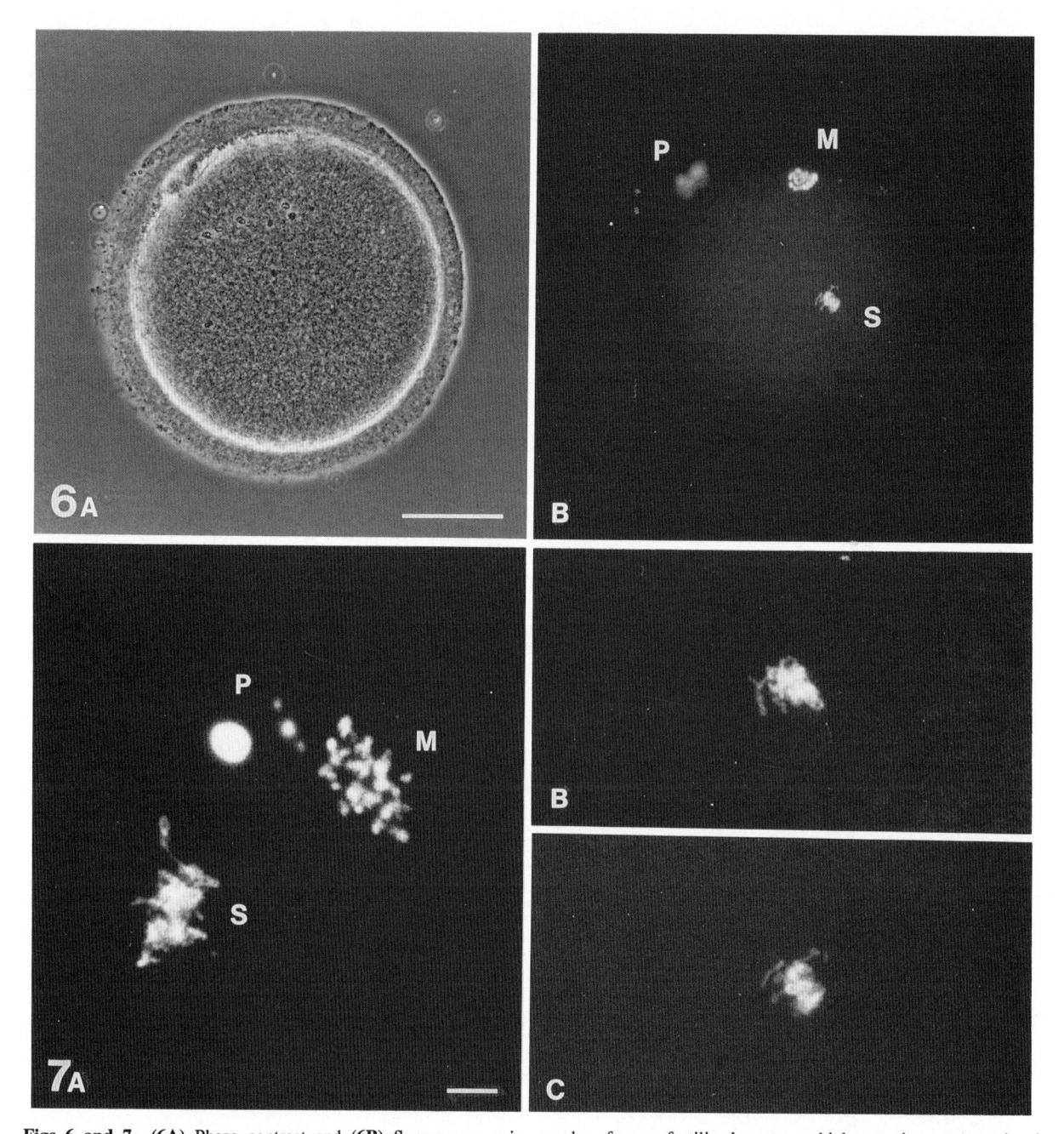

Figs 6 and 7. (**6A**) Phase contrast and (**6B**) fluorescence micrographs of an unfertilized oocyte which contains a sperm head (S) that has undergone premature chromosome condensation (PCC). M, metaphase chromosomes; P, polar body. Bar, 50 μm. (**7**) Higher magnifications of swollen sperm heads (S) which show the thin chromatin strands that are characteristic of PCC. M, metaphase chromosomes; P, polar body. Bar, 10 μm.

glutathione-like activity in the ooplasm (Perreault 1992) access to the nuclear compartment of the spermatozoon via the nuclear ring at the posterior base of the sperm head. Hence, in some cases the spermatozoon may be immobilized by stroking the tail but there may be insufficient damage to the sperm membrane, and in these instances, we would expect to see an undecondensed sperm head in the oocyte. Variations in the degree of damage to the sperm membrane during immobilization probably account for differences between our study and Dozortsev *et al.* (1994*a*) in the incidence of intact sperm heads in unfertilized ICSI oocytes.

One Pronuclear Oocytes

A similar pattern was seen in the 1 PN oocytes which comprised 18% of the unfertilized oocytes or 5% of the injected oocytes (Table 1). In each case the oocyte had activated after injection and had ejected a second polar

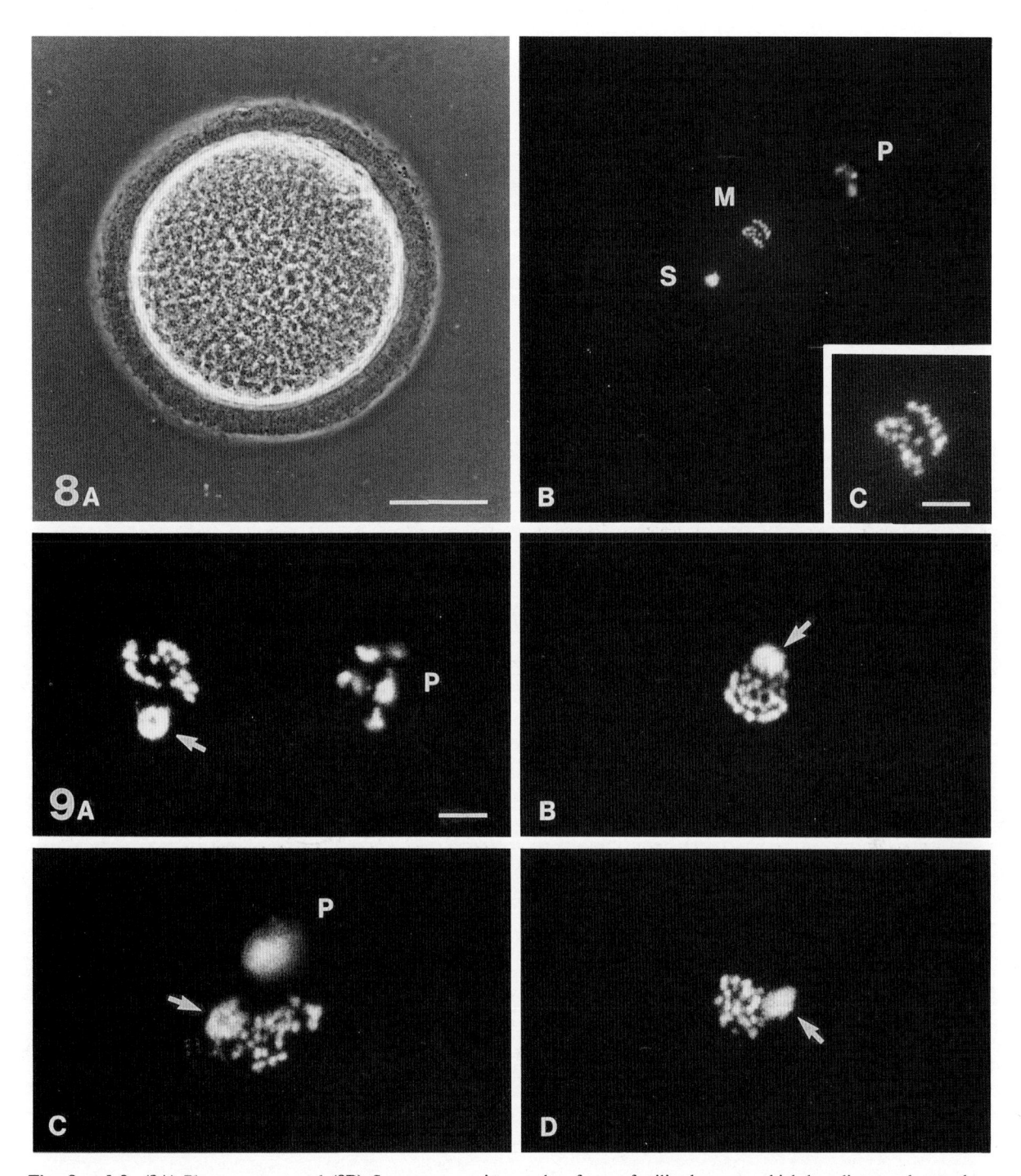

Figs 8 and 9. (**8A**) Phase contrast and (**8B**) fluorescence micrographs of an unfertilized oocyte which has disarrayed metaphase chromosomes (M) and a swollen sperm head (S). A higher magnification of the metaphase chromosomes is shown in 8C. P, polar body. Bars: 8A and 8B, 50 μm; 8C, 10 μm. (**9**) High magnification fluorescence micrographs of swollen sperm heads (arrows) which are closely associated with or enmeshed among the metaphase chromosomes of the oocyte. P, polar body. Bar, 10 μm.

body and formed a large PN with prominent nucleoli (Fig. 12). The incidence of 1 PN oocytes was similar (5% v. 2–6%) to that reported for routine IVF (Plachot and Crozet 1992; Staessen et al. 1993). A swollen sperm head was observed in 51% of these 1 PN oocytes (Table 1) whereas undecondensed sperm heads were seen in 31%. The ratio of these two aetiologies in 1 PN oocytes was different from metaphase oocytes, but as discussed later, this appears to be due to the epididymal sperm cases. The sperm ejection rate (19%) was the same

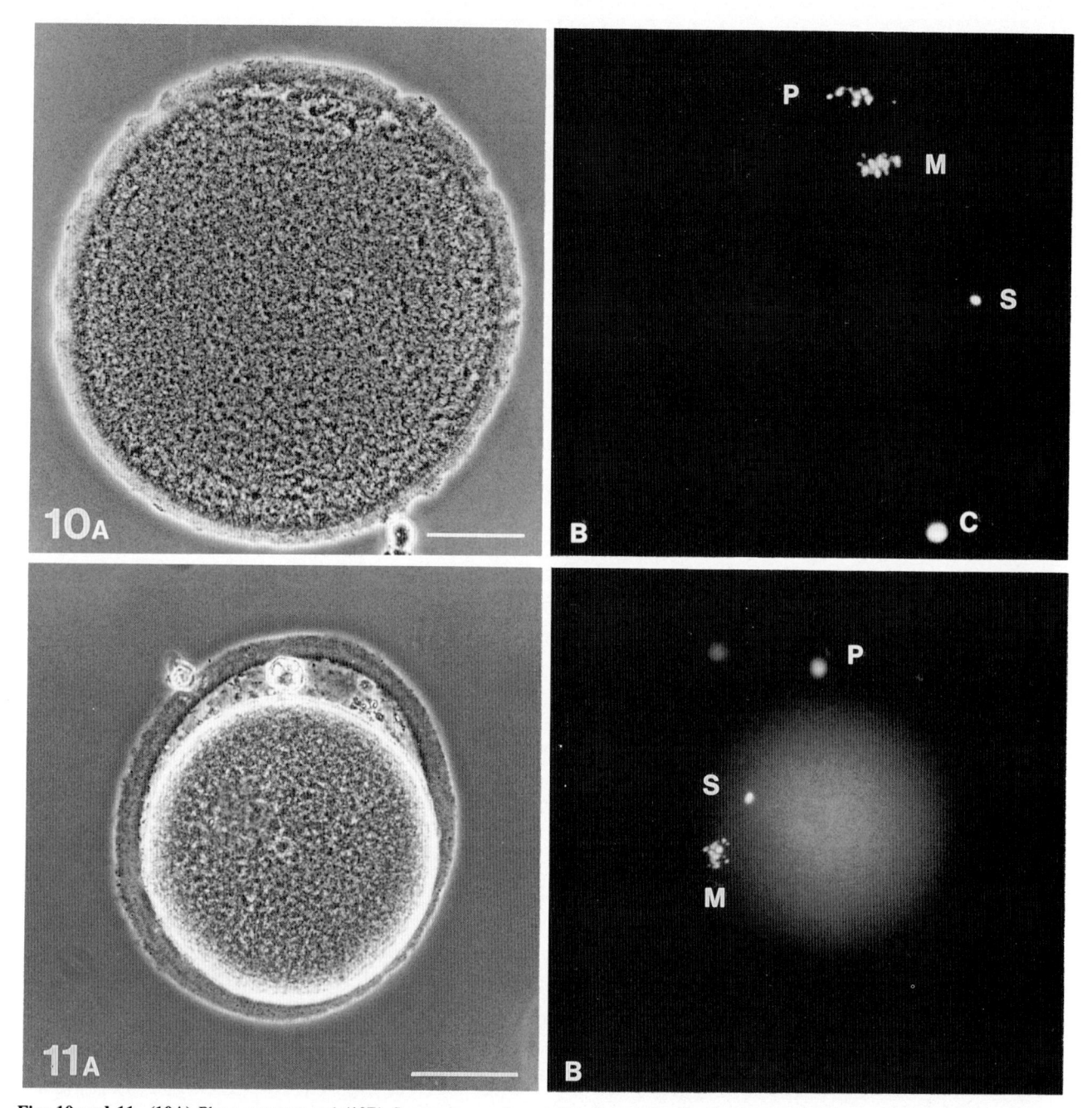

Figs 10 and 11. (10A) Phase contrast and **(10B)** fluorescence micrographs of an unfertilized oocyte which has a spermatozoon (S) in the PVS. C, coronal cell; M, metaphase chromosomes; P, polar body. Bar, 50 μm. **(11A)** Phase contrast and **(11B)** fluorescence micrographs of an unfertilized oocyte which contains an undecondensed sperm head (S) in the oocyte, at the same plane of focus as the metaphase chromosomes (M). P, polar body. Bar, 50 μm.

as for metaphase oocytes. Our results are comparable to those obtained by Dozortsev et al. (1994a), although our sperm ejection rate was higher.

Pronuclei appear about 5–6 h after ICSI (Nagy et al. 1994; Payne, unpublished observations), and yet these 1 PN oocytes showed no evidence of male PN formation when they were fixed at 17 h after injection. Hence, we do not believe that the single PN in these oocytes was merely due to asynchronous development of PN (Munné et al. 1993; Staessen et al. 1993), although it is possible that a small percentage of the oocytes might have developed a male PN later as observed by Staessen et al. (1993). Since parthenogenetic activation is more common in aged human oocytes (Balakier and Casper 1991; Plachot and Crozet 1992; Balakier et al. 1993), these 1 PN oocytes might represent a population

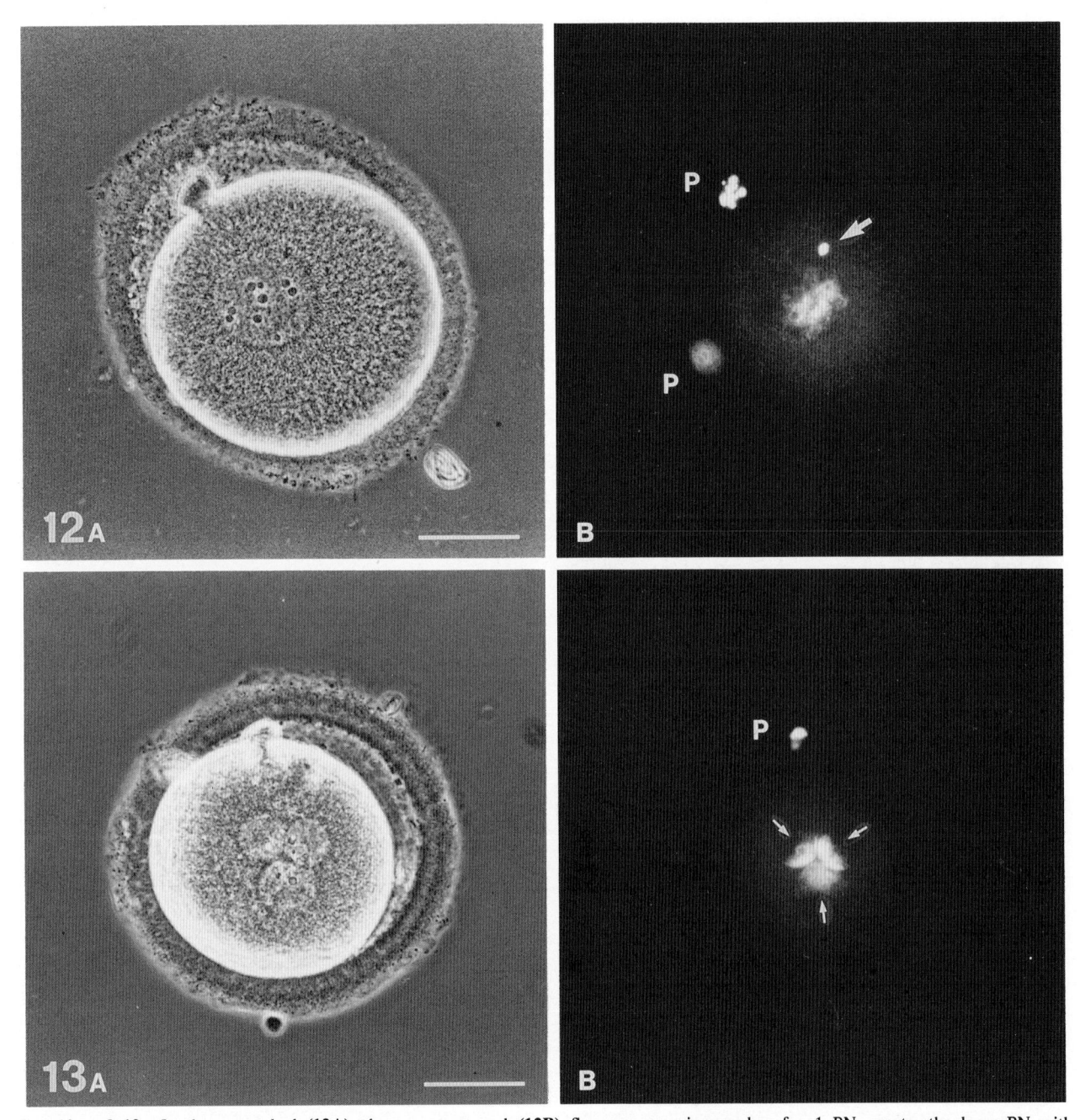

Figs 12 and 13. In these matched (**12A**) phase contrast and (**12B**) fluorescence micrographs of a 1 PN oocyte, the large PN with prominent nucleoli, a slightly swollen sperm head (arrow) and two polar bodies (P) are evident. Bar, 50 μm. **13A** Phase contrast and (**13B**) fluorescence micrographs of a typical 3 PN oocyte showing three closely associated PN (small arrows) in the centre of the oocyte and a single polar body (P). Bar, 50 μm.

of over-mature oocytes which activate very readily after ICSI but are defective in other respects because they are unable to induce or support male PN development.

Abnormally Fertilized Oocytes

A total of 70 abnormally fertilized oocytes were examined. Of these, 63 were 3 PN oocytes which all had a single polar body or a fragmented first polar body (Fig. 13). This indicates that the oocyte failed to extrude the second polar body at activation and both sets of maternal chromosomes developed into PN (Palermo et al. 1993). This phenomenon has also been reported after routine IVF (Selva et al. 1991; Plachot and Crozet 1992). It is intriguing why this only occurs in a small percentage of the injected oocytes and we speculate that it may be due to: *(1)* the orientation or position of the second meiotic spindle in the cortical cytoplasm; (2) damage to the oocyte cytoskeleton during injection; or (3) reorientation of the spindle during injection. Since spindle position and orientation is established during oocyte maturation (Sathananthan 1985), this might be a maturational defect.

The remaining 7 abnormally fertilized oocytes had abnormal PN. Some had two normal-sized PN, a third micro-PN and two polar bodies which suggests that they were fertilized but had undergone abnormal PN development or PN fragmentation. The other oocytes had two PN of grossly disproportionate sizes, one very large and the other very small.

Oocyte Activation and Nuclear Transformations after ICSI

Mature mammalian oocytes are arrested at metaphase of the second meiotic division. Meiotic arrest and the condensed state of the oocyte chromosomes is maintained by maturation promoting factor (MPF) which is a complex between the $p34^{cdc2}$ protein kinase and one of the cell cycle regulators, cyclin B. In turn, MPF is regulated by cytostatic factor (CSF) and the p39 protein product of the c-*mos* proto-oncogene (Kubiak et al. 1993; Pal et al. 1994). Entry of a spermatozoon into the oocyte initiates the degradation of cyclin B and a decrease in MPF activity, which leads to the completion of meiosis II (Lorca et al. 1991). This process is called activation, and it is mediated by an inositol 1,4,5-trisphosphate ($InsP_3$)-induced release of Ca^{2+} from intracellular stores which induces oscillatory Ca^{2+} waves throughout the oocyte (Miyazaki et al. 1993). This requires the stimulation of an intracellular messenger pathway, and there are currently two candidates. The first pathway involves receptor-mediated activation of G-proteins and phospholipase C, which in turn stimulates the production of $InsP_3$ and the release of Ca^{2+} (Miyazaki et al. 1993; Moore et al. 1993). The second pathway involves the release of a cytosolic component of the spermatozoon which directly triggers Ca^{2+} release in the oocyte (Swann 1990; Homa et al. 1993).

It is evident from the present study and other reports (Palermo et al. 1993; Van Steirteghem et al. 1993a; Payne et al. 1994b) that about 80% of human oocytes activate after ICSI. It is unclear why human oocytes activate so readily after ICSI, and it is even more intriguing because human oocytes do not readily activate in response to external stimuli (Abramczuk and Lopata 1990). Tesarik et al. (1994) reported that human oocytes undergo sperm-dependent Ca^{2+} oscillations after ICSI, and this supports the theory that a cytosolic sperm factor initiates oocyte activation (Swann et al. 1994). However, these results should be viewed cautiously for several reasons. First, Tesarik et al. (1994) used 48-h-old unfertilized human oocytes. Aged oocytes activate differently from fresh oocytes (Winston et al. 1991) so the pattern and timing of Ca^{2+} oscillations might be different. Second, Ca^{2+} oscillations did not commence until 4–12 h after injection, which is at the time of, or after, PN formation in injected human oocytes (Nagy et al. 1994; Payne, unpublished data). Ca^{2+} oscillations commence immediately after routine fertilization (Taylor et al. 1993). Third, in some preliminary experiments, we observed that injection of PVP alone activated 33–50% of fresh human oocytes (Flaherty and Payne, unpublished observations), which suggests that the process of injection, and in particular breakage of the oolemma, might initiate activation in some oocytes. Further studies are needed to confirm these results and to identify the mechanisms by which human oocytes activate after ICSI.

In the present study, 82% of the unfertilized oocytes (~20% of the injected oocytes) remained at metaphase II after injection, and the majority of these oocytes contained a swollen sperm head. Hence, the main block to fertilization after ICSI appears to be failure of oocyte activation. At present, it is unclear why activation did not occur, however, there are several explanations. First, the oocytes may be cytoplasmically immature and therefore unable to respond to injection of a spermatozoon. Evidence for this comes from studies which have shown that competence to undergo nuclear and cytoplasmic maturation are acquired independently during oocyte maturation (Eppig et al. 1994) and that mouse oocytes gradually develop the capacity for activation after they have reached metaphase II (Kubiak 1989). Second, if it eventuates that a cytosolic sperm factor activates the oocyte after ICSI (Swann et al. 1994), then deficiencies in or the absence of this factor could prevent activation. Third, the amplitude and frequency of the repetitive Ca^{2+} oscillations are important for oocyte activation (Vitullo and Ozil 1992; Collas et al. 1993). It has been reported that not all human oocytes exhibit multiple Ca^{2+} oscillations, and the periodicity of the transients varies between oocytes (Taylor et al. 1993; Tesarik et al. 1994), which indicates that oocytes respond differently to sperm penetration and injection and this might explain why 20% of the oocytes did not activate after ICSI.

We also observed the opposite phenomenon in which the oocyte activated and developed a female PN but the sperm head did not develop into a PN, despite the initiation of sperm head decondensation. Dozortsev et al. (1994a) also reported this phenomenon. We found that it occurred in 51% of the 1 PN oocytes (2·4% of the injected oocytes) and it was not simply a technical problem because the sperm head decondensed and therefore must have been correctly injected. Hence, oocyte or sperm defects must be involved to some degree. It is well known that ooplasmic factors regulate sperm

Table 2. Cytological observations on unfertilized oocytes in the epididymal sperm subgroup and the other patient subgroups (combined)

Metaphase and one pronuclear oocytes have been combined. Values in parentheses are percentages of the number of oocytes examined. n, number of oocytes examined

	Epididymal sperm $n = 41$	Other aetiologies $n = 384$
Swollen sperm head	20 (49%)	265 (69%)
Sperm ejected	6 (14%)	74 (19%)
Undecondensed sperm head	15 (37%)	45 (12%)

Table 3. Outcomes for three epididymal sperm cases

	Case 1	Case 2	Case 3
Oocytes injected	12	20	27
Oocytes fertilized	5	11	20
Fertilization rate	42%	55%	74%
Metaphase II oocytes:			
swollen sperm head	1	2	2
sperm ejected	1	2	—
undecondensed sperm head	2	3	—
One pronuclear oocytes:			
swollen sperm head	—	1	1
sperm ejected	—	1	—
undecondensed sperm head	2	—	1
Three pronuclear oocytes	—	—	6
Oocytes with abnormal pronuclei	—	—	—

Table 4. Outcomes for eight occasional motile sperm cases

	Case 1	Case 2	Case 3	Case 4	Case 5	Case 6	Case 7	Case 8
Oocytes injected	17	13	11	12	21	24	18	27
Oocytes fertilized	2	3	4	5	10	12	11	17
Fertilization rate	12%	23%	36%	42%	48%	50%	61%	63%
Metaphase II oocytes:								
swollen sperm head	11	7	2	7	6	4	—	9
sperm ejected	2	1	3	—	1	3	4	—
undecondensed sperm head	—	—	1	—	2	4	1	—
One pronuclear oocytes:								
swollen sperm head	—	—	—	—	—	—	—	—
sperm ejected	—	—	—	—	1	—	—	—
undecondensed sperm head	—	—	—	—	—	1	1	1
Three pronuclear oocytes	—	—	—	—	1	1	1	1
Oocytes with abnormal pronuclei	—	—	—	—	1	—	2	—

head decondensation, protamine–histone exchange and PN formation and that this in turn is dependent on oocyte maturity (Perreault 1992). Furthermore, there is a limited quantity of the factors which are responsible for PN formation (Tesarik and Kopecny 1989) and they are labile and have a limited half-life (Borsuk and Tarkowski 1989). Moreover, breakdown of the sperm nuclear envelope (NEBD) which is required for PN formation, can only occur at the end of metaphase II and is under oocyte control, although decondensation can occur without NEBD (Szollosi et al. 1994). These data suggest that the inability of these activated oocytes to transform the injected sperm head into a PN is indicative of oocyte immaturity or specific oocyte defects. However, the spermatozoon itself does contribute to PN formation by supplying the centrosome from which develops an aster of microtubules (Le Guen and Crozet 1989; Yllera-Fernandez et al. 1992; Navarra et al. 1994; Schatten 1994). Microtubule assembly from the sperm aster is required for the formation and migration of PN into the centre of the oocyte (Schatten 1994), so if the centriole or centrosome were absent or defective, this would prevent normal PN formation and fertilization after oocyte activation. Clearly, further investigations are required to establish whether or not the spermatozoon contributes to this type of fertilization failure.

Failed and Abnormal Fertilization in Patient Subgroups

In Table 2, the results for the epididymal sperm cases have been compared with the combined results for the other cases. The epididymal sperm subgroup demonstrated a lower proportion of oocytes with swollen sperm heads (49%) and a higher proportion containing an undecondensed sperm head (37%). A comparison of Tables 3 and 4 illustrates this on individual cases. These observations were based on a small number of oocytes and need to be confirmed in a larger series, however, they suggest that the aetiology of failed fertilization may be slightly different with epididymal sperm and this in turn might relate to a sperm factor that activates the oocyte (Swann *et al.* 1994).

Table 4 presents individual results for eight cases which achieved low to high fertilization rates after ICSI and shows the various patterns and the degree of variability we observed in cohorts of unfertilized and abnormally fertilized oocytes. In Cases 1, 2, 4 and 8, most of the unfertilized oocytes were still at metaphase II and contained a swollen sperm head, which as discussed earlier, suggests that a specific maturational defect exists in many of the oocytes from these patients. In other cases, however, failure of sperm head decondensation (Case 6) or ejection of the spermatozoon from the oocyte (Cases 3, 6, 7) were major causes of fertilization failure. Overall, there was considerable variability from one cycle to the next, and this illustrates that there are a variety of reasons for fertilization failure after ICSI.

Conclusions

Accurate assessment of fertilization and fertilization failure should be an important component of any ICSI programme. DNA staining of oocytes with Hoechst 33342 is a simple, efficient method for determining the causes of failed and abnormal fertilization after ICSI, and can be used during the training of new staff or as a quality control procedure if the fertilization rate is sub-optimal. We have shown that the majority (71%) of the unfertilized oocytes were still at metaphase II and contained a swollen sperm head, indicating that fertilization failure was associated with defective oocyte activation and not with poor injection technique. Ejection of the spermatozoon from the oocyte only accounts for 19% of the unfertilized oocytes in our ICSI programme and is therefore not a major cause of fertilization failure. Furthermore, we have demonstrated that 1 PN oocytes are either unfertilized or are at an arrested early stage of fertilization, and that 3 PN oocytes failed to extrude the second polar body which then developed into the third PN. The present study has also revealed some interesting and challenging phenomena that relate to the control of oocyte activation, sperm head decondensation and pronuclear formation after ICSI.

Acknowledgments

We thank the staff of the IVF Laboratory at The Queen Elizabeth Hospital, and in particular Regan Jeffrey, Michael Barry and Monica Briffa, the clinical and nursing staff of the Reproductive Medicine Units at The Queen Elizabeth Hospital and Wakefield Clinic, and Matthew Makinson for his help with the preparation of the micrographs.

References

Abramczuk, J. W., and Lopata, A. (1990). Resistance of human follicular oocytes to parthenogenetic activation: DNA distribution and content in oocytes maintained *in vitro*. *Hum. Reprod. (Oxf.)* **5**, 578–81.

Angell, R. R., Ledger, W., Yong, E. L., Harkness, L., and Baird, D. T. (1991). Cytogenetic analysis of unfertilized human oocytes. *Hum. Reprod. (Oxf.)* **6**, 568–73.

Balakier, H., and Casper, R. F. (1991). A morphologic study of unfertilized oocytes and abnormal embryos in human in vitro fertilization. *J. In Vitro Fertil. Embryo Transfer* **8**, 73–9.

Balakier, H., Squire, J., and Casper, R. F. (1993). Characterization of abnormal one pronuclear human oocytes by morphology, cytogenetics and *in-situ* hybridization. *Hum. Reprod. (Oxf.)* **8**, 402–8.

Bonduelle, M., Desmyttere, S., Buysse, A., Van Assche, E., Schietecatte, J., Devroey, P., Van Steirteghem, A. C., and Liebaers, I. (1994). Prospective follow-up study of 55 children born after subzonal insemination and intracytoplasmic sperm injection. *Hum. Reprod. (Oxf.)* **9**, 1765–9.

Borsuk, E., and Tarkowski, A. K. (1989). Transformation of sperm nuclei into male pronuclei in nucleate and anucleate fragments of parthenogenetic mouse eggs. *Gamete Res.* **24**, 471–81.

Calafell, J. M., Badenas, J., Egozcue, J., and Santalo, J. (1991). Premature chromosome condensation as a sign of oocyte immaturity. *Hum. Reprod. (Oxf.)* **6**, 1017–21.

Catt, J., Morton, M., and Saunders, D. (1994). Should all oocytes fertilise after intracytoplasmic sperm injection? *Proc. 26th Ann. Meet. Aust. Soc. Reprod. Biol.*, MP22 [Abstr.]

Collas, P., Sullivan, E. J., and Barnes, F. L. (1993). Histone H1 kinase activity in bovine oocytes following calcium stimulation. *Mol. Reprod. Dev.* **34**, 224–31.

Dozortsev, D., De Sutter, P., and Dhont, M. (1994*a*). Behaviour of spermatozoa in human oocytes displaying no or one pronuclei after intracytoplasmic sperm injection. *Hum. Reprod. (Oxf.)* **9**, 2139–44.

Dozortsev, D., De Sutter, P., and Dhont, M. (1994*b*). Damage to the sperm plasma membrane by touching the sperm tail with a needle prior to intracytoplasmic injection. *Hum. Reprod. (Oxf.)* **9** (Suppl. 4), 40 [Abstr.]

Eppig, J. J., Schultz, R. M., O'Brien, M., and Chesnel, F. (1994). Relationship between the developmental programs controlling nuclear and cytoplasmic maturation of mouse oocytes. *Dev. Biol.* **164**, 1–9.

Fishel, S., Timson, J., Lisi, F., and Rinaldi, L. (1992). Evaluation of 225 patients undergoing subzonal insemination for the procurement of fertilization in vitro. *Fertil. Steril.* **57**, 840–9.

Flaherty, S. P., Payne, D., Swann, N. J., and Matthews, C. D. (1995). Aetiology of failed and abnormal fertilization after intracytoplasmic sperm injection (ICSI). *Hum. Reprod. (Oxf.)* (In press.)

Gwatkin, R. B. L., Conover, J. C., Collins, R. L., and Quigley, M. M. (1989). Failed fertilization in human in vitro fertilization analyzed with the deoxyribonucleic acid-specific fluorochrome Hoechst 33342. *Am. J. Obstet. Gynecol.* **160**, 31–5.

Homa, S. T., Carroll, J., and Swann, K. (1993). The role of calcium in mammalian oocyte maturation and egg activation. *Hum. Reprod. (Oxf.)* **8**, 1274–81.

Kubiak, J. Z. (1989). Mouse oocytes gradually develop the capacity for activation during the metaphase II arrest. *Dev. Biol.* **136**, 537–45.

Kubiak, J. Z., Weber, M., de Pennart, H., Winston, N. J, and Maro, B. (1993). The metaphase II arrest in mouse oocytes is controlled through microtubule-dependent destruction of cyclin B in the presence of CSF. *EMBO J.* **12**, 3773–8.

Le Guen, P., and Crozet, N. (1989). Microtubule and centrosome distribution during sheep fertilization. *Eur. J. Cell Biol.* **48**, 239–49.

Lorca, T., Galas, S., Fesquet, D., Devault, A., Cavadore, J.-C., and Dorée, M. (1991). Degradation of the proto-oncogene product $p39^{mos}$ is not necessary for cyclin proteolysis and exit from meiotic metaphase: requirement for a Ca^{2+}-calmodulin dependent event. *EMBO J.* **10**, 2087–93.

Miyazaki, S., Shirakawa, H., Nakada, K., and Honda, Y. (1993). Essential role of the inositol 1,4,5-trisphosphate receptor/Ca^{2+} release channel in Ca^{2+} waves and Ca^{2+} oscillations at fertilization in mammalian eggs. *Dev. Biol.* **158**, 62–78.

Moore, G. D., Kopf, G. S., and Schultz, R. M. (1993). Complete mouse egg activation in the absence of sperm by stimulation of an exogenous G protein-coupled receptor. *Dev. Biol.* **159**, 669–78.

Munné, S., Tang, Y.-X., Grifo, J., and Cohen, J. (1993). Origin of single pronucleated human zygotes. *J. Assist. Reprod. Genet.* **10**, 276–9.

Nagy, Z. P., Liu, J., Joris, H., Devroey, P., and Van Steirteghem, A. C. (1994). Time-course of oocyte activation, pronucleus formation and cleavage in human oocytes fertilized by intracytoplasmic sperm injection. *Hum. Reprod. (Oxf.)* **9**, 1743–8.

Navara, C. S., First, N. L., and Schatten, G. (1994). Microtubule organization in the cow during fertilization, polyspermy, parthenogenesis, and nuclear transfer: the role of the sperm aster. *Dev. Biol.* **162**, 29–40.

O'Rand, M. G., Herman, B., Diguiseppi, J., Halme, J., Hammond, M. G., and Talbert, L. M. (1986). Analysis of deoxyribonucleic acid distribution in noncleaving oocytes from patients undergoing in vitro fertilization. *Fertil. Steril.* **46**, 452–60.

Ord, T., Patrizio, P., Marello, E., Balmaceda, J. P., and Asch, R. H. (1990). Mini-Percoll: a new method of semen preparation for IVF in severe male factor infertility. *Hum. Reprod. (Oxf.)* **5**, 987–9.

Pal, S. K., Torry, D., Serta, R., Crowell, R. C., Seibel, M. M., Cooper, G. M., and Kiessling, A. A. (1994). Expression and potential function of the c-mos proto-oncogene in human eggs. *Fertil. Steril.* **61**, 496–503.

Palermo, G., Joris, H., Devroey, P., and Van Steirteghem, A. C. (1992). Pregnancies after intracytoplasmic injection of single spermatozoon into an oocyte. *Lancet* **340**, 17–18.

Palermo, G., Joris, H., Derde, M.-P., Camus, M., Devroey, P., and Van Steirteghem, A. C. (1993). Sperm characteristics and outcome of human assisted fertilization by subzonal insemination and intracytoplasmic sperm injection. *Fertil. Steril.* **59**, 826–35.

Payne, D. (1995). Intracytoplasmic sperm injection: instrumentation and injection technique. In 'Intracytoplasmic Sperm Injection: the Revolution in Male Infertility'. *Reprod. Fertil. Dev.* **7**, 185–96.

Payne, D., and Matthews, C. D. (1995). Intracytoplasmic sperm injection: clinical results from the Reproductive Medicine Unit, Adelaide. In 'Intracytoplasmic Sperm Injection: the Revolution in Male Infertility'. *Reprod. Fertil. Dev.* **7**, 219–27.

Payne, D., McLaughlin, K. J., Depypere, H. T., Kirby, C. A., Warnes, G. M., and Matthews, C. D. (1991). Experience with zona drilling and zona cutting to improve fertilization rates of human oocytes in vitro. *Hum. Reprod.* **6**, 423–31.

Payne, D., Warnes, G. M., Flaherty, S. P., and Matthews, C. D. (1994a). Local experience with zona drilling, zona cutting and sperm microinjection. In 'The Infertile Male: Advanced Assisted Reproductive Technology'. *Reprod. Fertil. Dev.* **6**, 45–50.

Payne, D., Flaherty, S. P., Jeffrey, R., Warnes, G. M., and Matthews, C. D. (1994b). Successful treatment of severe male factor infertility in 100 consecutive cycles using intracytoplasmic sperm injection. *Hum. Reprod.* **9**, 2051–7.

Perreault, S. D. (1992). Chromatin remodeling in mammalian zygotes. *Mutat. Res.* **296**, 43–55.

Pieters, M. H. E. C., Geraedts, J. P. M., Dumoulin, J. C. M., Evers, J. L. H., Bras, M., Kornips, F. H. A. C., and Menheere, P. P. C. A. (1989). Cytogenetic analysis of in vitro fertilization (IVF) failures. *Hum. Genet.* **81**, 367–70.

Plachot, M., and Crozet, N. (1992). Fertilization abnormalities in human in-vitro fertilization. *Hum. Reprod. (Oxf.)* **7**, (Suppl 1), 89–94.

Quinn, P., Kerin, J. F., and Warnes, G. M. (1985). Improved pregnancy rate in human in vitro fertilization with the use of a medium based on the composition of human tubal fluid. *Fertil. Steril.* **44**, 493–8.

Sathananthan, A. H. (1985). Maturation of the human oocyte in vitro: nuclear events during meiosis (an ultrastructural study). *Gamete Res.* **12**, 237–54.

Schatten, G. (1994). The centrosome and its mode of inheritance: the reduction of the centrosome during gametogenesis and its restoration during fertilization. *Dev. Biol.* **165**, 299–335.

Schmiady, H., and Kentenich, H. (1989). Premature chromosome condensation after in-vitro fertilization. *Hum. Reprod. (Oxf.)* **4**, 689–95.

Schmiady, H., Sperling, K., Kentenich, H., and Stauber, M. (1986). Prematurely condensed human sperm chromosomes after in vitro fertilization (IVF). *Hum. Genet.* **74**, 441–3.

Selva, J., Martin-Pont, B., Hugues, J. N., Rince, P., Fillion, C., Herve, F., Tamboise, A., and Tamboise, E. (1991). Cytogenetic study of human oocytes uncleaved after in-vitro fertilization. *Hum. Reprod. (Oxf.)* **6**, 709–13.

Silber, S. J., Devroey, P., Tournaye, H., and Van Steirteghem, A. C. (1995). Fertilizing capacity of epididymal and testicular sperm using intracytoplasmic sperm injection (ICSI). In 'Intracytoplasmic Sperm Injection: the Revolution in Male Infertility'. *Reprod. Fertil. Dev.* **7**, 281–93.

Staessen, C., Janssenswillen, C., Devroey, P., and Van Steirteghem, A. C. (1993). Cytogenetic and morphological observations of single pronucleated human oocytes after in-vitro fertilization. *Hum. Reprod.* **8**, 221–3.

Swann, K. (1990). A cytosolic sperm factor stimulates repetitive calcium increases and mimics fertilization in hamster eggs. *Development* **110**, 1295–1302.

Swann, K., Homa, S., and Carroll, J. (1994). An inside job: the results of injecting whole sperm into eggs supports one view of signal transduction at fertilization. *Hum. Reprod. (Oxf.)* **9**, 978–80.

Szollosi, M. S., Borsuk, E., and Szollosi, D. (1994). Relationship between sperm nucleus remodelling and cell cycle progression of fragments of mouse parthenogenotes. *Mol. Reprod. Dev.* **37**, 146–56.

Taylor, C. T. (1994). Calcium signals and human oocyte activation: implications for assisted conception. *Hum. Reprod. (Oxf.)* **9**, 980–4.

Taylor, C. T., Lawrence, Y. M., Kingsland, C. R., Biljan, M. M., and Cuthbertson, K. S. R. (1993). Oscillations in intracellular free calcium induced by spermatozoa in human oocytes at fertilization. *Hum. Reprod. (Oxf.)* **8**, 2174–9.

Tejada, M. I., Mendoza, M. R., Corcostegui, B., and Benito, J. A. (1992). Factors associated with premature chromosome condensation (PCC) following *in vitro* fertilization. *J. Assist. Reprod. Genet.* **9**, 61–7.

Tesarik, J., and Kopecny, V. (1989). Developmental control of the human male pronucleus by ooplasmic factors. *Hum. Reprod. (Oxf.)* **4**, 962–8.

Tesarik, J., Sousa, M., and Testart, J. (1994). Human oocyte activation after intracytoplasmic sperm injection. *Hum. Reprod. (Oxf.)* **9**, 511–18.

Tournaye, H., Liu, J., Nagy, Z., Joris, H., Wisanto, A., Bonduelle, M., Van der Elst, J., Staessen, C., Smitz, J., Silber, S., Devroey, P., Liebaers, I., and Van Steirteghem, A. C. (1995) Intracytoplasmic sperm injection (ICSI): the Brussels experience. In 'Intracytoplasmic Sperm Injection: the Revolution in Male Infertility'. *Reprod. Fertil. Dev.* **7**, 269–79.

Urner, F., Bianchi, P. G., Campana, A., and Sakkas, D. (1993). Evidence of sperm entry into assumed unfertilized human oocytes after sub-zonal sperm microinjection. *Hum. Reprod. (Oxf.)* **8**, 2167–73.

Van Steirteghem, A. C., Liu, J., Joris, H., Nagy, Z., Janssenswillen, C., Tournaye, H., Derde, M.-P., Van Assche, E., and Devroey, P. (1993*a*). Higher success rate by intracytoplasmic sperm injection than by subzonal insemination. Report of a second series of 300 consecutive treatment cycles. *Hum. Reprod. (Oxf.)* **8**, 1055–60.

Van Steirteghem, A. C., Nagy, Z., Joris, H., Liu, J., Staessen, C., Smitz, J., Wisanto, A., and Devroey, P. (1993*b*). High fertilization and implantation rates after intracytoplasmic sperm injection. *Hum. Reprod. (Oxf.)* **8**, 1061–6.

Vitullo, A. D., and Ozil, J.-P. (1992). Repetitive calcium stimuli drive meiotic resumption and pronuclear development during mouse oocyte activation. *Dev. Biol.* **151**, 128–36.

Winston, N., Johnson, M., Pickering, S., and Braude, P. (1991). Parthenogenetic activation and development of fresh and aged human oocytes. *Fertil. Steril.* **56**, 904–12.

World Health Organization (1987). 'WHO Laboratory Manual for the Examination of Human Semen and Semen–Cervical Mucus Interaction'. 2nd Edn. (Cambridge University Press: Cambridge.)

Yllera-Fernandez, M. M., Crozet, N., and Ahmed-Ali, M. (1992). Microtubule distribution during fertilization in the rabbit. *Mol. Reprod. Dev.* **32**, 271–6.

Manuscript received 20 February 1995

Open Discussion

Bob Edwards (Cambridge):

Your presentation showed us all the anomalies that we would have predicted from the events that we discussed yesterday.

Simon Fishel (Nottingham):

Have you managed to correlate your data to any gross morphological features of the oocytes? For example we see eggs with inclusion bodies, vacuoles and unknown dark centres of varying sizes. They fertilize but their developmental potential is poor.

Flaherty:

No we haven't specifically looked at that. However, we see these fertilization anomalies in oocytes with various morphologies.

Janina Michalowska (Chicago):

Do you have any karyotype data on the men or characterization of sperm abnormalities by electron microscopy?

Flaherty:

No. There are many unanswered questions.

Alan Trounson (Melbourne):

Arif Bongso has been analyzing the chromosomes of these failed fertilization eggs and there is a very high proportion, about 80%, which are chromosomally abnormal. Have you looked at that? A problem I suppose is trying to separate oocyte and sperm factors. The other possibility on the sperm side would be to look at the ability of the sperm to decondense in dithiothreitol (DTT). Have you done either of those sorts of studies?

Flaherty:

We haven't looked at the chromosomal constitution of any of these oocytes but I believe that a lot of these problems are oocyte-related. Human sperm vary considerably in their response to disulfide reducing agents and there are differences in the degree of disulfide cross-linking in the nucleus. However, if you use a high enough concentration of DTT, you can make them all swell. So I suspect that in these oocytes, the glutathione-like reducing activity in the oocyte which decondenses the sperm head might be at a reduced level.

Sherman Silber (St Louis):

In Brussels they had a patient with many good-looking eggs but there was no fertilization with ICSI. There was still no fertilization after re-insemination of the eggs with donor sperm, so they performed ICSI with donor sperm and there was still no fertilization. So they were convinced that there is an egg factor when you don't get fertilization with ICSI.

Development and Implementation of Intracytoplasmic Sperm Injection (ICSI)

Gianpiero D. Palermo, Jacques Cohen,
Mina Alikani, Alexis Adler and Zev Rosenwaks

*The Centre for Reproductive Medicine and Infertility,
The New York Hospital–Cornell Medical Centre,
505 East 70th Street, New York, NY 10021, USA.*

Abstract. The purpose of this paper is to elucidate the experimental steps that led to the development of intracytoplasmic sperm injection (ICSI) and its application in the human. ICSI has become the most successful micromanipulation procedure for treating male infertility. A total of 355 *in vitro* fertilization (IVF) cycles utilizing ICSI are described; 180 couples were previously treated in 509 IVF cycles but achieved no fertilization and 175 couples could not be treated by IVF because of extremely poor semen parameters. Of the 3063 metaphase II (M II) oocytes retrieved, 2970 were injected with a survival rate of 93·6%, yielding 1917 bipronuclear zygotes (64·5%). In 148 patients, a foetal heart was evidenced by ultrasound; 11 of these patients miscarried between 7 and 13 weeks of gestation. The ongoing pregnancy rate was 38·6% (137/355) per retrieval and 40·5% (137/338) per embryo replacement. At the time of writing, there were 22 deliveries and one therapeutic abortion for a trisomy 21 chromosomal abnormality. In addition, 66 singleton, 37 twin, 10 triplet and 1 quadruplet pregnancies were ongoing. The concentration of motile spermatozoa in the ejaculate only slightly influenced the fertilization rate ($P < 0·001$) and the pregnancy outcome ($P < 0·01$). A preliminary injection procedure utilizing intracytoplasmic injection of isolated sperm heads was performed in 35 M II human oocytes with resultant fertilization and cleavage rates of 74% and 73% respectively. Skills in ICSI were acquired by injecting hamster and unfertilized human oocytes with human sperm. ICSI can be used to successfully treat couples who have failed IVF or who have too few spermatozoa for conventional *in vitro* insemination. Neither the semen parameters nor the origin of the sperm sample clearly influenced the outcome. The achievement of fertilization with only sperm heads suggests that the application of ICSI may be able to be extended to immature sperm cells, but further genetic evaluation concerning the effect of the centrosome on spindle formation is required.

Extra keywords: micromanipulation, hamster oocytes, human oocytes, sperm heads, male factor infertility.

Introduction

Intracytoplasmic sperm injection (ICSI) is the newest and most successful micromanipulation technique for treating male factor infertility. It entails the mechanical insertion of a chosen spermatozoon directly into the cytoplasm of a human oocyte. Initially, the technique was used in veterinary medicine for the purpose of clarifying the different steps of fertilization by investigating the fusion and penetration of animal gametes. The first procedure to inject sperm into an egg was done in the sea urchin by Hiramoto (1962), whereas the first mammalian egg injection procedure was reported by Lin (1966). Later, Uehara and Yanagimachi (1976) described the microinjection of human and golden hamster spermatozoa into hamster eggs. Despite the use of very fine micropipettes (4–6 μm in diameter) and a procedure performed under ideal conditions, only about 30% of the injected eggs survived the procedure (Thadani 1981). The injection of a spermatozoon into the egg cytoplasm bypassed the oolemma selection, but inevitably caused oocyte injury and consequent lysis (Markert 1983). Notwithstanding, Hosoi *et al.* (1988) obtained live offspring after the transfer of microfertilized rabbit eggs into the oviducts of pseudopregnant female rabbits.

Based on the successful fertilization of normal animal gametes using ICSI, the procedure was experimentally applied to human gametes. Injecting abnormal, round-headed human spermatozoa into the cytoplasm of hamster oocytes resulted in sperm nuclear decondensation (Lanzendorf *et al.* 1988*a*). This achievement suggested that it would be possible to successfully inject human spermatozoa into human oocytes (Lanzendorf *et al.* 1988*b*).

The subsequent fertilization of human oocytes by ICSI justified its clinical application for the treatment of infertile couples in whom the male partner had severely compromised semen parameters. Although this procedure was first applied to human gametes in 1988, there were no reports of human pregnancies until July 1992 (Palermo et al. 1992). Since that time, there have been additional reports of more extended series of pregnancies and deliveries obtained by ICSI (Palermo et al. 1993, 1995; Van Steirteghem et al. 1993). Use of the procedure has resulted in fertilization and pregnancy rates comparable to those obtained in patients with normal semen parameters undergoing standard in vitro fertilization (IVF). This relative independence of semen parameters has attracted attention to the procedure and many infertility centres have adopted ICSI as the treatment of choice for those couples afflicted with male factor infertility.

The present paper describes the comprehensive experimental work which contributed to the development and implementation of ICSI, including the definition of the optimal methodology and set-up for achieving fertilization, cleavage and pregnancies. Much of this early work was performed at the Centre for Reproductive Medicine of the Brussels Free University Hospital in Brussels, Belgium. In addition, this paper reports on 355 consecutive IVF cycles using ICSI performed at The Centre for Reproductive Medicine and Infertility at The New York Hospital–Cornell Medical Centre in New York, and indicates the specific differences in fertilization and pregnancy rates related to the different sperm parameters and semen collection and storage methods. Preliminary experimental data on the intracytoplasmic injection of isolated sperm heads (ICSHI) into human oocytes is also reported.

Materials and Methods

Preliminary ICSI Experiments

The human oocytes used for the preliminary intracytoplasmic injections were obtained from couples who had not achieved fertilization after standard in vitro insemination.

Hamster oocytes were collected from female golden hamsters superovulated by intraperitoneal injection of 25 I.U. of pregnant mare serum gonadotrophin (PMSG). About 56 h after PMSG administration, the hamsters were injected with 25 I.U. of human chorionic gonadotrophin (hCG) to induce ovulation. The animals were sacrificed by cervical dislocation 15–17 h post-hCG, and eggs were harvested from excised oviducts into a modified Tyrode's medium (T6) containing HEPES buffer (Bavister et al. 1983). Cumulus cells were removed by treatment with 0·1% hyaluronidase for 5–10 min.

Human spermatozoa from donors of proven fertility were collected by masturbation and then washed twice by centrifugation in T6 medium supplemented with 30 mg mL^{-1} of Fraction V bovine serum albumin (BSA). Details on the sperm selection methods have been described by Palermo et al. (1992).

Mouse spermatozoa and oocytes were collected, treated, and manipulated as previously reported by Palermo and Van Steirteghem (1991). The injection method, tool preparation and the set-up for micromanipulation (including media and reagents) have also been previously described (Palermo and Van Steirteghem 1991).

Patients

From September 1993 to June 1994, assisted fertilization by ICSI was performed in 355 cycles for couples with long-standing infertility. The mean age of the female partner was 35·1 years (range 26–44). The ICSI technique was reviewed and approved by the Committee on Human Rights of The New York Hospital–Cornell Medical Centre. The couples selected to participate in the assisted fertilization programme were patients with male factor or idiopathic infertility. The idiopathic indication included couples who were unable to achieve fertilization in vitro in a previous attempt ($n = 180$) as well as others with severely compromised semen parameters (severe oligozoospermia and/or asthenozoospermia, $n = 175$). The couples were counselled that ICSI was a new assisted reproductive technique and were informed of the many unknown aspects of this new treatment.

Semen Collection, Analysis, Classification and Sperm Selection

When possible, semen samples were collected by masturbation after at least three days of abstinence and they were allowed to liquefy for at least 20 min at 37°C before analysis. The other methods of semen collection used have been described elsewhere (Palermo et al. 1995).

Sperm concentration and motility were assessed in a Makler counting chamber according to criteria described previously (Cohen et al. 1992). Sperm morphology was then assessed by spreading 5 mL of semen or sperm suspension on prestained slides (Blustan-slides; Irvine Scientific, Santa Ana, CA, USA). Sperm morphology was evaluated and classified according to strict criteria (Kruger et al. 1986). Semen parameters were considered to be compromised when the sperm concentration was $<20 \times 10^6$ mL^{-1}, progressive motility was <40%, or <5% of the spermatozoa exhibited normal morphology.

The sperm sample was washed by centrifugation at 500g for 5 min in human tubal fluid (HTF) medium (Quinn et al. 1985) supplemented with 30 mg mL^{-1} of BSA (A-9647; Sigma, St Louis, MO, USA). Semen samples with $<5 \times 10^6$ sperm mL^{-1} or <20% motile spermatozoa were washed in HTF medium by a single centrifugation step at 1800g for 5 min. The resuspended pellet was layered on a discontinuous Percoll (Pharmacia, Uppsala, Sweden) gradient consisting of three layers (90%, 70%, 50%) and centrifuged at 300g for 20 min. A two-layer Percoll gradient (95%, 47·5%) was used when samples had a sperm concentration of $<5 \times 10^6$ mL^{-1} and <20% motility. The Percoll fraction containing the spermatozoa was washed twice in 4 mL of HTF medium by centrifugation at 1800g for 5 min to remove the silica gel particles. For spermatozoa with poor kinetic characteristics, the sperm suspension was exposed to 3 mM pentoxifylline and 3 mM 2-deoxy adenosine for 30 min and then washed again. The concentration of the final sperm suspension was adjusted to $1–1·5 \times 10^6$ mL^{-1}, when necessary, by the addition of HTF medium. The suspension was then incubated at 37°C in a gas atmosphere of 5% CO_2 in air.

Collection and Preparation of Oocytes

Female partners were down-regulated in the luteal phase with 1 mg day^{-1} (subcutaneous) of gonadotrophin-releasing hormone analogue (GnRHa) (Lupron; TAP Pharmaceutical, Chicago, IL, USA) followed by ovarian superovulation using human menopausal gonadotrophin (hMG) (Pergonal; Serono, Waltham, MA, USA) and/or pure follicle-stimulating hormone (FSH) (Metrodin; Serono) ($n = 220$ couples). Down-regulation with low-dose GnRHa (0·5 mg day^{-1}) was administered in 113 couples. In some cases, direct ovarian superovulation without GnRHa was performed by administering

FSH and/or hMG ($n = 10$ couples), or clomiphene citrate (CC) (Serophene; Serono) and hMG ($n = 10$ couples). When criteria for oocyte maturity were met, hCG was administered and oocytes were retrieved by vaginal ultrasound-guided puncture about 35 h after hCG administration.

Under the inverted microscope at 40× or 100× magnification, the cumulus–corona cell complexes were scored as mature, slightly immature, completely immature or slightly hypermature. Thereafter, the oocytes were further incubated for at least 4 h, and immediately before micromanipulation, the cumulus and corona cells were initially removed by exposure to HEPES-buffered HTF medium containing 80 I.U. mL^{-1} of hyaluronidase (Type VIII; Sigma) for up to 3 min. To enhance the enzymatic removal of the cumulus and corona cells, the oocytes were aspirated in and out of hand-drawn Pasteur pipettes with an inner diameter (ID) of ~ 200 μm. Each oocyte was washed twice in HTF medium supplemented with 10% patient serum and then examined under an inverted microscope at 200× magnification to assess integrity and maturity. The latter was performed by observing the presence of a germinal vesicle, germinal vesicle breakdown and the extruded first polar body. ICSI was performed on all oocytes that had reached metaphase II (M II).

Set-up and Procedure for Intracytoplasmic Injection

The preparation of the holding and injection micropipettes has already been extensively described (Palermo *et al.* 1995). In brief, the holding pipette had an ID of 20 μm and an outer diameter (OD) of 60 μm. The injection pipettes had a bevel angle of 30°, an ID of 5 μm, an OD of 6 μm and a sharp spike at the prominent edge of the bevelled tip.

Immediately before injection, 1 μL of sperm suspension was diluted with 4 μL of a 10% polyvinylpyrrolidone solution (PVP-K 90, molecular weight 360 000; ICN Biochemicals, Cleveland, OH, USA) in HEPES-buffered HTF medium in the centre of the Petri dish. When <500 000 spermatozoa were present in the ejaculate, the sperm suspension was concentrated in approximately 5 μL and transferred directly into the injection dish. The selected spermatozoon was aspirated from the concentrated 5 μL sperm suspension and transferred into the central droplet which contained PVP (to remove debris and facilitate aspiration control).

Each oocyte was placed in a 5 μL droplet of medium around the central drop of sperm in PVP. HEPES-buffered HTF medium supplemented with 5 mg mL^{-1} BSA (A-3156; Sigma) was used in the injection dish and the droplets were covered with lightweight paraffin oil (BDH, Poole, UK). The procedure was carried out using a heated stage (Easteach Laboratory, Centereach, NY, USA) on a Nikon Diaphot inverted microscope at 400× magnification using Hoffman modulation contrast optics. The microscope was equipped with two motor-driven, coarse-control manipulators and two hydraulic manipulators (MM-188 and MO-109; Narishige, Tokyo, Japan). The micropipettes were fitted to tool holders controlled by two IM-6 microinjectors (Narishige).

A spermatozoon with apparently normal morphology was chosen from the PVP drop and was aspirated tail first into the injection pipette. The injection pipette was introduced through the zona pellucida and the oolemma, deep into the cytoplasm, in a single motion without hesitation. The spermatozoon was injected using the smallest possible volume of medium (Palermo *et al.* 1995) because excessive medium reduces the chance of sperm decondensation.

The isolation of sperm heads was performed by lowering the injection pipette and pressing the spermatozoon with the bevelled edge of the tip in the region between the head and the midpiece. Rubbing the pipette against the bottom of the Petri dish caused the separation of the head from the tail. The injection of the sperm head into the cytoplasm was performed in a similar manner to the injection of intact sperm; the only difference was the difficulty of monitoring the delivery of the sperm head from the needle tip, between the cytoplasmic organelles of the oocyte.

Evaluation of Fertilization, Assisted Hatching and Rescue of Poor Quality Embryos

Oocytes were observed 12–17 h after injection, noting the integrity of the oocyte cytoplasm and the number and size of pronuclei. Cleavage of the fertilized oocyte was assessed 24 h after fertilization, and for each embryo, the number and size of the blastomeres were recorded as well as the percentage of anucleate fragments. After an additional 24 h ($\sim$63 h post-injection), the embryos were screened to determine the need for assisted hatching (AHA). An opening in the zona pellucida was made by zona drilling (ZD) using acidified Tyrode's solution (pH 2·35) and anucleate fragments were subsequently removed. The procedure was carried out in 10-mL droplets of HEPES-buffered HTF medium supplemented with 15% maternal serum (Cohen *et al.* 1992). Approximately 72 h after microinjection, up to 4 embryos ($\leq$30 years, up to 2–3 embryos; 31–42 years, up to 4 embryos) were transferred into the uterine cavity in HTF supplemented with 75% patient serum.

Therapeutic Implantation Support

For four days starting on the day of oocyte retrieval, methylprednisolone (16 mg day^{-1}) and tetracycline (250 mg 6 h^{-1}) were administered to all patients. Intramuscular supplementation with progesterone (25–50 mg day^{-1}) commenced one day after oocyte retrieval and was maintained throughout the luteal phase and up to the 7th week of gestation (Cohen *et al.* 1992).

Statistical Analysis

All statistical tests were performed using Statview 512+ (Brian-Power, Calabasas, CA, USA) and Microsoft Excel 4·0 (Microsoft, Redmond, WA, USA). All statistical tests were carried out two-tailed at the 5% level of significance. A χ^2-test was used to analyse the fertilization and ongoing pregnancy rates for each category of motile spermatozoa in the ejaculate and for each category of semen collection and storage method.

Results

Preliminary Experiments

In the initial experiments performed to assess the micromanipulation settings, 100% of the aged unfertilized human oocytes ($n = 10$) showed signs of oocyte activation after injection, indicated by the presence of pronuclei and/or early cleavage.

In an attempt to provide clearer proof of sperm nuclear decondensation, human spermatozoa were injected into the cytoplasm of 54 M II-stage hamster oocytes; 68% survived the procedure and 46% ($n = 17$) showed decondensation of the sperm nucleus on observation (4 h later) or after DNA staining with Giemsa. Sperm decondensation was not observed in 12 oocytes that were injected subzonally with a single sperm.

When 24 mouse oocytes were injected with a single intact mouse spermatozoon, only three of the oocytes (12%) survived the procedure and none fertilized. Of 23 mouse oocytes subzonally injected with a single sperm, 14 (61%) survived and 7 (50%) fertilized.

Clinical ICSI Results

The primary clinical indications for infertility involved subnormal semen parameters ($n = 231$) or antisperm antibodies bound to the spermatozoa ($n = 8$). The indications involving female partners were non-patent tubes ($n = 9$), the presence of serum antisperm antibodies ($n = 6$) and mild endometriosis ($n = 5$). In 12 couples, no clear reason for their infertility was identified. In the remaining 84 couples, the presence of male factor infertility was associated with other indications.

One hundred and eighty couples experienced complete fertilization failure in 509 prior IVF cycles (average number of attempts was 2·8). The mean semen parameters of these couples were as follows: sperm concentration of $28 \cdot 7 \times 10^6$ mL^{-1}, 31·6% progressive motility and 2·8% normal forms. Only 18 of the male partners presented with normal semen characteristics at the time of the attempt, and in the remaining semen samples, one or more parameters were impaired. Fertilization failure was assumed to be due to impaired sperm function which was not assessed by a routine semen analysis. Another 175 couples could not be treated by IVF due to extremely poor semen parameters (mean values: sperm concentration of $16 \cdot 9 \times 10^6$ mL^{-1}, 32·1% progressive motility and 2·2% normal forms).

All but 220 of the 3854 oocyte–cumulus cell complexes were recorded as mature at the time of retrieval. After removing the surrounding cumulus and corona cells, 3783 oocytes (98·2%) had an intact zona pellucida and a clear cytoplasm. Of these 3783 oocytes, 3063 had extruded the first polar body (80·9%), whereas 10·4% (393/3783) had a germinal vesicle and 8·6% (327/3783) had undergone germinal vesicle breakdown. Another 36 oocytes were degenerate and 35 were zona-free.

Table 1 describes the number of M II oocytes treated as well as the number of oocytes that survived and subsequently fertilized following ICSI. The degeneration rate was relatively low at 6·4% (190/2970). Eight other oocytes were injected by subzonal insemination in one patient and 66 oocytes (13 patients) were treated by conventional IVF.

Table 1. Survival and fertilization characteristics of the injected oocytes

M II, metaphase II; PN, pronuclei

No. of M II oocytes injected	2970	
No. of oocytes which survived injection	2780	(93·6%)
No. of oocytes with:		
2 PN	1917	(64·5%)[A]
1 PN	215	(9·6%)[B]
3 PN	110	(4·9%)[B]

[A] Value in parentheses is a percentage of the injected M II oocytes.
[B] Values in parentheses are percentages of the total number of pronuclear oocytes (1–3 PN).

From the 1917 bipronuclear oocytes, 1460 embryos were obtained (76·2%). Approximately 72 h after injection, 1025 embryos were transferred in 338 cycles (mean = 3·0 per cycle). A total of 790 (77·1%) embryos were micromanipulated by AHA before replacement. The remaining good quality embryos ($n = 314$) were cryopreserved in 77 cycles.

One hundred and ninety-one patients presented with a positive hCG titre, and of these, 28 pregnancies were biochemical, 14 patients had blighted ova and 1 patient had an ectopic pregnancy requiring a salpingectomy at 7 weeks of gestation. In 148 patients, a fetal heart was observed on ultrasonographic evaluation; 11 miscarried between 7 and 13 weeks of gestation. The ongoing pregnancy rate was 38·6% per oocyte retrieval (137/355) and 40·5% per embryo replacement (137/338). There were 81 singleton pregnancies (5 of which were vanishing twin pregnancies), 45 twin, 10 triplet and 1 quadruplet pregnancies. The frequency of sac formation per embryo transferred was 24·4 % (250/1025) and the implantation rate expressed as fetal hearts per embryo transferred was 21·7% (222/1025).

One therapeutic abortion was performed for a trisomy 21 fetus discovered at amniocentesis. At the time of writing, 22 pregnancies were delivered, two of which were premature (both singletons at 27 and 30 weeks respectively). The remaining 20 deliveries included 12 singleton and 8 twin pregnancies. The total number of babies born was 30, 11 males and 19 females. The remaining 114 ongoing pregnancies were as follows: 66 singleton, 37 twin, 10 triplet and 1 quadruplet.

Semen Parameters and ICSI Outcome

The relationship between semen parameters and the outcome of assisted fertilization was investigated. A semen score was calculated on the basis of the number of normal motile spermatozoa present in the fresh ejaculate: volume (mL) $\times$ concentration ($\times 10^6$ mL^{-1}) $\times$ total motility (%) $\times$ normal forms (%) $\times 10^6$. Based on the score, the cycles were divided into three groups: one group with immotile spermatozoa in the ejaculate, one group with the number of motile spermatozoa ranging from 39 to 500 000 and the last group with >500 000 motile spermatozoa. The first two groups of patients are generally considered unsuitable for treatment with standard IVF. Table 2 describes the number of cycles, fertilization rates and pregnancy results in terms of positive hCG as well as the presence of fetal hearts at ultrasound, according to the concentration of normal motile sperm cells.

Intracytoplasmic sperm injection can achieve fertilization regardless of sperm motility and the concentration of normal motile spermatozoa. Thus, spermatozoa can be collected for ICSI by masturbation, electro-ejaculation, or microsurgical epididymal sperm aspiration (MESA) and

Table 2. Fertilization and pregnancies obtained after intracytoplasmic sperm injection (ICSI) in relation to the total number of normal, motile spermatozoa in the ejaculate

hCG, human chorionic gonadotrophin

	No. of normal, motile spermatozoa			
	0	39–500 000	>500 000	Total
No. of cycles	115	158	82	355
Fertilization rate[A]	62·5%	70·1%	76·4%	68·9%
	(572/915)	(894/1275)	(451/590)	(1917/2780)
Pregnancies (hCG)	59	92	40	191
Ongoing pregnancies	36	71	30	137
Ongoing pregnancy rate[B]	31·2%	44·9%	36·6%	38·6%

[A] χ^2-test, 2×3, 2 d.f.; differences in normal, motile sperm concentration on fertilization, $P < 0.001$.
[B] χ^2-test, 2×3, 2 d.f.; differences in normal, motile sperm concentration on pregnancies, $P < 0.01$.

Table 3. Semen parameters, fertilization and pregnancies obtained with intracytoplasmic sperm injection (ICSI) according to the origin of the semen sample

hCG, human chorionic gonadotrophin

	Origin of semen			
	Fresh	Frozen	Electro-ejaculation	Epididymal
No. of cycles	308	17	7	23
Fertilization rate[A]	70·9%	67·8%	67·8%	47·1%
	(1677/2363)	(103/152)	(40/59)	(97/206)
Pregnancies (hCG)	166	8	3	14
Ongoing pregnancies	122	4	2	9
Ongoing pregnancy rate	39·5%	23·5%	28·6%	40·9%

[A] χ^2-test, 2×4, 2 d.f.; differences in semen origin on fertilization, $P < 0.001$.

can be processed or cryopreserved for future attempts (Table 3).

Intracytoplasmic Sperm Head Injection (ICSHI)

In 13 patients treated by ICSI, 35 M II sibling oocytes were injected with an isolated sperm head; 31 of the oocytes survived (89%) the injection procedure and 23 (74%) displayed two pronuclei. From 22 zygotes (one was cryopreserved), 16 embryos were obtained (73%), 5 with no fragments, 10 with 5–20% fragmentation, and only one with >20% fragmentation. In 4 patients, 4 embryos were replaced together with other ICSI-treated embryos and one patient established a twin pregnancy.

Of the 12 remaining embryos, 2 exhibited arrested cleavage, 4 displayed slow cleavage, and 2 exhibited irregularly-shaped blastomeres. A total of six embryos were analysed by fluorescence *in situ* hybridization (FISH). In 5 of these embryos, the injection of the sperm head was accompanied by the insertion of the dislodged tail. In all 6 embryos obtained from oocytes injected with isolated sperm heads ($n = 3$) and heads plus tails ($n = 3$), FISH analysis revealed a completely aneuploid distribution of the chromosomes.

Discussion

The experimental phase which was performed to perfect the skills needed for successful ICSI only succeeded when aged human oocytes and hamster oocytes were injected with human sperm. The reason for the limited success can be explained by the relative sizes of the gametes. Human oocytes have a diameter of ~120 μm whereas the spermatozoon is 3 μm wide and 55 μm long. This size permits the use of a pipette with an ID of 4–5 μm which results in a limited incidence of injury because of the large size of the egg. The same was true for hamster oocytes whose diameter is approximately 80 μm. When the same procedure was applied to mouse oocytes, however, it resulted in a remarkably high rate of injury (88%), and this high incidence of injury was attributed to the size of the injection pipette which had to be large enough to accommodate a spermatozoon with a perforatorium. The mouse model was important, however, because it offered the most convenient means of showing that the micromanipulation procedure, as performed, was not harmful to the embryos or to subsequent offspring. This experience suggested that we could inject single mouse sperm into the perivitelline space (PVS) of mouse oocytes after inducing the acrosome reaction. Of the 408 oocytes so injected, 70% fertilized and 97% cleaved to early blastocysts. The implantation rate was 46% (123/265) and 88 live offspring (71%) were delivered (Palermo and Van Steirteghem 1991). Based on these data, we can conclude that it is possible to develop micromanipulation techniques for use on all animal gametes, but that experimental ICSI can only succeed when human sperm are injected into hamster oocytes or unfertilized human oocytes (Tesarik *et al.* 1994).

Prior to the establishment of the first pregnancies after ICSI, 187 human oocytes had been injected from 56 patients whose sibling oocytes were treated by SUZI. Of these ICSI oocytes, 86% survived and 46% (73/160) fertilized (Palermo et al. 1992).

In the present study, 324 couples were treated in 355 consecutive cycles of assisted fertilization by ICSI. Injection of a single spermatozoon into the cytoplasm was performed in 2970 oocytes, of which 1917 fertilized normally. The frequency of fetal hearts per embryo transferred exceeded 21%. Previous papers have reported that patients treated by this technique could indeed achieve pregnancies and give birth to normal babies (Palermo et al. 1992). It has also been shown that ICSI consistently surpasses subzonal insemination in terms of fertilization (Palermo et al. 1993; Van Steirteghem et al. 1993). Subzonal insemination requires only a few spermatozoa but its success is highly dependent upon the ability of those spermatozoa to fuse with the oolemma. In the process, penetration of more than one sperm cell often occurs, rendering the embryo genetically abnormal (Cohen et al. 1991).

In the study described herein, mechanical damage resulting from the injection procedure was relatively low (6·4%) compared with previous reports (Palermo et al. 1993; Van Steirteghem et al. 1993). The improvement probably results from the repositioning of the oocyte in relation to the polar body to avoid the area of polar granularity during insertion of the injection pipette. The area of polar granularity is considered to be the locus of germinal vesicle breakdown and the chromosomes and meiotic spindle. This redefined ICSI technique achieved a consistent fertilization rate of 64·5% (68·9% of the intact oocytes), and only two couples had complete fertilization failure, one occurring with semen obtained by MESA.

The number of motile sperm generally needed to perform standard *in vitro* insemination is approximately 500 000. Patients with ≥500 000 motile sperm had a fertilization rate of 76·4% with ICSI. When the procedure was performed with samples containing <500 000 motile sperm, the fertilization rate was 66·9%. Although significantly lower ($P = 0·01$), this fertilization rate was similar to that obtained using standard IVF in selected patients. When a semen analysis showed no normal, motile spermatozoa in the ejaculate, the fertilization rate was 62·5%. These findings demonstrate that the consistency with which the ICSI technique achieves fertilization does not strictly depend on semen parameters and they are consistent with a previous study which illustrated the absence of any clear correlation between semen characteristics and outcome of ICSI (Palermo et al. 1993).

The absence of a correlation between sperm characteristics (concentration, motility and morphology) and eventual fertilization following ICSI raises the question of whether sperm integrity is indeed necessary to achieve fertilization in the human. A preliminary study was therefore performed in our laboratory involving intracytoplasmic injection of only sperm heads after mechanical separation of the midpiece and tail. The fertilization rate (74%) obtained after sperm head injection demonstrated that the midpiece is unnecessary for sperm nuclear decondensation, however, further experiments are required to investigate whether the embryos will develop normally. This follow-up is especially important in light of our recent report that the first embryonic spindle is organized by the male sperm centrosome and centriole, which is located in the midpiece (Palermo et al. 1994). These findings must be confirmed from more extensive cytogenetic studies. The centriole appears to be necessary for the zygote to progress in cleavage while maintaining a normal euploid status.

To clarify whether it is necessary to maintain the integrity of the spermatozoon or the presence of the anatomical substructures of the sperm cell (chromatin and centrioles), we injected mechanically-separated sperm heads and tails into 5 human oocytes. Four of these oocytes survived and all showed normal fertilization. The 3 oocytes that had normal cleavage patterns have all been analysed by FISH and the outcome was a completely aneuploid distribution of the chromosomes. From this finding it appears that, in order to allow normal bipolar spindle formation, it is necessary to maintain the integrity of the spermatozoon or at least the close proximity of the centriole to the male pronucleus.

Conclusions

For the purpose of acquiring and refining the skills necessary for the ICSI procedure, it is preferable to begin by injecting human spermatozoa into human or hamster oocytes. The ICSI technique appears to be a powerful micromanipulation tool for achieving fertilization and pregnancy independent of the semen characteristics, collection methods and storage. The fertilization and pregnancy rates obtained after injecting a single spermatozoon into the cytoplasm are comparable to those obtained with standard *in vitro* insemination in non-male factor patients. The evidence that ICSI can achieve fertilization with sub-fertile spermatozoa, epididymal sperm, testicular sperm (Schoysman et al. 1993) and sperm heads suggests the possible application of this procedure to more immature forms such as round spermatids (Ogura and Yanagimachi 1995). However, the question remains whether abnormal spindle formation occurs due to the absence or misplacement of the centrosome. As stated earlier, further cytogenetic studies are required to ascertain whether the injection of isolated sperm heads or spermatid nuclei will allow normal and healthy conception.

Acknowledgments

We thank the clinical and scientific staff of The Centre for Reproductive Medicine and Infertility for their expert assistance. We thank Sasha Sadowy, Adrienne Reing, Toni Ferrara and Elena Kissin for technical assistance, and Donna Espenberg for editorial assistance.

References

Bavister, B. D., Leibfried, M. L., and Lieberman, G. (1983). Development of preimplantation embryos of the golden hamster in a defined culture medium. *Biol. Reprod.* **28**, 235–47.

Cohen, J., Alikani, M., Adler, A., Berkeley, A., Davis, O., Ferrara, T., Graf, M., Grifo, J., Liu, H. C., Malter, H. E., Reing, A., Suzman, M., Talansky, B. E., and Rosenwaks, Z. (1992). Microsurgical fertilization procedures: the absence of stringent criteria for patient selection. *J. Assist. Reprod. Genet.* **9**, 197–206.

Cohen, J., Alikani, M., Malter, H. E., Adler, A., Talansky, B. E., and Rosenwaks, Z. (1991). Partial zona dissection or subzonal sperm insertion: microsurgical fertilization alternatives based on evaluation of sperm and embryo morphology. *Fertil. Steril.* **56**, 696–706.

Hiramoto, Y. (1962). Microinjection of the live spermatozoa into sea urchin eggs. *Exp. Cell. Res.* **27**, 416–26.

Hosoi, Y., Miyake, M., Utsumi, K., and Iritani, A. (1988). Development of rabbit oocytes after microinjection of spermatozoa. *Proc. 11th Int. Congr. Anim. Reprod. Artif. Insem.*, 331. [Abstr.]

Kruger, T. F., Menkveld, R., Stander, F. S. H., Lombard, C. J., Van der Merwe, J. P., Van Zyl, J. A., and Smith, K. (1986). Sperm morphologic features as a prognostic factor in *in vitro* fertilization. *Fertil. Steril.* **46**, 1118–23.

Lanzendorf, S., Maloney, M., Ackerman, S., Acosta, A., and Hodgen, G. (1988*a*). Fertilizing potential of acrosome-defective sperm following microsurgical injection into eggs. *Gamete Res.* **19**, 329–37.

Lanzendorf, S. E., Maloney, M. K., Veeck, L. L., Slusser, J., Hodgen, G. D., and Rosenwaks, Z. (1988*b*). A preclinical evaluation of pronuclear formation by microinjection of human spermatozoa into human oocytes. *Fertil. Steril.* **49**, 835–42.

Lin, T.P. (1966). Microinjection of mouse eggs. *Science* **151**, 333–7.

Markert, C.L. (1983). Fertilization of mammalian eggs by sperm injection. *J. Exp. Zool.* **228**, 195–201.

Ogura, A., and Yanagimachi, R. (1995). Spermatids as male gametes. In 'Intracytoplasmic Sperm Injection: the Revolution in Male Infertility'. *Reprod. Fertil. Dev.* **7**, 155–9.

Palermo, G., and Van Steirteghem, A. (1991). Enhancement of acrosome reaction and subzonal insemination of a single spermatozoon in mouse eggs. *Mol. Reprod. Dev.* **30**, 339–45.

Palermo, G., Joris, H., Devroey, P., and Van Steirteghem, A. C. (1992). Pregnancies after intracytoplasmic injection of single spermatozoon into an oocyte. *Lancet* **340**, 17–18.

Palermo, G., Joris, H., Derde, M.-P., Camus, M., Devroey, P., and Van Steirteghem, A. (1993). Sperm characteristics and outcome of human assisted fertilization by subzonal insemination and intracytoplasmic sperm injection. *Fertil. Steril.* **59**, 826–35.

Palermo, G., Munné, S., and Cohen, J. (1994). The human zygote inherits its mitotic potential from the male gamete. *Hum. Reprod. (Oxf.)* **9**, 1220–5.

Palermo, G. D., Cohen, J., Alikani, M., Adler, A., and Rosenwaks, Z. (1995). Intracytoplasmic sperm injection: a novel treatment for all forms of male factor infertility. *Fertil. Steril.* (In press.)

Quinn, P., Warnes, G. M., Kerin, J. F., and Kirby, C. (1985). Culture factors affecting the success rate of *in vitro* fertilization and embryo transfer. *Ann. N.Y. Acad. Sci.* **442**, 195–204.

Schoysman, R., Vanderzwalmen, P., Nijs, M., Segal, L., Segal-Bertin, G., Geerts, L., van Roosendaal, E., and Schoysman, D. (1993). Pregnancy after fertilisation with human testicular spermatozoa. *Lancet* **342**, 1237.

Tesarik, J., Sousa, M., and Testart, J. (1994). Human oocyte activation after intracytoplasmic sperm injection. *Hum. Reprod. (Oxf.)* **9**, 511–18.

Thadani, V. M. (1981). A study of oocyte interactions using *in vitro* fertilization and sperm microinjection'. Ph.D. Thesis. Yale University, New Haven.

Uehara, T., and Yanagimachi, R. (1976). Microsurgical injection of spermatozoa into hamster eggs with subsequent transformation of sperm nuclei into male pronuclei. *Biol. Reprod.* **15**, 467–70.

Van Steirteghem, A. C., Liu, J., Joris, H., Nagy, Z., Janssenswillen, C., Tournaye, H., Derde, M.-P., Van Assche, E., and Devroey, P. (1993). Higher success rate by intracytoplasmic sperm injection than by subzonal insemination. Report of a second series of 300 consecutive treatment cycles. *Hum. Reprod. (Oxf.)* **8**, 1055–60.

Manuscript received 27 March 1995

Open Discussion

Sherman Silber (St Louis):

Two technical questions. First, when you have a very flexible egg membrane, is there a special trick to puncturing it without pushing the pipette all the way through to the other side? Second, even though sperm morphology supposedly doesn't matter, is it important to select sperm with good morphology?

Palermo:

Yes, there is a way to overcome the membrane problem. Once you have gone deep into the egg, you make a funnel, and then you go back and hook the border of this funnel with the spike on the injection pipette. The trick is to go in VERY slowly without extending the membrane.

With regard to sperm morphology, I select the best looking sperm. We have a better fertilization rate with normal sperm.

Alan Trounson (Melbourne):

I disagree with you regarding injection of motile sperm. We did a study in which we injected motile sperm and the fertilization rate was exactly the same.

Palermo:

I have tried motile and immotile sperm. The fertilization rate was much better with immobilized sperm. At Cornell, we record if the sperm is motile or starts to move again in the injection pipette because the fertilization rate is not as good.

Robert McLachlan (Melbourne):

Your triplet and higher ongoing pregnancy rate was 10%. Has that figure led you to reduce the number of embryos you're willing to transfer?

Palermo:

I agree with you that it is high. In the United States, patients are very concerned about achieving a pregnancy and perhaps less concerned about the incidence of multiple pregnancies. It is a major issue.

Yvonne Du Plessis (Stockholm):

Do you have any data on the effect of the type of ovarian stimulation on the implantation rate with ICSI?

Palermo:

I don't see any clear relationship with pregnancy. I'm trying to investigate the relationship between the type and length of stimulation, the characteristic response of the patient and the incubation time between oocyte retrieval and injection on the membrane, whether it breaks right away and whether it is difficult to pierce. I think it's also important to determine the incidence of 3 pronuclei and the damage rate after different stimulation regimes.

Intracytoplasmic Sperm Injection — Clinical Results from the Reproductive Medicine Unit, Adelaide

Dianna Payne[A] and Colin D. Matthews

Reproductive Medicine Laboratories, Department of Obstetrics and Gynaecology, The University of Adelaide, The Queen Elizabeth Hospital, Woodville, SA 5011, Australia.
[A] *To whom correspondence should be addressed.*

Abstract. The clinical results of 391 cycles of intracytoplasmic sperm injection (ICSI) performed between June 1993 and July 1994 are presented in this report. A total of 4797 oocytes were collected, of which 3792 were injected. Of these, 2603 (69%) fertilized, with normal and three pronuclear fertilization rates of 65% and 4% respectively. About 6% of the oocytes were destroyed while denuding and during ICSI. There were 373 (95%) embryo transfers from which 119 pregnancies arose, giving pregnancy rates of 32% per transfer and 30% per cycle, and an implantation rate of 15% per embryo. Of the pregnancies, 98 (82%) were ongoing. Supernumerary embryos were frozen in 44% of the cycles and 61 subsequent transfers of 130 frozen–thawed embryos produced 11 pregnancies (18%). Only 47 (12%) patients had less than 50% of their oocytes fertilized (mean 31%) after ICSI, and of these, 8 had no fertilization of 13 eggs. Nevertheless, 37 of these 47 patients had an embryo transfer and 9 achieved a pregnancy with an implantation rate of 14% per embryo. The percent normal sperm morphology weakly correlated with percent fertilization ($r^2 = 0.027$, $P < 0.02$) but not with the implantation rate ($r^2 = 0.003$, $P > 0.05$). Fifty-nine patients with only occasional motile sperm in the ejaculate and 23 patients in whom epididymal sperm were aspirated were treated. The fertilization rates (66% and 70% respectively) and pregnancy rates per transfer (32% and 24% respectively) were comparable in these two subgroups. The overall ICSI results were also compared with 515 cycles of routine *in vitro* fertilization (IVF) which were performed at the same time. The fertilization rate (69% v. 71%), percent of cycles with freezing (46% v. 52%) and percent of embryos either frozen or transferred (64% v. 71%) were significantly lower after ICSI, whereas the number of cycles reaching transfer (95% v. 89%), pregnancy rate per transfer (32% v. 25%) and implantation rate (15% v. 12%) were significantly higher after ICSI. It appears that, overall, the results from ICSI are similar to or better than those from routine IVF, even among patients with occasional motile or epididymal sperm.

Extra keywords: ICSI, sperm morphology, epididymal sperm, pregnancy, implantation rate.

Introduction

Intracytoplasmic sperm injection (ICSI) has been in clinical use since 1992 (Palermo *et al.* 1992) and has revolutionized the treatment of severe male factor infertility. Although earlier micro-assisted fertilization techniques such as zona drilling, zona cutting and subzonal injection (SUZI), increased the fertilization rate, they suffered from a number of disadvantages such as relatively low fertilization rates, high polyspermy rates and an inability to treat very severe oligozoospermia (reviewed by Payne 1995*b*). Because only one viable sperm per oocyte is required for ICSI, patients with occasional motile sperm can now be admitted to clinical ICSI programmes, whereas before their only option was the use of donor sperm.

ICSI was instituted on a trial basis in our unit in June 1993, but it immediately became obvious that it was far superior to SUZI, and so ICSI was adopted shortly thereafter as the only micro-assisted fertilization technique. As the success of ICSI became widely known, the number of patients presenting with severe oligozoospermia has more than quadrupled and at present 44% of our *in vitro* fertilization (IVF) patient base comprises couples with severe male factor infertility who require ICSI (Fig. 1). This report details the outcome of 391 ICSI cycles performed in our unit between June 1993 and July 1994.

Materials and Methods

Patient Selection and Treatment

Patients were offered ICSI for one of the following reasons: (i) semen was too poor for routine IVF in the first instance with <200 000 motile sperm recovered per ejaculate, including patients with only occasional sperm; (ii) fertilization previously failed or was <25% in at least one cycle of routine IVF and/or SUZI; (iii) new patients with < 20% morphologically normal sperm in their ejaculate had ICSI on half of their oocytes and routine insemination of the others, as Duncan et al. (1993) showed that these patients have particularly poor fertilization rates after routine IVF in our programme; (iv) patients with obstructive azoospermia in whom we could only collect epididymal sperm.

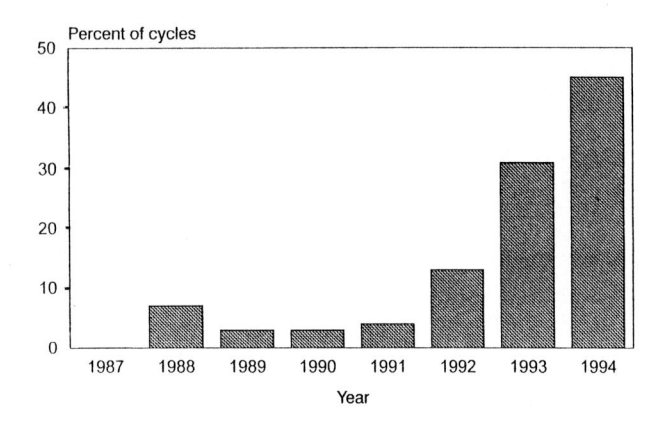

Fig. 1. The percent of IVF cycles in our unit requiring micromanipulative techniques since the introduction of zona drilling in 1987.

Informed written consent was obtained from each couple and the study had the approval of the Ethics of Human Research Committees at The Queen Elizabeth Hospital and The University of Adelaide.

The ovarian stimulation protocols have been described in detail elsewhere (Payne et al. 1994a, 1994b). Briefly, patients were downregulated in the previous luteal phase with leuprorelin acetate (Lucrin; Abbott Australasia, Kurnell, NSW, Australia) before stimulation with human menopausal gonadotrophin (hMG) (Humegon; Organon, Lane Cove, NSW or Pergonal; Serono, Frenchs Forest, NSW) and ovulation induction with human chorionic gonadotrophin (hCG) (Profasi; Serono).

Semen Preparation

Semen preparation has been described elsewhere (Payne et al. 1994b). Briefly, depending on the severity of oligozoospermia, motile sperm were isolated or concentrated using discontinuous Percoll gradients (Ord et al. 1990; Kirby et al. 1991) or by repeated centrifugation and resuspension in culture medium (Payne et al. 1994b).

Preparation of Epididymal Sperm

Epididymal sperm aspiration was performed approximately 2–3 h after oocyte retrieval so that the oocytes were denuded and ready for injection by the time the sperm were collected. Spermatozoa from the rete testis and proximal regions of the epididymis were aspirated into multiple aliquots (200 μL) of warm HEPES-buffered human tubal fluid (HTF) medium (Quinn et al. 1985) which did not contain serum. Each aspirate was checked for the presence of motile sperm and when an adequate sample was recovered it was taken back to the laboratory for immediate preparation. Sperm were maintained at 35°C during transit. Further samples were collected for cryopreservation. The sperm were washed twice by centrifugation at 300 g and resuspension in bicarbonate-buffered HTF containing 5% maternal serum, then resuspended in 200 μL of medium and immediately used for ICSI. Cryopreservation of sperm was carried out as soon as possible after collection, using a 1:1 dilution with citrate–glycerol–egg yolk buffer before cooling to $-70°C$ then plunging into liquid nitrogen N_2.

Evaluation of Sperm Morphology

Sperm smears from the ejaculate used for ICSI were fixed in 95% ethanol, stained by the modified Papanicolaou procedure, and then the morphology of 200 sperm from each sample was scored according to criteria set out by the World Health Organization (1987).

Oocyte Preparation

Cumulus cells were removed by brief exposure (30 s) to 1 mg mL^{-1} ovine hyaluronidase (Type III; Sigma, St Louis, MO, USA), then the oocyte was washed through four changes of medium before mechanical removal of coronal cells. Oocytes were maintained at all times at 37°C in an atmosphere of 5% CO_2 in air.

Intracytoplasmic Sperm Injection

ICSI micropipettes were manufactured as described by Payne (1995a) and were similar to those described by Van Steirteghem et al. (1993a). The microinjection procedure was performed as described by Van Steirteghem et al. (1993a, 1993b) and Payne et al. (1994b) with the modification that the polar body was always oriented at 12 o'clock and the opening of the injection pipette always faced towards 6 o'clock.

Control oocytes were denuded in exactly the same manner and were inseminated with approximately 50 000 motile sperm mL^{-1}.

Assessment of Fertilization and Cleavage

Approximately 17 h after ICSI, oocytes were examined for fertilization (two pronuclei and two polar bodies) using Nomarski optics. Embryo development was assessed at approximately 41 h and 63 h post-injection and suitable embryos were transferred to the uterus at about 68 h post-injection (Day 3). Supernumerary good quality embryos were frozen according to the method of Testart et al. (1986).

Pregnancy Testing

A quantitative serum β-hCG of >25 I.U. on Day 15 and Day 22 post-embryo transfer was considered a positive pregnancy test. Clinical pregnancies were confirmed by ultrasound at 8 weeks of gestation. The implantation rate was calculated by dividing the number of embryos transferred by the number of implantations. Pregnancies that did not reach 8 weeks (scan) were assumed to have had one implanted embryo.

Statistical Analysis

InStat (Graph Pad, San Diego, CA, USA) was used for all statistical analyses. A χ^2-test with Yates correction or a Fisher's Exact test was used depending on the sample size. $P < 0.05$ was considered significant.

Results

A total of 4797 oocytes were recovered in 391 ICSI cycles and, of these, 3792 were injected and 2603 (69%) fertilized (Table 1). Overall, 65% of the oocytes fertilized

Table 1. A comparison of intracytoplasmic sperm injection (ICSI) and routine *in vitro* fertilization (IVF) cycles between June 1993 and July 1994

n.s., not significant; ORP, oocyte recovery procedure; PN, pronuclei

	ICSI	Routine IVF	Significance
No. of cycles	391	511	—
No. of oocytes	4797	5236	—
No. of oocytes injected or inseminated	3792	5051	—
No. of fertilized oocytes[A]:	2603 (69%)	3582 (71%)	$P = 0.0224$
2 PN[A]	2469 (65%)	3395 (67%)	n.s.
3 PN[A]	134 (4%)	187 (4%)	n.s.
No. of 1 PN oocytes[A]	173 (5%)	131 (3%)	$P < 0.0001$
No. of embryo transfers	373 (95%)	456 (89%)	$P = 0.0008$
No. of embryos transferred (average)	972 (2.6)	1179 (2.6)	—
Day of embryo transfer (post-ORP)	3	2	—
No. of pregnancies	119	115	
Pregnancy rate per transfer	32%	25%	$P = 0.0074$
No. of implantations	146	139	—
Implantation rate per embryo	15%	12%	$P = 0.0327$
No. of cycles with freezing	173 (44%)	266 (52%)	$P = 0.0233$
No. of embryos frozen	616	1229	—
No. of embryos transferred or frozen	1588 (64%)	2408 (71%)	$P < 0.0001$

[A] Values in parentheses are percentages of the injected or inseminated oocytes.

normally (2 pronuclei and 2 polar bodies) and 4% had three pronuclei. A further 5% of the oocytes showed 1 large pronucleus and 2 polar bodies and were activated but not fertilized (see Flaherty *et al.* 1995). A total of 972 embryos were transferred in 373 transfers (average of 2.6 embryos per transfer) and 119 pregnancies were established giving pregnancy rates of 32% per transfer and 30% per cycle, and an implantation rate per embryo of 15%.

A preliminary life table analysis after 3 cycles indicated that patients are just as likely to become pregnant after their third cycle as their first, and that 73% of patients embarking on ICSI should be pregnant at the end of their third cycle (Fig. 2).

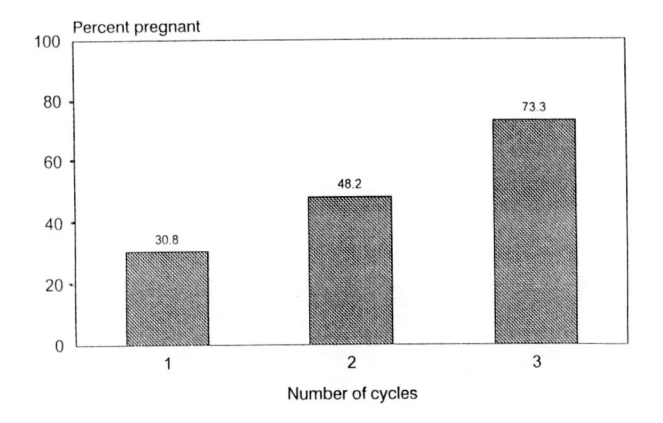

Fig. 2. A life table analysis of 391 ICSI cycles to show the expectation of pregnancy after 1, 2 or 3 cycles. The pregnancy rate is shown above each bar.

Frozen Embryo Transfers

Supernumerary embryos (616) were frozen in 173 (44%) cycles at an average of 3.6 embryos per cycle. To date, we have performed 74 frozen–thawed embryo transfer cycles in 61 patients. In all, 130 of the 223 (58%) embryos survived the freeze–thaw procedure. There were 13 cycles in which no embryos survived and 61 cycles in which 130 embryos were transferred. Eleven pregnancies were established including one twin pregnancy, giving a pregnancy rate of 18% per transfer and an implantation rate per embryo of 9%.

Comparison of ICSI and Routine IVF

The percent of morphologically good embryos was calculated by adding the number of transferred embryos to the number of embryos frozen and dividing by the total number of 2 pronuclear embryos created. After ICSI, 64% of embryos were either frozen or transferred (Table 1). For comparison, 511 routine IVF cycles performed during the same period have been included and the results are also outlined in Table 1. The overall, 2 pronuclear and 3 pronuclear fertilization rates were not significantly different between ICSI and IVF, although the percent of 1 pronuclear oocytes was significantly higher after ICSI (5% v. 3%, $P < 0.0001$). The pregnancy rate per transfer (32% versus 25%, $P = 0.0074$) and implantation rate per embryo (15% v. 12%, $P = 0.0327$) were significantly higher after ICSI than IVF. In contrast, the percent of cycles which had embryos frozen ($P = 0.0233$) and the percent of embryos that were transferred or frozen ($P < 0.0001$) were significantly higher after IVF.

Uninjected Oocytes

Of the 4797 oocytes that were collected, 1006 were not injected. There were 339 (7%) immature oocytes, of which 160 (3·3%) had a prominent germinal vesicle (GV) and 179 (3·7%) had not extruded the first polar body and were therefore either at prophase I or metaphase I. There were 79 (1·6%) morphologically abnormal oocytes (grossly vacuolated, fragmented or degenerate) that were not injected, 268 (5·6%) oocytes that were destroyed during denuding or injection, and 32 (0·8%) oocytes that were lost. Hence, 718 (15%) oocytes were unsuitable for ICSI or were lost or destroyed. The remaining 288 oocytes were allocated to a control group for routine insemination.

Fertilization Failure

Overall, 95% of cycles resulted in an embryo transfer. Of the 18 patients who did not have an embryo transfer, 8 had no fertilization. Of these, 6 patients had a single oocyte and 1 patient had 2 oocytes that were injected but failed to fertilize, and one patient had 5 oocytes in which the spermatozoa were all ejected into the perivitelline space. A further 6 patients had poor embryo development, 4 due to toxic paraffin oil and 2 due to failure of a single embryo to cleave. Two patients had all their embryos frozen due to hyperstimulation, one had no sperm on the day of injection and one had only one immature oocyte that was not injected.

Patient Subgroups

During this study, 59 patients had only occasional motile sperm in their semen. In these cases, the entire ejaculate was centrifuged and the resulting sperm were resuspended in approximately 200 μL of medium. Sufficient motile sperm were recovered to inject all of the oocytes in all but 3 of these cases, although finding motile sperm was often a very time consuming exercise. The results from this subgroup are presented in Table 2. The fertilization rate (66%), percent of patients receiving an embryo transfer (92%), pregnancy rate per transfer (32%), implantation rate per embryo (13%) and percent of patients with frozen embryos (44%) were all comparable to the overall ICSI results.

Table 2. Intracytoplasmic sperm injection (ICSI) results for patients with occasional motile sperm

No. of cycles	59
No. of oocytes injected	575
No. of oocytes fertilized	377 (66%)
No. of embryo transfers	54 (92%)
No. of embryos transferred (average)	146 (2·7)
No. of pregnancies	17
Pregnancy rate per transfer	32%
No. of implantations	19
Implantation rate per embryo	13%
No. of cycles with freezing	26 (44%)
No. of embryos frozen	83

The results of ICSI with rete testis and proximal epididymal sperm from patients with obstructive azoospermia are shown in Table 3. The overall fertilization rate was 70%. Twenty-one patients had 51 embryos transferred and 5 (24%) pregnancies occurred. Another pregnancy occurred after the transfer of 2 frozen embryos in a patient who had all her embryos frozen because of the risk of hyperstimulation. In 3 of the 23 cycles, epididymal sperm which had been frozen in a previous cycle were used, and 50% of these oocytes fertilized, 9 embryos were transferred in 3 transfers and one ongoing twin pregnancy was established.

Table 3. Intracytoplasmic sperm injection (ICSI) results using rete testis and epididymal sperm for patients with obstructive azoospermia

No. of cycles	23
No. of oocytes injected	210
No. of oocytes fertilized	148 (70%)
No. of embryo transfers	21 (91%)
No. of embryos transferred (average)	51 (2·4)
No. of pregnancies	5
Pregnancy rate per transfer	24%
No. of implantations	7
Implantation rate per embryo	14%
No. of cycles with freezing	10 (43%)
No. of embryos frozen	35

Although the overall ICSI fertilization rate was about 70%, 12% of patients had <50% fertilization after ICSI. The cycle details for the <50% fertilization group were compared with the $\geq$50% fertilization group (Table 4). There were no differences in the mean values for female age at the time of treatment, maximum oestradiol at the time of hCG injection, ampoules of hMG used, or the number of oocytes collected. The fertilization rates were 31% and 77%, respectively, and the average number of embryos transferred was correspondingly lower in the <50% fertilization group (2·1 v. 2·7). There were no significant differences in the pregnancy rates (24% v. 33%) or implantation rates per embryo (14% v. 15%).

Effect of Sperm Morphology

The percent normal sperm morphology in the neat semen was correlated with the fertilization rate and implantation rate per embryo in 206 ICSI cycles performed up to April 1994. The average implantation rate per embryo was calculated by dividing the number of implantations in a particular pregnancy by the number of embryos transferred, thus giving a percent implantation rate per embryo per transfer. There was a weak correlation between the fertilization rate after ICSI and percent normal sperm morphology (Fig. 3) but no such relationship existed between sperm morphology and the implantation rate per embryo (Fig. 4).

Table 4. A comparison of results in patients who achieved <50% or ≥50% fertilization after intracytoplasmic sperm injection (ICSI)

hMG, human menopausal gonadotrophin

	<50%	≥50%
No. of cycles	47	344
Mean age[A]	32·5 (22·9–46·3)	33·4 (21·2–47·8)
Mean maximum oestradiol[A]	6·7 (0·9–18·1)	7·0 (1·3–38·6)
Mean ampoules of hMG	39·6	35·3
Mean no. of oocytes collected[A]	10·8 (1–28)	12·4 (1–38)
No. of oocytes for ICSI	339	3169
No. of oocytes fertilized	106 (31%)	2453 (77%)
No. of embryo transfers	37 (79%)	335 (97%)
No. of embryos transferred (average)	78 (2·1)	894 (2·7)
No. of pregnancies	9 (24%)	109 (33%)
No. of implantations	11	134
Implantation rate per embryo	14%	15%

[A] Values in parentheses are ranges.

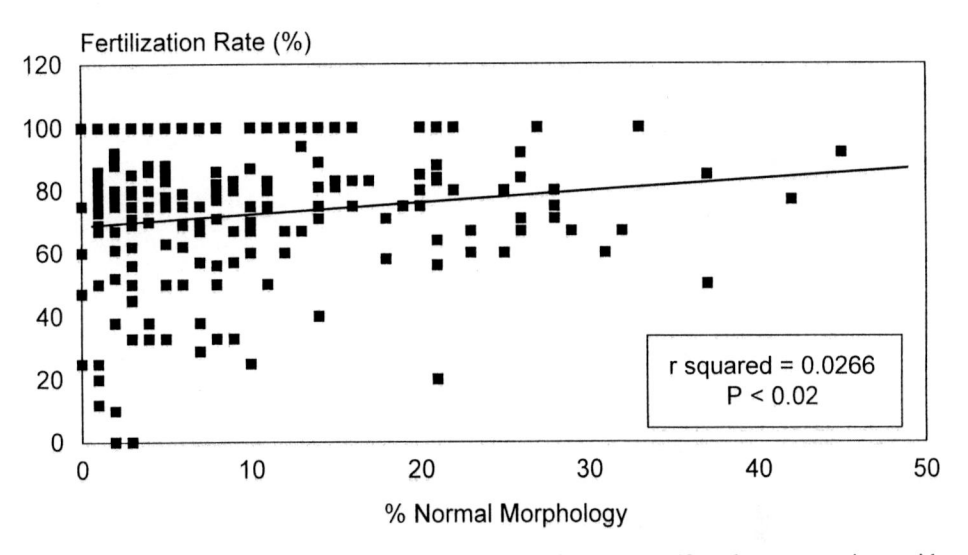

Fig. 3. Normal morphology (%) correlated with the fertilization rate. Note that many patients with very poor sperm morphology achieve high fertilization rates.

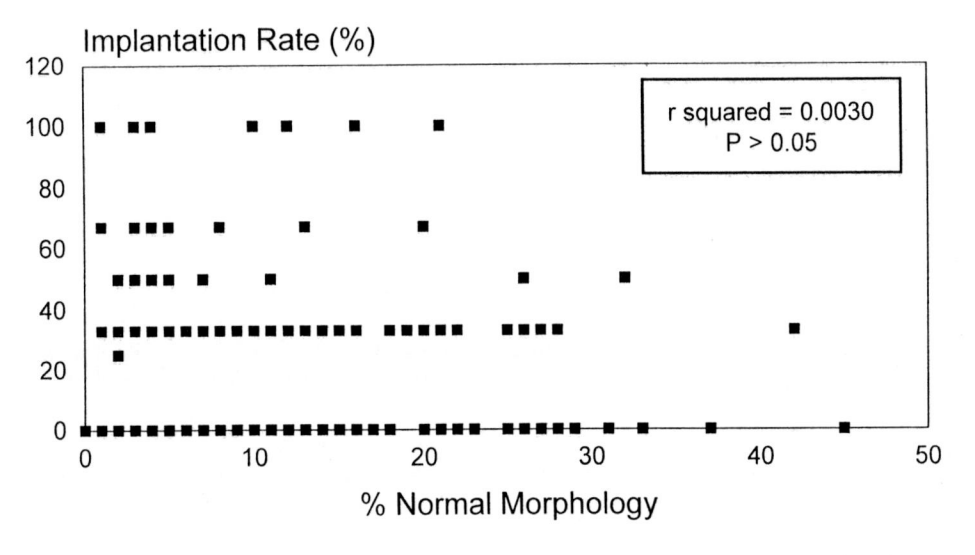

Fig. 4. Normal morphology (%) correlated with implantation rate per embryo transferred.

Table 5. Comparison of pregnancy outcomes from intracytoplasmic sperm injection (ICSI) and routine *in vitro* fertilization (IVF)

	ICSI	Routine IVF	Significance
Biochemical	6 (5%)	6 (5%)	
Ectopic	2 (2%)	1 (1%)	
Miscarriage	11 (9%)	25 (22%)	$P = 0.0106$
Blighted ovum	3 (3%)	—	
Singleton	72 (61%)	63 (55%)	
Twin	23 (19%)	17 (15%)	
Triplet	3 (3%)	3 (3%)	
Total	119	115	

Table 6. Follow-up of 23 babies (19 pregnancies) born after intracytoplasmic sperm injection (ICSI)

Average age of mother (years)[A]	32·1 (26·1–40·6)
Average gestation length (weeks)[A]	38·2 (34·4–41·6)
Average birth weight (g)[A]	2909 (1630–4160)
Delivery method	8 vaginal
	3 elective caesarean
	4 emergency caesarean
Sex ratio	15 male (65%)
	8 female (35%)
Special care	23 days (1 set of twins)
Congenital abnormality (1 baby)	Small ventricular septal defect, hypospadias

[A] Values in parentheses are ranges.

Pregnancy Outcomes

A breakdown of the 119 ICSI pregnancies is presented in Table 5 and is compared with 115 routine IVF pregnancies from the same period. Of the 119 ICSI pregnancies, 114 (96%) were clinical, and 98 (82%) are ongoing or have delivered compared with 83 (72%) of the 115 routine IVF pregnancies. The miscarriage rate was significantly lower after ICSI compared with routine IVF ($P = 0.0106$).

Up until July 1994 there have been 23 babies delivered from 19 pregnancies following ICSI and brief obstetric details are given in Table 6. There was one minor congenital abnormality reported, a small ventricular septal defect and hypospadias.

Discussion

Severe male factor infertility has limited the effectiveness of routine IVF in resolving all forms of infertility. Since 1986, various micromanipulative techniques have been used in an attempt to improve the *in vitro* fertilization rate for couples who have very poor semen. Techniques such as zona drilling (Gordon and Talansky 1986), zona cutting or partial zona dissection (Tsunoda *et al.* 1986; Malter and Cohen 1989) and SUZI (Ng *et al.* 1988) effectively removed the zona pellucida as a barrier to the fertilizing spermatozoon and resulted in increased fertilization rates. However, inconsistent results from patient to patient, low fertilization rates compared with routine IVF and high polyspermy rates, particularly after SUZI, were insurmountable problems associated with these techniques (Payne *et al.* 1994a). Nevertheless, their application demonstrated that normal pronuclear formation, embryo development and pregnancies could result from the sperm of patients with severe male factor infertility.

Initial reports on ICSI (Palermo *et al.* 1992, 1993) showed that if a spermatozoon were injected into the oocyte cytoplasm, consistently high rates of fertilization could be obtained. We have found that fertilization after ICSI is consistently 65–70% and that this compares favourably with fertilization after routine IVF (67%). The two figures are not quite equivalent as all the immature oocytes have been eliminated from the ICSI figures, whereas in routine IVF, oocyte maturity is not scored at insemination due to the presence of the cumulus cells. If we assume that 7% of the routine IVF oocytes were immature, then the corrected number of mature oocytes at insemination in Table 1 would be 4697 and the corrected fertilization rate would be about 76%. Even with this correction factor, the ICSI and IVF fertilization rates are still comparable.

Interestingly, the polypronuclear fertilization rate after routine IVF and ICSI is the same (5%). It is generally assumed that the presence of three pronuclei in routine IVF oocytes means that the oocyte was fertilized dispermically whereas the presence of three pronuclei after ICSI is due to the retention of the second polar body (Palermo et al. 1993; Flaherty et al. 1995). However, there is no reason to assume that the derivation of the third pronucleus is different between the two groups. ICSI produces good embryos and a pregnancy rate which is comparable to routine IVF, so it is unlikely that the injection procedure is having such a detrimental effect on the oocyte that it retains the second polar body. Dispermic fertilization does occur but usually when more than one sperm has easy access to the oocyte plasma membrane (e.g. SUZI) or if the zona pellucida has been cracked through increased aspiration pressure. Additionally, 24-h-old polar bodies are very often fragmented and unless they are stained with a DNA stain, it is difficult to state with absolute certainty that 2 polar bodies exist. Hence, we feel that it may be incorrect to assume different causes for the appearance of three pronuclei in ICSI and IVF oocytes and that retention of the second polar body may also be a cause of three pronuclear IVF oocytes, rather than just dispermic fertilization.

The frequency of one pronuclear oocytes was significantly lower after routine IVF than ICSI, suggesting that something in the treatment of ICSI oocytes predisposes them to activation without male pronucleus formation. Fishel et al. (1992) suggested that exposure to hyaluronidase may artificially activate the oocyte. We expose oocytes to hyaluronidase with a specific activity of 690 I.U. mL^{-1} for about 30 s which is considerably higher activity than that used by Van Steirteghem et al. (1993a, 1993b) (80 I.U. mL^{-1}), yet the percentage of one pronuclear oocytes in both programmes is similar (5% v. 3%). The presence of decondensing sperm heads in a significant proportion of both routine IVF one pronuclear oocytes (Balakier et al. 1993) and one pronuclear ICSI oocytes (Flaherty et al. 1995) suggests that both groups of oocytes display a similar aetiology. It is interesting to speculate on the cytoplasmic mechanisms that differentiate between male and female pronuclear formation even after the sperm head has undergone the initial step of decondensation.

The pregnancy rate and implantation rate were significantly higher after ICSI than routine IVF, yet the number of cycles with freezing and the percentage of embryos transferred or frozen was significantly lower. These apparently contradictory observations may be explained by taking into account the day of transfer. In our unit, routine IVF embryos are transferred and frozen on Day 2 after oocyte recovery whereas embryos from ICSI cycles are transferred and frozen on Day 3. Initially, it was thought that the partners of men with severe male factor infertility were generally more fertile than patients undergoing routine IVF, in that there were probably fewer female factors compounding the severe male factor infertility and that this contributed to the higher pregnancy rate after ICSI. It is generally considered that the uterus contributes to the implantation rate by being in a receptive condition when embryos are present. Other data suggests that if an embryo has pregnancy potential it will implant into any tissue; ectopic pregnancies in the human support this view. Therefore the potential for pregnancy may be more a function of embryo viability than uterine receptivity, although we acknowledge that this is a contentious issue. By culturing embryos for an extra day we are allowing the embryos to 'declare their intentions'. Often embryos which have been graded highly on Day 2 may look much poorer on Day 3 and those embryos which look good on Day 3 may not have been selected for transfer on Day 2. Day 3 transfers allow an extra 24 h of growth and, hence, more proficient selection of viable embryos. Moreover, there is a marked attrition rate among all extra corporeally fertilized oocytes with only 20% reaching the blastocyst stage (Bolton et al. 1989; Hardy et al. 1989). An additional 24 h in culture may account for lower numbers of embryos being acceptable for freezing after ICSI, but conversely, it may also account for the significantly higher pregnancy rate and the reduced miscarriage rate after ICSI.

Sperm from patients with occasional motile sperm and obstructive azoospermia did equally well after ICSI with fertilization rates of 66% and 70% respectively. Pregnancy rates and, more significantly, implantation rates per embryo were also similar and compare very favourably with routine IVF. Similarly, patients with <50% fertilization produced embryos which implanted at a rate of 14% indicating that, once fertilization occurs, embryo viability appears to be independent of semen variables. This is supported by the lack of correlation between percent normal morphology and the implantation rate.

Percent normal morphology weakly correlated with the fertilization rate although this is of little clinical significance as over half the patients with morphologies of less than 5% had fertilization rates >50%. In cases in which the fertilization rate after ICSI is <50%, there could be some intrinsic abnormality in the sperm which prevents nuclear decondensation and pronuclear formation, or it may simply be that the oocyte is deficient in the factors that control these processes. Whatever the cause, most of these patients had an embryo transfer and a good proportion (24%) of them became pregnant. Of the 18 patients who did not have embryos transferred, 10 had only one or two oocytes collected which either failed to fertilize, were immature, or failed to cleave after fertilization. A poor response to ovarian stimulation indicates a female factor and therefore it is not surprising that the outcome was poor among these patients. Other reasons for no embryo were extraordinary events such as a batch of embryo-toxic paraffin oil, and hyperstimulation which necessitated freezing all the embryos. The only patient in whom ICSI can be said to have failed was a patient with 5 oocytes injected in which every sperm was subsequently ejected from the cytoplasm. This patient now has an ongoing pregnancy after a single ICSI embryo was transferred in a subsequent cycle.

To date, we have encountered one minor congenital abnormality in 23 babies born after the transfer of ICSI embryos. These data are too preliminary to draw any conclusions, although it is encouraging and compares favourably with the national Australian average of 2·2% for major congenital malformations among babies born after assisted reproduction techniques (National Perinatal Statistics Unit 1991). A larger study in which 130 babies have been assessed following ICSI found no increase in congenital abnormalities compared with routine IVF (Bonduelle et al. 1994). These initial figures suggest that the ICSI technique is safe, however, conscientious follow-up of babies must be maintained.

ICSI has revolutionized the treatment of male factor infertility and is possibly the single most significant breakthrough in the treatment of infertility since the advent of IVF itself. A few live sperm situated somewhere in the male reproductive tract is the only requirement for ICSI and many patients, including paraplegics and those who wish to store semen before cancer therapy, now have a very good chance of having their own biological children.

Acknowledgments

We thank Dr Sean Flaherty for his critical appraisal of the manuscript. Our thanks also go to Regan Jeffrey, Michael Barry, Monica Briffa and the staff of the Routine IVF and Andrology laboratories. We acknowledge the assistance of the clinical, nursing and general staff of the Reproductive Medicine Units at the Queen Elizabeth Hospital and Wakefield Clinic.

References

Balakier, H., Squire, J., and Caspar R. F. (1993). Characterization of abnormal one pronuclear human oocytes by morphology, cytogenetics and *in-situ* hybridization. *Hum. Reprod. (Oxf.)* **8**, 402–8.

Bolton, V. N., Hawes, S. M., Taylor, C. T., and Parsons, J. H. (1989). Development of spare human preimplantation embryos *in vitro*: an analysis of the correlations among gross morphology, cleavage rates, and development to the blastocyst. *J. In Vitro Fertil. Embryo Transfer* **6**, 30–5.

Bonduelle, M., Legein, J., Buysse, A., Devroey, P., Van Steirteghem, A. C., and Liebaers, I. (1994). Comparative follow-up study of 130 children born after ICSI and 130 children born after IVF. *Hum. Reprod. (Oxf.)* **9**, (Suppl. 4), 38 [Abstr.].

Duncan, W. W., Glew, M. J., Wang, X.-J., Flaherty, S. P., and Matthews, C. D. (1993). Prediction of *in vitro* fertilization rates from semen variables. *Fertil. Steril.* **59**, 1233–8.

Fishel, S., Timson, J., Lisi, F., and Rinaldi, L. (1992). Evaluation of 225 patients undergoing subzonal insemination for the procurement of fertilization *in vitro*. *Fertil. Steril.* **57**, 840–9.

Flaherty, S. P., Payne, D., Swann, N. J., and Matthews, C. D. (1995). Assessment of fertilization failure and abnormal fertilization after intracytoplasmic sperm injection (ICSI). In 'Intracytoplasmic Sperm Injection: the Revolution in Male Fertility'. *Reprod. Fertil. Dev.* **7**, 197–210.

Gordon, J. W., and Talansky, B. E. (1986). Assisted fertilization by zona drilling: a mouse model for correction of oligospermia. *J. Exp. Zool.* **239**, 347–54.

Hardy, K., Handyside, A. H., and Winston, R. M. L. (1989). The human blastocyst: cell number, death and allocation during late preimplantation development *in vitro*. *Development* **107**, 597–604.

Kirby, C. A., Flaherty, S. P., Godfrey, B. M., Warnes, G. M., and Matthews, C. D. (1991). A prospective trial of intrauterine insemination of motile spermatozoa *versus* time intercourse. *Fertil. Steril.* **56**, 102–7.

Malter, H. E., and Cohen, J. (1989). Partial zona dissection of the human oocyte: a nontraumatic method using micromanipulation to assist zona pellucida penetration. *Fertil. Steril.* **51**, 139–48.

National Perinatal Statistics Unit (1991). 'Assisted Conception in Australia and New Zealand 1989'. p. 14. (Fertility Society of Australia: Sydney.)

Ng. S.-C., Bongso, A., Ratnam, S. S., Sathananthan, H., Chan, C. L. K., Wong, P. C., Haggland, L., Anandakumar, C., Wong, Y. C., and Goh, V. H. H. (1988). Pregnancy after transfer of sperm under zona. *Lancet* **2**, 790.

Ord, T., Patrizio, P., Marello, E., Balmaceda, J. P., and Asch, R. H. (1990). Mini-Percoll: a new method of semen preparation for IVF in severe male factor infertility. *Hum. Reprod. (Oxf.)* **5**, 987–9.

Palermo, G., Joris, H., Devroey, P., and Van Steirteghem, A. C. (1992). Pregnancies after intracytoplasmic injection of single spermatozoon into an oocyte. *Lancet* **340**, 17–18.

Palermo, G., Joris, H., Derde, M.-P., Camus, M., Devroey, P., and Van Steirteghem, A. (1993). Sperm characteristics and outcome of human assisted fertilization by subzonal insemination and intracytoplasmic sperm injection. *Fertil. Steril.* **59**, 826–35.

Payne, D. (1995a). Intracytoplasmic sperm injection: instrumentation and injection technique. In 'Intracytoplasmic Sperm Injection: the Revolution in Male Fertility'. *Reprod Fertil. Dev.* **7**, 185–96.

Payne, D. (1995b). Micro-assisted fertilization. *Reprod Fertil. Dev.* **7**. (In press.)

Payne, D., Warnes, G. M., Flaherty, S. P., and Matthews, C. D. (1994a). Local experience with zona drilling, zona cutting and sperm microinjection. In 'The Infertile Male: Advanced Assisted Reproductive Technology'. *Reprod. Fertil. Dev.* **6**, 45–50.

Payne, D., Flaherty, S. P., Jeffrey. R., Warnes, G. M., and Matthews, C. D. (1994b). Successful treatment of severe factor infertility in 100 consecutive cycles using intracytoplasmic sperm injection. *Hum Reprod. (Oxf.)* **9**, 2051–7.

Quinn P., Kerin, J. F., and Warnes, G. M. (1985). Improved pregnancy rate in human *in vitro* fertilization with the use of a medium based on the composition of human tubal fluid. *Fertil. Steril.* **44**, 493–8.

Testart, J., Lassalle, B., Belaisch-Allart, J., Hazout, A., Forman, R., Rainhorn, J. D., and Frydman, R. (1986). High pregnancy rate after early human embryo freezing. *Fertil. Steril.* **46**, 268–72.

Tsunoda, Y., Yasui, T., Nakamura, K., Uchida, T., and Sugie, T. (1986). Effect of cutting the zona pellucida on the pronuclear transplantation in the mouse. *J. Exp. Zool.* **240**, 119–25.

Van Steirteghem, A. C., Liu, J., Joris, H., Nagy, Z., Janssenswillen, C., Tournaye, H., Derde, M.-P., Van Assche, E., and Devroey, P. (1993*a*). Higher success rate by intracytoplasmic sperm injection than by subzonal insemination. Report of a second series of 300 consecutive treatment cycles. *Hum. Reprod. (Oxf.)* **8**, 1055–60.

Van Steirteghem, A. C., Joris, H., Liu, J., Nagy, Z., Bocken, G., Vankelecom, A., Desmet, B., and Van Ranst, H. (1993*b*). Protocol intracytoplasmic sperm injection (ICSI). In 'First International Course on Assisted Fertilization by Intracytoplasmic Sperm Injection'. pp. 1–10. (ESHRE Campus Workshop: Brussels.)

World Health Organization (1987). 'Laboratory Manual for the Examination of Human Semen and Semen–Cervical Mucus Interaction'. 2nd Edn. (Cambridge University Press: Cambridge.)

Manuscript received 13 January 1995

Factors Affecting Success With Intracytoplasmic Sperm Injection

M. J. Tucker[A], P. C. Morton, G. Wright,
P. E. Ingargiola, A. E. Jones and C. L. Sweitzer

Reproductive Biology Associates, 5505 Peachtree Dunwoody Road, Suite 400, Atlanta, GA 30342, USA.
[A] *To whom correspondence should be addressed.*

Abstract. In this study, 141 couples underwent 163 cycles of *in vitro* fertilization (IVF) and embryo transfer in which the eggs were inseminated by intracytoplasmic sperm injection (ICSI). Overall, 41% of the injected eggs were normally fertilized and 81% of the resulting embryos were suitable for cryopreservation (91 embryos) or uterine transfer. From 153 fresh embryo transfers, 45 ongoing or delivered pregnancies (27·6% per cycle) were achieved, and of the 507 embryos transferred, 54 successfully implanted giving an implantation rate per embryo of 10·7%. Five additional pregnancies did not yield a viable fetus or underwent a spontaneous abortion, giving a miscarriage rate of 10% (5/50). Increased maternal age or a prior diagnosis of failed fertilization after conventional IVF had a significantly negative impact on success. Sperm from the testis and epididymis, those retrieved by electro-ejaculation, and completely immotile ejaculated sperm all gave rise to pregnancies. ICSI reinsemination was used with limited success to rescue failed fertilization cycles, although the implantation rate per embryo was poor (5%). ICSI has greatly improved the ability to use IVF for treating couples with a poor fertilization potential.

Extra keywords: male infertility, micromanipulation, testis, epididymis, fertilization failure, reinsemination, ICSI.

Introduction

Since its introduction (Palermo *et al.* 1992), intracytoplasmic sperm injection (ICSI) has gained wide acceptance as the method of choice for micromanipulation assisted fertilization in human *in vitro* fertilization (IVF). A need has, however, arisen to better understand the true potential of this technique in differing clinical circumstances. In general, there is a firm recognition of the impact that age, gamete quality and quantity, and patient diagnosis can have on conventional IVF success. Not surprisingly, these factors might also influence ICSI success rates.

In terms of patient diagnosis, the most obvious categories of couples referred for assisted fertilization with ICSI are those with a significant male factor and those who have experienced significant fertilization failure. As well as having significant differences in semen quality, these two groups also present with differing potential in terms of fertilization history. Given that ICSI bypasses many of the processes involved in normal fertilization, it would seem that conventional fertilization status may have little relevance to ICSI outcome. Nevertheless, failed fertilization couples have a known fertilization defect, whereas male factor couples, if sufficient sperm can be harvested for ICSI, have an unknown fertilization potential.

This paper presents overall ICSI data collected during a two-year period, and this data is analysed with respect to patient age and diagnosis. In the context of failed fertilization, consideration is also given to reinsemination by assisted fertilization in an attempt to rescue failed cycles. Although late fertilized embryos may exhibit poor implantation potential (Tucker *et al.* 1991a), reinsemination by ICSI may at least yield some chance of pregnancy, and may provide additional information of value in subsequent cycles.

Materials and Methods

Patients

During the period from September 1992 to July 1994, 141 couples underwent 163 cycles of IVF in which all the eggs were inseminated by ICSI. Twenty of these couples had previously experienced a minimum of two cycles of complete fertilization failure, including some cycles in which subzonal insemination (SUZI) had been used without success. The aggregate semen profile (mean±s.d.) during the 25 ICSI cycles undertaken by these failed fertilization patients was $65·7\pm30·1\times10^6$ sperm mL^{-1}, $42·0\pm20·3\%$ motility and $9·6\pm6·6\%$ normal forms (strict criteria; Kruger *et al.* 1988). A further 107 couples had some form of significant male factor infertility, and the aggregate seminal parameters in this male factor group were $3·8\pm4·7\times10^6$ sperm mL^{-1}, $18·8\pm6·3\%$ motility and $4·1\pm6·0\%$ normal forms. This group included 14 couples from whom sperm were retrieved either by epididymal aspiration ($n = 8$), testicular biopsy ($n = 5$) or electro-ejaculation ($n = 1$). The seminal parameters in the electro-ejaculation case were 13×10^6 sperm mL^{-1}, 7% motility and 5% normal forms. The epididymal and testicular samples all possessed low numbers of sperm (from 200 to 2×10^6 sperm harvested) with poor motility (< 20%). In 43 other cycles, SUZI was used for reinsemination purposes (Tucker *et al.* 1993a), and the results from these cycles are presented for comparison with the ICSI reinsemination data.

All the women received ovarian stimulation with either gonadotrophin-releasing hormone analogue down-regulation in conjunction with human menopausal gonadotrophin (hMG) and/or follicle-stimulating hormone (FSH), or in a few cases, clomiphene citrate alone. No cycles with donated eggs are reported.

ICSI and in vitro Culture

All gametes and embryos were handled in Earle's balanced salt solution (EBSS) with the addition of 8% (v/v) plasmatein (Pool and Martin 1994) or maternal serum during the insemination stage, followed by transfer at the zygote stage into EBSS containing 15% serum. ICSI was performed as previously described (Tucker *et al.* 1993a) using straight glass tools prepared using a programmable P-97 pipette puller (Sutter Instrument, Novato, CA, USA), and a microgrinder and microforge (Narishige Instrument, Tokyo, Japan). Micromanipulation procedures were carried out on an IMT-2 inverted microscope (Olympus Optical, Tokyo, Japan) fitted with a heated stage and either Nomarski differential interference contrast optics or Hoffman modulation contrast optics. Two droplets (approximately 5 μL each) of medium containing eggs or sperm were placed on a warmed glass depression well slide and covered with mineral oil. The holding pipette and injection needle entered these droplets at 10° from the horizontal, with the angle of travel of the injection needle adjusted to parallel this angle of approach in order to minimize potential egg membrane damage.

Semen samples were routinely processed by separation on a single 90% layer of Percoll, unless the sperm count was $<1 \times 10^6$ mL^{-1} or the sperm were all immotile, in which case the Percoll concentration was reduced to 70% to increase the sperm harvest. Centrifugation through the Percoll layer was at 100–300g for 15–25 min; the centrifugal force was varied according to the initial sperm concentration. The harvested sperm were washed three times before resuspension in a minimal volume of EBSS containing 25% serum or plasmatein to achieve easy harvesting for injection. This final sperm sample was allowed to sediment under oil for several hours at 37°C to enhance the motile sperm population in the upper layer. If the sperm exhibited progressive motility, small numbers (100–500) of sperm were placed centrally in a droplet of 10% polyvinylpyrrolidone (PVP) (ICSI-100; Scandinavian IVF Science, Göteborg, Sweden) on the depression well glass slide. Otherwise, a very dilute sperm sample was added to EBSS without HEPES buffer and then placed on the depression well slide.

Shortly after collection, the eggs were manually dissected free of most of their cumulus cells, followed 1 h later by placement into 0·05% hyaluronidase (Type III or VIII; Sigma, St Louis, MO, USA) for 1 min to digest the remaining cumulus mass. Tenacious coronal cells were subsequently removed by mechanical dissection using heat-pulled glass pipettes. About 3–6 h after collection, the mature eggs were batched into a clean droplet of EBSS containing 8% serum or plasmatein on the depression well glass slide and individually injected with a single sperm. Of key importance to the success of the ICSI procedure was the confirmation of sperm placement into the ooplasm. This was accomplished either by stirring the ooplasm with the needle tip coupled with aspiration of the ooplasm into the needle lumen, or by a repeated stab. Fine control of the injection procedure was achieved throughout by filter-isolated mouth aspiration. Eggs were rarely exposed to periods of more than 4–5 min on the stage of the inverted microscope.

Following ICSI, eggs were either returned to EBSS containing 8% serum or plasmatein (116 cycles) or placed directly onto partial monolayers of virally-screened bovine oviductal epithelial cells (Tucker *et al.* 1994; 1995) in EBSS containing 15% serum (47 cycles). This distribution was not randomized, but took place according to the availability of suitable cell monolayers during the first 105 ICSI cycles. Fertilization checks were performed at 14–18 h post-ICSI, and all normally fertilized embryos were placed into EBSS containing 15% serum if they were not already on co-culture cells. Co-cultured zygotes were left on the same cells until cryopreservation or transfer. Up to four embryos were transferred to the uterus on day 3 of development, and excess embryos were frozen at the 2–6-cell stage in propanediol and sucrose (Tucker *et al.* 1991a). About 1–4 h before transfer, ICSI embryos underwent zona drilling with acidic Tyrode's medium to enhance blastocyst hatching (Tucker *et al.* 1994).

Electro-ejaculation, Epididymal and Testicular Sperm Retrieval

In one cycle, semen was collected by electro-ejaculation as previously described (Toledo *et al.* 1992). In 8 cycles, sperm were retrieved from the epididymis by aspiration with a 25 G intravenous catheter (Critikon, Tampa, FL, USA). In a further 5 cycles, sperm were obtained directly from testicular tissue, either from a peripheral biopsy or by fine needle puncture. The samples were collected into EBSS containing 8% serum or plasmatein. The addition of pentoxifylline and 2-deoxyadenosine to the collection medium in 7 of these cycles appeared to be of little advantage and neither motility nor fertilization were increased in comparison with the 7 cycles undertaken without these chemicals (data not shown). Consequently, the use of pentoxifylline and 2-deoxyadenosine has been discontinued. After collection, the sperm were either separated on a 70% or 45% Percoll layer, or prepared by washing, resuspension and sedimentation under oil if sperm numbers were too low to risk losing significant numbers of sperm in the Percoll layer. The harvested sperm were used directly for ICSI without further processing, and in four epididymal sperm cases, small aliquots of sperm were also cryopreserved for later use.

Pregnancy Assessment

All patients underwent an initial serum test for β-human chorionic gonadotropin (β-hCG) about 12–14 days after embryo transfer. Cycles in which the β-hCG level remained elevated for a minimum of three consecutive tests at 5-day intervals, but failed to progress to a full pregnancy, are reported as biochemical pregnancies. All the other pregnancies are reported as viable, and include ongoing pregnancies at 14 weeks and beyond of gestation with a minimum of one healthy fetus, and those which have gone to term.

Statistical Analysis

Statistical comparisons were performed by a χ^2-test with Yate's correction using the InStat programme (Graph Pad, San Diego, CA, USA).

Results

Tables 1 and 2 outline the overall fertilization and pregnancy data for the 163 ICSI cycles. A total of 2157 eggs were retrieved in 163 egg collections, of which 1794 (83·2%) were mature and underwent sperm injection; 1537 (85·7%) survived injection. Normal fertilization occurred in 735 of the intact eggs (47·8%), and 598 (81·4%) of the resulting embryos were suitable for either cryopreservation or fresh uterine transfer. An embryo transfer was not performed in 10 cycles, due to total fertilization failure (4 cycles), cleavage arrest (5 cycles), or in one case in which all the embryos were frozen due to severe ovarian hyperstimulation. From 153 fresh transfers of 507 embryos, we achieved 50 pregnancies

Table 1. Overall fertilization data after intracytoplasmic sperm injection (ICSI)

ET, fresh embryo transfer; PN, pronuclei

No. of egg collections	163
No. of injected eggs	1794
No. of intact eggs (survival rate)	1537 (86%)
No. of 2 PN eggs	735
2 PN fertilization rate per injected egg (per intact egg)	41% (48%)
No. of 1 PN eggs[A]	112 (7·3%)
No. of 3 PN eggs[A]	19 (1·2%)
No. of embryos suitable for ET or cryopreservation[B]	598 (81%)
No. of embryos cryopreserved	91

[A] Values in parentheses are the percentage of the intact eggs.
[B] Value in parentheses is the percentage of the 2 PN fertilized eggs.

Table 2. Pregnancy outcomes after intracytoplasmic sperm injection (ICSI)

Viable pregnancies were ongoing or delivered at the time of writing. hCG, human chorionic gonadotrophin

Patient age in years (mean±s.d.)(range)	34·3±6·0 (25–44)
No. of egg collections	163
No. of embryo transfers	153 (94%)
No. of embryos transferred	507
Mean no. of embryos transferred (range)	3·3 (1–4)
No. of pregnancies (β-hCG positive)	50
Pregnancy rate (β-hCG) per egg collection	30·6%
Pregnancy rate (β-hCG) per transfer	32·7%
No. of viable pregnancies	45
Viable pregnancy rate per egg collection	27·6%
Implantation rate per embryo	10·7% (54/507)
Normal deliveries	9 (5 males, 4 females)
Ongoing pregnancies	36[A]
Multiple pregnancy rate	16%
Miscarriage rate	10% (5/50)

[A] Comprises 29 singleton, 5 twin and 2 triplet ongoing pregnancies.

Table 3. Age-related outcome after intracytoplasmic sperm injection (ICSI)

Viable pregnancies were ongoing or delivered at the time of writing. ET, fresh embryo transfer; hCG, human chorionic gonadotrophin; PN, pronuclei

	<36 years old	≥36 years old
No. of egg collections	103	60
No. of embryo transfers	100 (97%)	53 (88%)
Total no. of eggs collected	1395	762
Mean no. of eggs per cycle	13·5	12·7
No. of injected eggs	1179	615
No. of intact eggs (survival rate)	1101 (93%)	436 (71%)[A]
No. of 2 PN eggs (fertilization rate)	539 (49%)	196 (45%)
No. of embryos suitable for ET or cryopreservation	460 (85%)	138 (70·5%)[B]
No. of embryos cryopreserved	74	17
No. of embryos transferred	386	121
Mean no. of embryos transferred	3·9	2·3[B]
No. of pregnancies (β-hCG positive)[C]	40 (40%)	10 (19%)
No. of viable pregnancies[C]	37 (37%)	8 (15%)[B]
Implantation rate per embryo	11·7% (45/386)	7·4% (9/121)

[A] χ^2-test, $P < 0·001$. [B] χ^2-test, $P < 0·05$. [C] Pregnancy rates per embryo transfer are given in parentheses.

(32·7% per transfer; 30·6% per cycle). There was a pregnancy loss of 10%, which yielded a viable pregnancy rate of 29·4% per transfer or 27·6% per cycle. To date, 9 singleton pregnancies have gone to term (5 male, 4 female), with a further 36 pregnancies ongoing at 14 weeks and beyond. The multiple pregnancy rate was 15·6%. In 5 cycles in which frozen-thawed ICSI embryos were transferred, one viable singleton pregnancy has arisen to date.

The mean female age was 34·3 years, with a range of 25–44 years (Table 2). When the overall ICSI data

Table 4. The use of epididymal or testicular sperm and intracytoplasmic sperm injection (ICSI)

Viable pregnancies were ongoing or delivered at the time of writing

	Epididymal sperm	Testicular sperm
No. of patients	8	5
No. of injected eggs	88	54
No. of intact eggs (survival rate)	82 (93%)	50 (93%)
No. of fertilized eggs	32	19
Fertilization rate[A]	39%	38%
No. of embryo transfers	8	5
No. of viable pregnancies[B]	4 (50%)	3 (60%)
Implantation rate per embryo	25% (7/28)	19% (3/16)

[A] Percentage of the intact eggs.
[B] Pregnancy rates per cycle are given in parentheses.

Table 5. Three cases in which immotile sperm were used for intracytoplasmic sperm injection (ICSI)

	Case 1	Case 2	Case 3
Patient age (years)	40	32	31
Sperm viability	20%	22%	25%
Fertilization rate	42% (8/19)	40% (6/15)	33% (5/15)
No. of embryos cryopreserved	2	—	—
No. of embryos transferred	4	4	4
Pregnancy[A]	No	Triplets	No

[A] Overall implantation rate per embryo was 25% (3/12).

were analysed in relation to female age, an interesting divergence in results was found (Table 3). In 60 cycles in which the woman was ≥36 years, egg survival after ICSI, adequate embryonic development for cryopreservation or transfer, the mean number of embryos transferred and the viable pregnancy rate were all significantly poorer than in the 103 cycles performed in the younger (<36 years) patient group.

In 13 cycles in which epididymal or testicular sperm were used, the fertilization rate was reduced compared with the general ICSI results (Table 4). Nevertheless, the implantation rate of embryos generated from epididymal and testicular sperm (25% and 19% respectively) was good. In one cycle (data not shown), sperm were retrieved by electro-ejaculation for ICSI, and this resulted in the delivery of a male child.

There were 3 cycles in which totally immotile sperm were used for ICSI (Table 5). Based on a live:dead dye exclusion assessment, 20–25% of the sperm were viable. The fertilization rates nevertheless markedly exceeded this and a triplet pregnancy (now at 18 weeks) was established in one of the cycles.

ICSI outcome was analysed in relation to the principal patient diagnosis, which was male factor infertility (138 cycles) or previous idiopathic fertilization failure (25 cycles). The results are presented in Table 6. Although the sample sizes were unequal, there was a significantly lower fertilization rate, viable pregnancy rate and implantation rate in the fertilization failure group.

When fertilization failure occurs during an IVF cycle, one response is to apply or repeat assisted fertilization techniques to rescue what would otherwise be a failed cycle. Our previous experience with reinsemination by SUZI is summarized in Table 7. There were 43 separate cycles of IVF in which SUZI was used for reinsemination. In 14 cycles in which SUZI failed initially, we achieved fertilization after SUZI reinsemination, and there were 5 delivered pregnancies. In 14 cycles in which conventional insemination failed, we obtained fertilization after SUZI reinsemination, and this resulted in 2 delivered pregnancies. Mixed transfers of Day 1 and reinseminated SUZI embryos in 9 cycles gave rise to 3 delivered pregnancies, whereas mixed transfers of conventional IVF day 1 embryos and reinseminated SUZI embryos in 6 cycles gave rise to one delivery.

Table 8 presents similar data for cycles in which ICSI was utilized for reinsemination. In 22 cycles, conventional fertilization failed completely, but ICSI reinsemination allowed transfers to occur in 17 of the cycles, yielding two viable pregnancies. In 4 cycles in which ICSI failed initially, the eggs were successfully reinseminated by ICSI, embryo transfer was possible in 2 of these cycles and a viable pregnancy resulted. The data from these 26 reinsemination cycles are combined in the third column of Table 8 to provide an overall impression of the efficacy of ICSI reinsemination (fertilization rate, 41%; pregnancy rate per cycle, 12%; implantation rate, 5%). Table 8 also shows 10 mixed transfers of Day-1

Table 6. Treatment of fertilization failure and male factor infertility by intracytoplasmic sperm injection (ICSI)

Viable pregnancies were ongoing or delivered at the time of writing. hCG, human chorionic gonadotrophin; PN, pronuclei

	Fertilization failure	Male factor
No. of patients	20	121
No. of egg collections	25	138
Patient age in years (mean±s.d.)	35.3±3.8	33.8±5.3
No. of eggs injected	317	1477
Mean no. of eggs injected	12.7	10.7
No. of intact eggs (survival rate)	283 (89%)	1254 (85%)
No. of 2 PN eggs (fertilization rate)	86 (30.4%)	649 (52%)[A]
No. of embryos transferred	76	431
Mean no. of embryos transferred	3.0	3.4
No. of pregnancies (β-hCG positive)[B]	4 (16%)	46 (33.3%)
No. of viable pregnancies[B]	3 (12%)	42 (30.4%)[C]
Implantation rate per embryo	5.3% (4/76)	11.6% (50/431)[D]

[A] χ^2-test, $P < 0.001$. [B] Pregnancy rates per cycle are given in parentheses.
[C] χ^2-test, $P < 0.05$. [D] χ^2-test, $P < 0.01$.

Table 7. Reinsemination by subzonal insemination (SUZI) of unfertilized eggs resulting from SUZI or conventional *in vitro* fertilization (IVF) insemination

Viable pregnancies were ongoing or delivered at the time of writing. D1, inseminated on Day 1; D2, reinseminated by SUZI on Day 2; PN, pronuclei

	No initial SUZI fertilization	Some initial SUZI fertilization	No initial IVF fertilization	Some initial IVF fertilization
No. of egg collections	14	9	14	6
No. of eggs injected	112	143	120	134
No. of 2 PN eggs (fertilization rate)	33 (29%)	17 (21%)[A], 13 (21%)[B]	22 (18%)	12 (13%)[C], 6 (16%)[B]
No. of eggs with ≥3 PN	9 (8%)	2 (1.5%)	11 (9%)	—
Zygotes which failed to cleave	3 (9%)	1	3 (14%)	1
No. of cryopreserved embryos	3	—	—	5
No. of embryo transfers	13	9	6	4
No. of embryos transferred	27	29	19	12 (8 IVF, 4 SUZI)
Origin of the transferred embryos	D2 SUZI	D1 SUZI+D2 SUZI	D2 SUZI	D1 IVF+D2 SUZI
No. of viable pregnancies	5 (36%)	3 (33%)	2 (14%)	1 (17%)
Implantation rate per embryo	22% (6/27)	10% (3/29)	11% (2/19)	8% (1/12)

[A] SUZI insemination on Day 1. [B] Reinsemination by SUZI on Day 2. [C] Conventional IVF insemination on Day 1.

Table 8. Reinsemination by intracytoplasmic sperm injection (ICSI) of unfertilized eggs resulting from initial insemination by conventional *in vitro* fertilization (IVF) or ICSI

Viable pregnancies were ongoing or delivered at the time of writing. PN, pronuclei

	IVF	ICSI	Total	IVF/ICSI[A]
No. of egg collections	22	4	26	10
No. of eggs injected	236	21	257	76
No. of intact eggs (survival rate)	199 (84%)	16 (76%)	215 (84%)	70 (92%)
No. of 2 PN eggs[B]	84 (42%)	5 (31%)	89 (41%)	27 (39%)
No. of 1 PN eggs[B]	8 (4%)	2 (13%)	10 (5%)	5 (7%)
No. of 3 PN eggs[B]	4 (2%)	—	4 (2%)	—
No. of cleaved embryos	58 (69%)	3 (60%)	61 (69%)	20 (74%)[C]
No. of embryo transfers	17	2	19	10
No. of viable pregnancies[D]	2 (9%)	1 (25%)	3 (12%)	2 (20%)
Pregnancy outcomes	female, ongoing	male	—	male, ongoing
Implantation rate per embryo	4% (2/58)	33% (1/3)	5% (3/61)	6% (2/35)

[A] Mixed transfers of Day 1 IVF embryos and ICSI reinseminated embryos.
[B] Values in parentheses are percentages of the intact eggs.
[C] An additional 15 embryos from conventional IVF insemination were available.
[D] Pregnancy rates per cycle are given in parentheses.

conventionally fertilized embryos and ICSI reinseminated embryos in which the pregnancy rate was 20% and the implantation rate per embryo was 6%.

Discussion

With increasing experience comes greater appreciation of which infertile couples are most appropriately treated using ICSI during their IVF therapy. The results presented in this paper show a distinct worsening of outcome from ICSI with increasing age of the female partner, an observation not dissimilar to the situation in routine IVF (Navot et al. 1991). However, this poorer outcome may well be exacerbated by the need for optimal egg quality to survive the invasiveness of the intracytoplasmic sperm injection procedure. Older women who yield poor quality eggs have a significantly higher rate of egg degeneration after injection, even before fertilization, a fact which inevitably will have an impact on the overall success rate for these patients. Moreover, cleavage failure is higher in these older women, possibly due to a higher incidence of cytoskeletal damage caused during injection of the poor quality eggs. This will also have a further negative effect on the outcome in this group.

Our overall ICSI results indicate an adequate outcome relative to our general IVF population, although the marginally lower fertilization rate and higher incidence of cleavage failure means that the viable pregnancy rate was slightly lower and fewer embryos were cryopreserved per couple. Most of the women in the <36 years group received 4 embryos at transfer, and although up to 4 embryos were transferred in the older group in some instances, there were not always 4 morphologically suitable embryos available for transfer, consequently the average number of embryos transferred per patient was lower in the ≥36 years group. In spite of the slightly higher overall numbers of embryos transferred in these ICSI cycles compared with our conventional IVF programme, the multiple pregnancy rate was not high.

ICSI is the most successful form of micromanipulation assisted fertilization so far developed, and suffers from none of the weaknesses of previous approaches. Results from partial zona dissection (PZD) were often clinically poor and inconsistent (Tucker et al. 1991b). SUZI of multiple sperm allowed about 70% of couples to have an embryo transfer and embryonic implantation rates were adequate (Tucker et al. 1993a). However, the most severe male factor cases could not be treated, polyspermy was often a problem, and the number of embryos generated for cryopreservation was minimal. The only principal drawbacks of ICSI are egg degeneration and cleavage arrest. These problems notwithstanding, ICSI does come close to guaranteeing an embryo transfer for each couple who has an egg collection. During 1993, only 6·5% of all the couples (540 cycles) in our clinic who underwent an egg collection for conventional IVF did not have an embryo transfer, and our ICSI results in this report compare very favourably (6·1%) in a patient group with a similar age distribution.

Our ICSI results compare adequately with those previously reported by other groups (Palermo et al. 1993; Van Steirteghem et al. 1993a; Fishel et al. 1994; Redgment et al. 1994). Although there have been limited comparisons of ICSI and SUZI (Van Steirteghem et al. 1993b; Fishel et al. 1994; Redgment et al. 1994), the larger issue of how ICSI compares on a routine basis with conventional insemination (Tucker et al. 1993b) remains to be answered. The significance of this should determine whether or not ICSI can totally replace conventional insemination (Tucker et al. 1995).

The extremes of male factor infertility which can now be treated with ICSI, hinge largely on the need to collect only a few sperm. Sperm can be relatively easily retrieved from severe oligozoospermic samples (e.g. retrograde ejaculates collected following electro-ejaculation), as well as directly from the epididymis and testis (Devroey et al. 1994; Tournaye et al. 1994). The advantage of testicular biopsy over epididymal aspiration is that it can be simply performed under local anaesthesia. The overall quality of the testicular sperm recovered, however, is generally poor, and the ability to cryopreserve some of the sample for later use, as can be done with epididymal sperm, is not currently feasible. Regardless of which source is used, however, the fertilization and implantation rates per embryo were comparable. Whether sperm viability is even a prerequisite for a successful ICSI outcome is very much in question given our results using immotile sperm with depressed sperm viability. Fertilization and implantation rates were both higher than might have been anticipated if sperm viability were essential for fertilization and development of a healthy fetus.

Central to our understanding of a successful outcome when a sperm is injected directly into an egg is how the gametes fuse following this unnatural procedure. While fertilization rates may average 40–70%, some couples achieve significantly poorer results after ICSI, regardless of egg quality. It is of great interest that couples who experience idiopathic fertilization failure had, in this series, a significantly poorer outcome following ICSI compared with those couples with male factor infertility. The fertilization rate was significantly lower in the failed fertilization group, and this correlates with the observation that these couples have a known poor fertilization potential following conventional insemination. The assumption then is that male factor cases have in essence a better fertilization potential in conventional IVF terms than the unexplained fertilization failure cases. The situation may, however, be a little more complicated than merely being a matter of fertilization potential. Although the fertilization potential of either or both gametes may in some way be compromised, the fact that the pregnancy rate and the implantation rate per embryo are lower in the idiopathic fertilization failure group strongly suggests that even if fertilization occurred, the viability of the resulting embryos would be compromised. Chromosomal abnormalities might occur at a higher than expected rate in either or both gametes from these patients, and this could account for the higher rate of embryonic demise. Consequently, gamete donation may be a more cost effective option for many of these couples.

Beyond the occurrence of fertilization failure or a reduced fertilization rate is the question of whether or not to attempt to redress this problem by reinsemination, either to increase the number of embryos for transfer or cryopreservation, or to salvage a cycle in which no fertilization occurred initially. Traditionally, reinsemination has not been considered a particularly fruitful strategy for the creation of viable embryos (Tucker *et al.* 1991*a*), but more recently, reports in which reinsemination was performed using SUZI (Tucker *et al.* 1993*a*; Wiker *et al.* 1993) or ICSI (Nagy *et al.* 1993) suggest that assisted fertilization techniques can have a more beneficial impact on reinsemination success rates on the day after egg collection. Updated SUZI reinsemination data was presented in the present paper and partially confirms this, however, the results from our own clinic indicate that the ability of ICSI to rescue failed fertilization cycles is limited. Nonetheless, the observation that no abnormal children have been born after this form of reinsemination does help, in a small way, to justify the use of ICSI reinsemination to rescue failed cycles, to increase the number of embryos for transfer or cryopreservation, and to enable some diagnosis of the fertilization potential with ICSI in subsequent cycles. This policy, however, does little to address why the fertilization outcome is still inconsistent for all patients following ICSI. Furthermore, concerns over increased rates of aneuploidy in such late-fertilized ICSI embryos may strongly detract from the widespread use of reinsemination, although with fluorescent *in situ* hybridization technology it is now feasible to screen for embryonic abnormalities before embryo replacement (Grifo *et al.* 1994).

It is now over two years since the first successful report on the use of ICSI in human IVF (Palermo *et al.* 1992), and over one year since testicular sperm were proven to be able to generate a human pregnancy (Schoysman *et al.* 1993). Our results confirm and help to further establish that ICSI is currently the optimal form of micromanipulation assisted fertilization, and also illustrate that any man with some degree of complete spermatogenesis can be treated using testicular biopsy and ICSI.

Acknowledgments

We are grateful to the following physicians for their clinical assistance during these studies: Carlene Elsner, Hilton Kort, Joe Massey, Dorothy Mitchell-Leef, Andrew Toledo, James Bennett, Jenelle Foote, Bruce Green and Michael Witt.

References

Devroey, P., Liu, J., Nagy, Z., Tournaye, H., Silber, S. J., and Van Steirteghem, A. C. (1994). Normal fertilization of human oocytes after testicular sperm extraction and intracytoplasmic sperm injection. *Fertil. Steril.* **62**, 639–41.

Fishel, S., Timson, J., Lisi, F., Jacobson, M., Rinaldi, L., and Gobetz, L. (1994). Micro-assisted fertilization in patients who have failed subzonal insemination. *Hum. Reprod. (Oxf.)* **9**, 501–5.

Grifo, J., Rosenwaks, Z., Cohen, J., and Munné, S. (1994). Implantation failure of morphologically normal human embryos is due largely to aneuploidy. *Proc. Am. Fertil. Soc.* S2. [Abstr.]

Kruger, T. F., Acosta, A. A., Simmons, K. F., Swanson, R. J., Matta, J. F., and Oehninger, S. (1988). Predictive value of abnormal sperm morphology in *in vitro* fertilization. *Fertil. Steril.* **49**, 112–17.

Nagy, Z. P., Joris, H., Liu, J., Staessen, C., Devroey, P., and Van Steirteghem, A. C. (1993). Intracytoplasmic single sperm injection of 1-day-old unfertilized human oocytes. *Hum. Reprod. (Oxf.)* **8**, 2180–4.

Navot, D., Bergh, P. A., Williams, M. A., Garrisi, G. J., Guzman, I., Sandler, B., and Grunfeld, L. (1991). Poor oocyte quality rather than implantation failure as a cause of age-related decline in female fertility. *Lancet* **337**, 1375–7.

Palermo, G., Joris, H., Devroey, P., and Van Steirteghem, A. C. (1992). Pregnancies after intracytoplasmic injection of single spermatozoon into an oocyte. *Lancet* **340**, 17–18.

Palermo, G., Joris, H., Derde, M.-P., Camus, M., Devroey, P., and Van Steirteghem, A. (1993). Sperm characteristics and outcome of human assisted fertilization by subzonal insemination and intracytoplasmic sperm injection. *Fertil. Steril.* **59**, 826–35.

Pool, T. B., and Martin, J. E. (1994). High continuing pregnancy rates after *in vitro* fertilization–embryo transfer using medium supplemented with a plasma protein fraction containing alpha- and beta-globulins. *Fertil. Steril.* **61**, 714–19.

Redgment, C. J., Yang, D., Tsirigotis, M., Yazdani, N., Al Shawaf, T., and Craft, I. L. (1994). Experience with assisted fertilization in severe male factor infertility and unexplained failed fertilization *in vitro*. *Hum. Reprod. (Oxf.)* **9**, 680–3.

Schoysman, R., Vanderzwalmen, P., Nijs, M., Segal, L., Segal-Bertin, G., Geerts, L., Van Roosendaal, E., and Schoysman, D. (1993). Pregnancy after fertilization with human testicular spermatozoa. *Lancet* **342**, 1237.

Toledo, A. A., Tucker, M. J., Bennett, J. K., Green, B. G., Kort, H. I., Wiker, S. R., and Wright, G. (1992). Electro ejaculation in combination with *in vitro* fertilization and gamete micromanipulation for treatment of anejaculatory male infertility. *Am. J. Obstet. Gynecol.* **167**, 322–6.

Tournaye, H., Devroey, P., Liu, J., Nagy, Z., Lissens, W., and Van Steirteghem, A. (1994). Microsurgical epididymal sperm aspiration and intracytoplasmic sperm injection: a new effective approach to infertility as a result of congenital bilateral absence of the vas deferens. *Fertil. Steril.* **61**, 1045–51.

Tucker, M., Elsner, C., Kort, H., Massey, J., Mitchell-Leef, D., and Toledo, A. (1991*a*). Poor implantation of cryopreserved reinsemination-fertilized human embryos. *Fertil. Steril.* **56**, 1111–6.

Tucker, M. J., Bishop, F. M., Cohen, J., Wiker, S. R., and Wright, G. (1991b). Routine application of partial zona dissection for male factor infertility. *Hum. Reprod. (Oxf.)* **6**, 676–81.

Tucker, M. J., Wiker, S. R., Wright, G., Morton, P. C., and Toledo, A. A. (1993a). Treatment of male infertility and idiopathic failure to fertilize *in vitro* with under zona insemination and direct egg injection. *Am. J. Obstet. Gynecol.* **169**, 324–32.

Tucker, M., Wiker, S., and Massey, J. (1993b). Rational approach to assisted fertilization. *Hum. Reprod. (Oxf.)* **8**, 1778.

Tucker, M. J., Ingargiola, P. E., Massey, J. B., Morton, P. C., Wiemer, K. E., Wiker, S. R., and Wright, G. (1994). Assisted hatching with or without bovine oviductal epithelial cell co-culture for poor prognosis *in-vitro* fertilization patients. *Hum. Reprod. (Oxf.)* **9**, 1528–31.

Tucker, M. J., Wright, G., Morton, P. C., Mayer, M. P., Ingargiola, P. E., and Jones, A. E. (1995). Practical evolution and application of direct intracytoplasmic sperm injection for male factor and idiopathic fertilization failure infertilities. *Fertil. Steril.* (In press.)

Van Steirteghem, A. C., Nagy, Z., Joris, H., Liu, J., Staessen, C., Smitz, J., Wisanto, A., and Devroey, P. (1993a). High fertilization and implantation rates after intracytoplasmic sperm injection. *Hum. Reprod. (Oxf.)* **8**, 1061–6.

Van Steirteghem, A. C., Liu, J., Joris, H., Nagy, Z., Janssenswillen, C., Tournaye, H., Derde, M.-P., Van Assche, E., and Devroey, P. (1993b). Higher success rate by intracytoplasmic sperm injection than by subzonal insemination. Report of a second series of 300 consecutive treatment cycles. *Hum. Reprod. (Oxf.)* **8**, 1055–60.

Wiker, S. R., Tucker, M. J., Wright, G., Malter, H. E., Kort, H. I., and Massey, J. B. (1993). Repeated sperm injection under the zona following initial fertilization failure. *Hum. Reprod. (Oxf.)* **8**, 467–9.

Manuscript received 7 March 1995

Open Discussion

Bob Edwards (Cambridge):

Reinsemination has had a dubious reputation. Do you think it's worth it?

Tucker:

It has been mentioned previously that reinsemination might be inappropriate on the basis of egg aging, which in turn may give rise to a high rate of chromosomal abnormalities and obstetric problems. I'm very honest and up front, and tell the couple that the implantation potential of the embryos is limited and we counsel them that problems may occur obstetrically. So given all those provisions, I think it's a worthwhile approach.

Edwards:

It's my impression that the meiotic spindle in the human egg is very stable, even after 24 h. So you probably won't risk quite as many chromosomal abnormalities as you might think. Have you done any studies on this?

Tucker:

No, I've not studied that.

David Edgar (Melbourne):

Was the embryo morphology any different after reinsemination?

Tucker:

Cleavage failure, or at least the development of embryos which were suitable for freezing or transfer was lower. In our general ICSI programme, about 83% of the embryos arising from two pronuclear eggs are suitable for transfer or freezing. However, only about 69% of those arising from reinsemination were suitable for transfer of freezing. It's not a problem with fragmentation of the embryos, they are just delayed in development. So on Day 3 when we do embryo transfers, they are at the 2–4-cell stage instead of the 6–12-cell stage. We apply assisted hatching to all these embryos in an attempt to accelerate their potential to reach the hatched blastocyst stage.

Debra Gook (Melbourne):

What do you do if you reinseminate an ICSI egg and then see cleavage without seeing pronuclei?

Tucker:

I'm pretty conservative. The reinsemination embryos get inspected thoroughly to ensure that they have extruded two polar bodies and they have only two pronuclei with nucleoli. We don't transfer an embryo just because it cleaves.

Sean Flaherty (Adelaide):

A comment about the men with immotile sperm. We had one case of a man who had 100% immotile sperm; occasionally you would find one that just twitched very slightly. He had 29% viable sperm by Hoechst dye exclusion. They had a cycle of ICSI and a pregnancy resulted which was subsequently lost. They returned and had a transfer of frozen-thawed embryos and now have a 20-week ongoing pregnancy.

The Use of Intracytoplasmic Sperm Injection for the Treatment of Severe and Extreme Male Infertility

Harold Bourne[AE], Nadine Richings[B],
Offer Harari[ABD], William Watkins[A], Andrew L. Speirs[AB],
W. Ian H. Johnston[AB] and H. W. Gordon Baker[C]

[A] Reproductive Biology Unit, Royal Women's Hospital, 132 Grattan Street, Carlton, Vic. 3053, Australia.
[B] Melbourne IVF, 320 Victoria Parade, East Melbourne, Vic. 3002, Australia.
[C] Department of Obstetrics and Gynaecology, University of
Melbourne, Royal Women's Hospital, Carlton, Vic. 3053, Australia.
[D] Current address: Bnai Zion Medical Center, Department of Obstetrics and Gynaecology,
Faculty of Medicine, Technion, PO Box 4940, Haifa 31048, Israel.
[E] To whom correspondence should be addressed.

Abstract. The outcome of treatment by intracytoplasmic sperm injection (ICSI) is described for patients with severe male infertility. In 296 consecutive cycles, a normal fertilization rate of 69% was achieved with 288 cycles (97%) resulting in embryos suitable for transfer. A total of 32 clinical pregnancies were achieved from the transfer of fresh embryos (clinical pregnancy rate of 12% per transfer) and an additional 44 clinical pregnancies were obtained after the transfer of frozen–thawed embryos (clinical pregnancy rate of 16% per transfer). Overall, 57 of the 76 pregnancies were ongoing or delivered. An analysis of outcome in 5 male factor subgroups revealed no significant differences in pregnancy and implantation rates between the categories. However, the fertilization rate was significantly lower in patients with oligoasthenoteratozoospermia and significantly higher in those patients for whom epididymal sperm were used for insemination. The treatment of patients with extreme male infertility is also described; normal fertilization and embryo development were obtained using ICSI in patients with mosaic Klinefelter's syndrome, severe sperm autoimmunity, round-headed acrosomeless sperm (globozoospermia), completely immotile sperm selected by hypo-osmotic swelling and sperm isolated from testicular biopsies. Three ongoing pregnancies were obtained from 6 patients for whom testicular sperm were used. These results demonstrate the value of ICSI in the management of severe male infertility, however, the treatment of some types of extreme male infertility using ICSI may be limited.

Extra keywords: micromanipulation, ICSI, epididymal sperm, testicular sperm, hypo-osmotic swelling.

Introduction

The use of standard *in vitro* fertilization (IVF) for treating male infertility has been successful when the sperm defects are not severe (Baker *et al.* 1993), however, its success is limited with severe male infertility in which the fertilization rates are usually low. Various techniques have been utilized in an attempt to improve the outcome of insemination with poor quality sperm, including the use of Percoll density gradient centrifugation (Ord *et al.* 1990), increasing the number of sperm at insemination (Oehninger *et al.* 1988), using motility stimulants (Yovich *et al.* 1990), insemination in small volumes (Cohen *et al.* 1985), and removal of the cumulus cells before insemination (Ord *et al.* 1993). However, fertilization rates are still unpredictable and frequently lower than for couples with normal semen.

In addition, there is a large group of patients whose semen is too poor to be considered for standard IVF or who fail to achieve fertilization after insemination *in vitro* even with the use of the above mentioned insemination techniques. This may be due to too few sperm in the ejaculate or an extremely abnormal semen profile, such as very poor or absent motility or very severe teratozoospermia. There is also a significant population of patients with apparently normal semen but with persistent failure of fertilization *in vitro*. Although the cause of this failure is often unknown, a defect in the acrosome reaction of sperm after binding to the zona pellucida has recently been reported as a cause of reduced fertilization in patients with apparently normal semen (Liu and Baker 1994*a*). Another group of patients who have a poor result with standard IVF are those with a male genital tract obstruction. Initial results using epididymal sperm and standard insemination were promising, but these results have not been maintained (Silber et al. 1990, 1994).

In an attempt to improve the outcome for patients with severe male infertility, methods were developed to bypass the barrier of the zona pellucida. Mechanical or chemical dissolution of part of the zona pellucida by zona-drilling or zona-cutting gave sperm direct access to the oolemma after insemination, but required sperm to swim through the opening (Cohen et al. 1988; Gordon et al. 1988; Payne et al. 1991). Microinjection of sperm into the perivitelline space by sub-zonal insemination (SUZI) (Laws-King et al. 1987; Ng et al. 1988; Fishel et al. 1990) generally required fewer sperm, and fertilization could be obtained with completely immotile sperm (Bongso et al. 1989). However, with all these approaches, the sperm had to spontaneously acrosome react before binding to the oolemma (Liu and Baker 1994b) and the fertilization rates were still low. In addition, polyspermy was a frequent problem and, although pregnancies were achieved, the pregnancy rates in most cases were poor (reviewed in Schmutzler et al. 1994).

The initial report of pregnancies after intracytoplasmic sperm injection (ICSI) by Palermo et al. (1992) demonstrated that fertilization and pregnancies could be achieved after the injection of single sperm directly into oocytes. Subsequent reports have confirmed high fertilization and pregnancy rates and many normal, healthy babies have been born (Van Steirteghem et al. 1993a, 1993b). This technique has overcome many of the problems of treating male infertility and has created a treatment option for patients with semen profiles who previously were considered unlikely to be successful by IVF.

In this report we describe our experience with ICSI. We characterize the outcome of treatment based on male infertility type and we also describe the use of ICSI in a group of patients with specific problems to assess the potential of ICSI in treating severe and extreme male infertility.

Materials and Methods

Patients

Data were collated from 263 patients undergoing 296 consecutive oocyte retrieval cycles at the Royal Women's Hospital and Melbourne IVF between June 1993 and May 1994, with the inclusion of an additional 5 oocyte retrieval cycles performed after this period for patients with extreme indications. The results of embryo thaw cycles performed up to September 1994 were included in the analysis.

The outcome of a subgroup of 205 oocyte retrieval cycles were analysed in 5 major diagnostic categories based on semen characteristics or the results of previous IVF cycles. Semen quality was based on the average of at least 2 semen analyses performed according to guidelines set out by the World Health Organization (1992) in the previous three years. For sperm morphology, the acrosomal area of the sperm head was also taken into account and any doubtfully normal sperm were classified as abnormal (Liu and Baker 1994b). Ninety-six oocyte retrieval cycles were not able to be classified into these groups due to insufficient semen analysis data, variable results or extreme indications for their infertility (see below).

The diagnostic categories were defined as follows:

(1) Severe oligozoospermia: average sperm concentration $<2 \times 10^6$ mL^{-1}.

(2) Oligoasthenoteratozoospermia: average sperm concentration $<20 \times 10^6$ mL^{-1} with $<25\%$ progressive motility and/or $<40\%$ total motility, and $>85\%$ abnormal sperm morphology.

(3) Asthenoteratozoospermia: average sperm concentration $>20 \times 10^6$ mL^{-1} with $<25\%$ progressive motility and/or $<40\%$ total motility, and $>85\%$ abnormal sperm morphology.

(4) Low IVF: well or poorly defined causes of fertilization failure *in vitro* which were not related to sperm defects described in Categories 1–3. These included patients with disordered zona-induced acrosome reactions (Liu and Baker 1994a), other disorders of sperm–zona pellucida binding or penetration, poor oolemma binding, isolated defects of sperm chromatin (acridine orange staining abnormality) and currently unexplained defects which might involve sperm, oocytes or both.

(5) Epididymal sperm: patients requiring either microsurgical epididymal sperm aspiration (MESA) or percutaneous epididymal cyst aspiration for sperm retrieval due to bilateral congenital absence of the vas deferens, Young's syndrome, failed vasectomy reversal or post inflammatory epididymal obstruction. Only cases in which motile sperm could be retrieved were included in this category.

Patients with extreme indications for their infertility were described as follows:

(1) Mosaic Klinefelter's syndrome (1 patient, 3 cycles): sperm count $<1 \times 10^3$ sperm mL^{-1} and a peripheral blood chromosomal analysis of 100 cells showing 96 47 XXY cells, 2 48 XXXY cells and 2 46 XY cells. The results of 2 ICSI cycles in this patient have been reported previously (Harari et al. 1994).

(2) Round-headed acrosomeless sperm (1 patient, 1 cycle): 100% acrosomeless sperm as assessed by light microscopy, and with no sperm binding to either the zona pellucida or the oolemma (Bourne et al. 1995).

(3) Completely immotile sperm (2 patients, 2 cycles): 1 patient with a structural sperm defect and 1 patient in whom no motile sperm were isolated from a testicular biopsy. In both these cases, sperm were selected for injection by observing tail coiling in hypo-osmotic medium.

(4) Untreated severe sperm autoimmunity (2 patients, 3 cycles): both patients had normal semen analyses but had high levels of sperm antibodies (immunobead test, $>80\%$ binding of IgA antibodies to the sperm head) and severely impaired cervical mucus penetration (Kremer test, <2 cm penetration over 1 h).

(5) Testicular biopsy (6 patients, 6 cycles): in these patients, sperm retrieval either by fine needle or open biopsy was performed due to an intratesticular blockage (Young's syndrome, post small-pox infection or of unclear origin) or failure to obtain sperm by MESA.

Cystic fibrosis gene studies of four of the major mutations including ΔF508 were undertaken in men with congenital absence of the vas and in their partners if this was abnormal. Approximately half of the men tested positive for ΔF508, but none of their partners were positive. Any couple with a positive result was given genetic counselling.

The ICSI procedure was introduced with the approval of the relevant institutional ethics committees. All patients were counselled about the procedures by the attendant medical staff and a specialist infertility counsellor, and informed written consent was obtained prior to the commencement of treatment.

Ovarian Stimulation and Oocyte Collection

In most cases, a short ovarian stimulation protocol was used which consisted of human menopausal gonadotrophin (hMG) (Humegon;

Organon, Lane Cove, NSW, or Pergonal; Serono, Frenchs Forest, NSW, Australia) and gonadotrophin releasing hormone analogue (Lucrin; Abbott Australasia, Kurnell, NSW, Australia). Oocytes were collected by ultrasound guided transvaginal ovarian puncture 36 h after the administration of human chorionic gonadotrophin (hCG) (Pregnyl; Organon). Luteal phase support was given in the form of progesterone pessaries (100 mg day^{-1}; Royal Women's Hospital, Melbourne, Australia) or hCG injections (1000 I.U. every 3 days) for 12 days after oocyte retrieval. In a few cases, oocytes were collected in natural cycles.

Preparation of Sperm

Sperm were isolated from ejaculates produced on the day of oocyte retrieval or from a sample which was cryopreserved before treatment. Epididymal sperm samples were obtained by MESA or percutaneous epididymal cyst aspiration and were either used fresh or after cryopreservation. Testicular sperm were isolated from tissue samples obtained by open or fine needle biopsy of the testis (Mallidis and Baker 1993).

In most cases, samples were diluted with HEPES-buffered human tubal fluid (HTF) medium (Irvine Scientific, Irvine, CA, USA) which was supplemented with 10% patient serum or 4 mg mL^{-1} human serum albumin (Fraction V; Irvine Scientific) (supplemented HEPES-HTF) and centrifuged at 1800g for 5 min before separation on a mini-Percoll gradient (Ord et al. 1990). The resultant sperm pellet was washed by one or two centrifugation steps of 1800g for 5 min to remove the Percoll. The final pellet was resuspended in a small volume (<0.5 mL) of supplemented HEPES-HTF. A simple swim-up was used in some cases in which there were $>5 \times 10^6$ progressively motile sperm in the sample. If only a few sperm were found (<10 sperm in the entire haemocytometer chamber), then the sample was centrifuged once (1800g for 5 min) and resuspended in a small volume of supplemented HEPES-HTF.

Testicular biopsy samples were prepared by dissection in supplemented HEPES-HTF using fine scissors or 25 G needles. The resultant coarse suspension was transferred to a 5 mL tube (Falcon 2003; Becton Dickinson, Lincoln Park, NJ, USA) and left standing to allow the large tissue clumps and debris to settle out. The top layer of the suspension was then either separated on a mini-Percoll gradient or centrifuged once (700g for 10 min) and then resuspended in a small volume of supplemented HEPES-HTF. Samples were then plated onto the injection dish as described below and left at 37°C until injection.

Preparation of Oocytes

Cumulus cells were removed form oocytes by brief exposure (<1 min) to 100 I.U. mL^{-1} hyaluronidase (Bovine Type VI; Sigma, St Louis, MO, USA or Hyalase; Fisons, Castle Hill, NSW, Australia) in supplemented HEPES-HTF followed by aspiration through a fine bore glass pipette. Oocytes which exhibited a polar body after cumulus removal or after a few hours *in vitro* were injected on the day of collection. A small number of immature oocytes were cultured overnight and injected the following day after they had extruded a polar body.

Microinjection Procedure

For injection, a small drop (5-20 μL) of the final sperm suspension and small drops (5-10 μL) of fresh supplemented HEPES-HTF were spread onto a large Petri dish (Falcon 1006; Becton Dickinson) and covered with approximately 6 mL of temperature-equilibrated light paraffin oil (BDH, Poole, UK) or mineral oil (Sigma). Sperm injection was performed using ML-188 micromanipulators and IM-6 injectors (Narishige, Tokyo, Japan) attached to a Diaphot TMD inverted microscope (Nikon, Tokyo, Japan) equipped with a heated stage (LEC Instruments, Melbourne, Australia) set at 37°C.

Microinjection was based on the methodology described by Palermo et al. (1992) but without the use of polyvinylpyrrolidone (PVP). Motile sperm were aspirated from the suspension into a fine injection pipette (outer diameter of 6-10 μm), transferred to a drop containing an oocyte and immobilized by crushing the tail between the injection pipette and the dish. The freshly immobilized spermatozoon was re-aspirated into the injection pipette and released into the cytoplasm of a mature oocyte after pushing the pipette through the zona pellucida and puncturing the oolemma. Prior to expelling the spermatozoon, rupture of the oolemma was confirmed by aspiration of a small volume of the oocyte cytoplasm into the injection pipette. After injection, oocytes were transferred to fresh HTF containing 10% patient serum for culture.

Hypo-osmotic medium was used to select viable sperm in patients with completely immotile sperm. It was prepared by diluting (1:2) supplemented HEPES-HTF with high quality, purified water (Nanopure; Sybron/Barnstead, Boston, MA, USA) followed by filtration through a 0.2-μm filter. The resultant medium ($\sim$100 mOsm) was spread onto the dish for injection along with fresh drops of medium and the sperm suspension. Immotile sperm were aspirated from the sperm suspension and transferred to the hypo-osmotic medium. Some sperm exhibited tail coiling within seconds of contacting the solution, and these sperm were immediately transferred to the iso-osmotic HTF medium containing an oocyte and used for injection. Prior to injection, the injection pipette was washed by repeated aspiration of fresh HTF to ensure removal of the hypo-osmotic solution.

Survival, Fertilization and Embryo Cleavage

Oocytes were deemed to have survived ICSI if they remained intact and failed to show any obvious signs of lysis or degeneration over the 2 days following injection. Oocytes were assessed for the presence of pronuclei (PN) about 15-20 h after injection and were examined for cleavage after a further 40 h and 60 h.

Embryo Transfer and Cryopreservation

In most cases, fresh embryos were transferred 3 days after microinjection and surplus embryos were frozen in 1, 2-propanediol and sucrose (Lassalle et al. 1985). In a small number of cases, embryos were transferred or frozen on Day 2 post-injection. Routinely, only 2 embryos were transferred to minimize the risk of a multiple pregnancy, although up to 3 embryos were transferred if the embryo quality or post-thaw survival was poor. The allocation of embryos to fresh transfer or freezing was based on their morphology. If only a small number of embryos were suitable for freezing, or embryo quality varied significantly, then the poorer embryos or a mixture of embryo qualities were transferred fresh to maximize embryo utilization.

Embryos were transferred after thawing in either a natural or artificial cycle. In natural cycles, embryos were replaced 2 or 3 days (depending on the age of the embryos) after ovulation had occurred as determined using a urine dip-stick test for luteinizing hormone (LH; Clearplan One Step; Fisons). For artificial cycles, endometrial growth was stimulated by oestradiol valerate (2-6 mg day^{-1}). Progesterone pessaries (100 mg day^{-1}) were commenced when the endometrial thickness was $\geq$7 mm and embryos were transferred 2 or 3 days after the start of progesterone treatment. In these artificial cycles, luteal phase support was continued using progesterone pessaries.

Pregnancy Assessment

A serum β-hCG measurement was planned for 14-18 days after embryo transfer (ET). A β-hCG concentration >10 I.U. L^{-1} was considered positive. Clinical pregnancies were confirmed by the presence of a gestational sac on ultrasound scan 4 weeks after ET.

Statistical Analysis

Differences in the fertilization, implantation and pregnancy rates were compared using χ^2-tests for significance, or by Fisher's Exact Test for smaller contingency tables.

Results

A total of 3636 oocytes were collected in 296 consecutive retrieval cycles (average 12·3 per cycle) and 2858 oocytes (79%) were inseminated by ICSI and a further 175 oocytes were inseminated by standard IVF as a comparison in patients with borderline or variable semen quality. The remaining oocytes were either immature, degenerate, damaged during cumulus removal or used for approved research. In the first 4 ICSI cases, 20 oocytes were inseminated by SUZI as a trial during the introduction of ICSI, however, these oocytes have been excluded from the analysis.

Twenty patients had some of their oocytes inseminated by standard IVF. In 18 of these cases, 26 out of 135 oocytes fertilized normally after standard IVF (19%) compared with 116 out of 163 oocytes from the same patients after ICSI (71%) (χ^2-test, $P < 0.001$). Only 6 of these patients (33%) achieved normal fertilization with standard IVF whereas all achieved fertilization with ICSI. One patient had 22 oocytes inseminated with donor sperm and another had all the oocytes (18) inseminated by standard IVF with 1 oocyte fertilizing normally but failing to cleave. Six of the remaining oocytes which had failed to fertilize were injected the following day; one fertilized normally but failed to cleave. The remaining results deal only with those oocytes which were originally inseminated by ICSI.

The results on fertilization and embryo development following ICSI are summarized in Table 1. A high survival rate (90%) was achieved with 69% of these oocytes fertilizing normally (2 PN). The pronuclear stage was missed in a small number of oocytes (1·9%). In some oocytes, PN were seen as early as 6 h after injection but were no longer evident by 18 h. Therefore, oocytes in which the PN were missed but which cleaved to morphologically normal embryos at the same time as sibling 2 PN oocytes were classified as normally fertilized. Abnormal fertilization (1 PN or >2 PN) occurred at a similar rate (5–6%) to that found in patients undergoing routine IVF treatment. A total of 582 embryos were transferred fresh and 1031 embryos were frozen, together representing 91% of the oocytes which had fertilized normally after ICSI. Only 511 frozen embryos have been thawed and transferred to date, leaving a large number of embryos still frozen and available for future use.

Embryos suitable for transfer or cryopreservation were obtained in 288 out of the 296 consecutive oocyte retrieval cycles (97%). In 19 cycles (6·4%), all the embryos were frozen because of the risk of ovarian hyperstimulation syndrome. No embryos were available for transfer in 8 cycles (2·7%). In 6 of these cycles, only 1–3 oocytes were collected, and in 2 of these cycles, only abnormal fertilization occurred. Another patient achieved fertilization of one oocyte by ICSI after the injection of oocytes which had failed to fertilize by standard IVF but it failed to cleave, and in another cycle, all the oocytes which survived injection developed with only 1 PN.

Embryo transfer results are summarized in Table 2. A total of 32 clinical pregnancies resulted from the transfer of fresh embryos (12% per transfer) and an additional 44 clinical pregnancies were obtained after the transfer of frozen–thawed embryos (16% per transfer). An overall ongoing or delivered pregnancy rate of 19% per oocyte retrieval cycle was obtained from the transfer of fresh and/or frozen embryos. Eight sets of twins occurred out of 69 intrauterine fetal heart gestations (12%) and 12 fetal heart pregnancies were lost as first or second trimester spontaneous abortions (9 fresh transfer pregnancies and 3 thaw transfer pregnancies; 30% and 7·5% of intrauterine fetal heart gestations respectively).

Fertilization, implantation and pregnancy results based on male infertility category are described in Table 3. The normal fertilization rates in the different male infertility groups were not uniform due to the low fertilization rate in the oligoasthenoteratozoospermia group and the high fertilization rate in those cycles inseminated with epididymal sperm. There were no statistically significant differences in the implantation rates (fetal hearts per total number of embryos transferred) between the groups, although the cycles using epididymal sperm had the highest implantation rate of 11%. This group also had the highest ongoing or delivered pregnancy rate of 46% per oocyte retrieval cycle.

Normal fertilization and the development of embryos suitable for transfer or cryopreservation was achieved in all cases of extreme male infertility (Table 4). A high fertilization and pregnancy rate was achieved with testicular sperm. A high rate of cleavage failure was seen in the patient with mosaic Klinefelter's syndrome, while the fertilization rate was low (27%) in the 2 patients having sperm selected by hypo-osmotic swelling.

Discussion

In this report, we have demonstrated high rates of oocyte survival, normal fertilization and embryo development after the use of ICSI for treating severe male infertility. The survival and fertilization rates achieved in this study are similar to those in the initial reports of Van Steirteghem *et al.* (1993*a*, 1993*b*), however, the percentage of normally

Table 1. Oocyte survival, fertilization rates and embryo utilization after intracytoplasmic sperm injection (ICSI)

ET, embryo transfer; PN, pronuclei

No. of oocytes injected	2858
No. of oocytes surviving	2561 (90%)
Normal fertilization[A]:	
total	1774 (69%)
2 PN	1725 (67%)
0 PN, cleaved[B]	49 (1·9%)
Abnormal fertilization[A]:	
1 PN	140 (5·5%)
>2 PN	153 (6·0%)
Embryo utilization:	
transferred fresh	582 (average 2·2 per ET)
frozen	1031 (3·6 per cycle with embryos)
total embryos used clinically	1613 (91% of normally fertilized)
thawed and transferred	511 (average 1·9 per ET)
total no. transferred	1093

[A] Values in parentheses are percentages of oocytes which survived injection.
[B] PN were not observed, but the oocytes cleaved 1 day after injection.

Table 2. Embryo transfer outcome in 296 consecutive cycles of intracytoplasmic sperm injection (ICSI)

ET, embryo transfer; hCG, human chorionic gonadotrophin

	Fresh ET[A]	Frozen–thaw ET[B]	Oocyte retrievals[C]
No. of cycles	269	268	296
hCG positive pregnancies	41 (15%)	62 (23%)	103 (35%)
Clinical pregnancies:			
ectopic	2 (0·7%)	—	2 (0·7%)
blighted ovum	—	5 (1·9%)	5 (1·7%)
fetal heart	30 (11%)	39 (15%)	69 (23%)
Ongoing or delivered pregnancies	21 (7·8%)	36 (13%)	57 (19%)

[A] Values in parentheses are percentages of 269 fresh ETs.
[B] Values in parentheses are percentages of 268 frozen-thaw ETs.
[C] Values in parentheses are percentages of 296 oocyte retrievals.

Table 3. Fertilization, implantation and pregnancy rates based on male infertility category in 205 intracytoplasmic sperm injection (ICSI) cycles

hCG, human chorionic gonadotrophin; PN, pronuclei

	Severe oligozoospermia	Oligoasthenoteratozoospermia	Asthenoteratozoospermia	Low IVF	Epididymal sperm
Oocyte retrieval cycles	65	41	36	35	28
Oocytes surviving ICSI	548	397	331	226	285
Normally-fertilized (2 PN) oocytes[AB]	374 (68%)	250 (63%)	240 (73%)	156 (69%)	215 (75%)
Implantation rate per embryo[C]	13/242 (5·4%)	11/158 (7%)	9/161 (5·6%)	8/113 (7·1%)	14/131 (11%)
hCG-positive pregnancies[D]	21 (32%)	16 (39%)	12 (33%)	8 (23%)	18 (64%)
Clinical pregnancies[D]	13 (20%)	12 (29%)	9 (25%)	7 (20%)	14 (50%)
Ongoing or delivered pregnancies[D]	11 (17%)	8 (20%)	5 (14%)	5 (14%)	13 (46%)

[A] Values in parentheses are fertilization rates expressed as percentages of the oocytes that survived injection.
[B] 5×2 χ^2-test, $P = 0.006$; non-uniformity of results was due to low fertilization rate in the oligoasthenoteratozoospermia group compared with the other groups ($P < 0.003$) and the high fertilization rate for epididymal sperm compared with the other groups ($P = 0.01$).
[C] Number of fetal hearts per total number of embryos transferred. Includes the transfer of fresh and frozen–thawed embryos.
[D] Pregnancy rates in parentheses are expressed per oocyte retrieval cycle.

Table 4. Fertilization, embryo development and pregnancies using intracytoplasmic sperm injection (ICSI) in patients with extreme male infertility

	Mosaic Klinefelter's	Severe sperm autoimmunity	100% immotility	Round-headed acrosomeless sperm	Testicular sperm
Oocyte retrieval cycles	3	3	2	1	6
Oocytes surviving ICSI	19	26	11	7	72
Normally fertilized (2 PN) oocytes[A]	18 (95%)	22 (85%)	3 (27%)	3 (43%)	51 (71%)
Normal embryos[B]	10 (56%)	22 (100%)	3 (100%)	2 (67%)	50 (98%)
Embryos frozen	4	15	2	—	27
Fresh embryos transferred	6	7	1	2	14
Frozen-thawed embryos transferred	1	—	—	—	12
Pregnancies	—	—	—	—	3[C]

[A] Values in parentheses are fertilization rates expressed as percentages of the oocytes which survived injection.
[B] Values in parentheses are percentages of the 2 PN oocytes which developed normally.
[C] Two pregnancies resulted from transfer of fresh embryos and one from frozen embryos. All were clinical (fetal heart) singleton pregnancies.

fertilized oocytes which were used clinically (transferred or frozen) was higher in the present study (91% v. 71%). This may be due to the high usage of embryo freezing in our programme and a tendency to transfer poorer or mixed quality embryos in the initial fresh transfer.

Since introducing freezing into routine clinical practice, we have progressively adopted a policy of maximizing embryo utilization and reducing the risk of multiple pregnancy. Embryos are allocated to fresh transfer or cryopreservation based on morphological quality. Poorer quality embryos are less likely to survive freezing, but if they are transferred fresh, they have a low, but not zero, chance of producing a pregnancy. Therefore, if embryo quality varied significantly or there was only a small number of embryos suitable for freezing, the poorer quality embryos, or a mixture of embryo qualities, were transferred fresh. This approach was used to maximize the cumulative chance of obtaining a singleton pregnancy from that retrieval cycle. Using embryos in this way may explain the lower implantation rate that was obtained in this study compared to earlier reports (Van Steirteghem et al. 1993b).

The results from the use of frozen embryos in our routine IVF programme have been consistent and in many cases better than those obtained from the transfer of fresh embryos. This is also our experience with ICSI, in which a large percentage of the pregnancies resulted from the transfer of frozen-thawed embryos (see Table 2). In addition, many ICSI embryos remain frozen and therefore additional pregnancies can be expected from their future use.

A clinical pregnancy rate of 16% per transfer was obtained using frozen-thawed embryos which suggests that the injection procedure does not compromise the ability of embryos to survive freezing and thawing. The higher pregnancy rate per transfer obtained with frozen-thawed embryos compared to fresh embryos in this study may reflect the tendency to transfer the poorer quality embryos and reserve the better quality embryos for freezing because of their increased chance of cryosurvival.

Our results demonstrate that high fertilization rates and pregnancies can be achieved in the different male factor infertility catergories. The significantly lower fertilization rate in the oligoasthenoteratozoospermia group may be related to the consistently high percentage of morphologically abnormal sperm in these patients. A correlation between abnormal morphology and fertilization after SUZI has been reported (Payne et al. 1994) although it requires further study to determine whether or not a similar relationship exists after ICSI.

The fertilization rate we obtained in cycles in which epididymal sperm were injected was higher than in previous reports (Silber et al. 1994; Tournaye et al. 1994) and highlights the potential of ICSI in treating male genital tract obstruction. In these earlier studies, the oocytes in some patients were injected with immotile sperm which could account for the lower fertilization rate relative to our study. However, this would not explain the difference in the fertilization rate for the remaining patients. The relationship between epididymal length, cystic fibrosis mutation status and fertilization by standard IVF was reported by Patrizio et al. (1994a, 1994b), but this may not be of importance with ICSI because the fertilization rate in this study was consistently high and therefore confirms the findings of Silber et al. (1994). There was a significantly higher normal fertilization rate in those cycles inseminated with epididymal sperm compared to the other male infertility groups (Table 3), and furthermore, there was a high ongoing or delivered pregnancy rate and a low incidence of clinical abortions in these patients. Whether these results are due to the use of inherently better quality sperm or a higher fecundity in the partners of these patients requires further study. However, the use of ICSI has completely revolutionized the management of male genital tract obstruction, an aetiology for which fertilization and pregnancy rates were previously low and unpredictable, even after the use of partial zona dissection or SUZI for insemination (Garrisi et al. 1993).

Our results for patients with extreme male factor indications suggest that there may be limits to the effectiveness of ICSI. The patient with mosaic Klinefelter's syndrome obtained a very high normal fertilization rate, however, there was a high rate of cleavage arrest and 8 out of the 18 fertilized oocytes (44%) failed to cleave after PN were observed. It is assumed that there is no genetic risk in treating this condition, as it is thought that only germ cells with an XY karyotype are capable of producing sperm (Lyon 1974). Fluorescence *in situ* hybridization (FISH) with specific X and Y probes could be used to confirm that only X- or Y-bearing sperm are produced, and not XY- or XX-bearing sperm. The use of embryo biopsy and FISH to determine the sex chromosome content of the embryos may also be of benefit in this category. Whether the high incidence of cleavage failure is related to the karyotype, or to dysfunctional oocytes in the partner (only one patient was treated in this study group) remains unclear and requires further investigation.

A high fertilization and cleavage rate was obtained in the patients with severe sperm autoimmunity. Many of the embryos obtained from these patients remain frozen and a pregnancy is still possible in these cases. The results from the use of completely immotile sperm demonstrate that fertilization is possible with sperm selected by hypo-osmotic swelling. The ability of sperm to swell under hypo-osmotic conditions is related to the presence of a functional membrane (Jeyendran *et al.* 1984) and so it is feasible to use it as a method for selecting viable, immotile sperm for ICSI. However, the fertilization rate was low and this may indicate that either the method was inefficient in selecting sperm with the capacity to fertilize or that sperm viability was compromised by exposure to the hypo-osmotic solution. Alternatively, the sperm in these patients may have had additional defects unrelated to their immotility which made them less likely to fertilize no matter which sperm were selected for injection. Additional work is needed to evaluate the usefulness of this technique.

The injection of round-headed, acrosomeless sperm (globozoospermia) resulted in normal fertilization. The treatment of this condition, however, may prove to be difficult. Fishel *et al.* (1994) have also reported fertilization with this type of sperm defect using ICSI. However, the fertilization rate was low (18%) and only 38% of those patients having treatment achieved fertilization. Absence of the acrosome can be associated with other structural defects such as ultrastructural abnormalities of the midpiece and flagellum. However, these additional defects would probably not interfere with sperm decondensation. In addition, the patient in our study had normal sperm motility and was therefore likely to have normal tail morphology. It is presumed that sterility due to this type of sperm defect has a genetic basis but whether this reduces the capacity of these sperm to fertilize after ICSI is unknown. Recently, a pregnancy and live birth were reported following the transfer of embryos fertilized with acrosomeless sperm (Lundin *et al.* 1994). However, the efficiency of ICSI for treating this condition remains to be fully evaluated. It is unknown whether there is a risk of this condition being expressed in any offspring and patients should be advised accordingly.

The fertilization and pregnancy rates in those patients having sperm retrieval by testicular biopsy were similar to those obtained with epididymal sperm. This confirms that testicular sperm can fertilize and produce viable pregnancies after ICSI as reported by Schoysman *et al.* (1993) and Silber (1994). Although the number of treatments of this type are still low, it is possible that these patients will perform as well as those in whom epididymal sperm are used.

The incidence of cycles in which no normal embryos were produced was very low (2·7%), and in most of these, only a small number of oocytes were injected and so it was difficult to assign an exact cause for the failure. However, the role of oocyte defects cannot be overlooked as many of the oocytes in these cycles fertilized abnormally.

The results that can be obtained with ICSI question the role of the non-nuclear components of sperm in fertilization. A recent study in mice has demonstrated the birth of normal, live young by the electrofusion of round spermatids and oocytes (Ogura *et al.* 1994). This, combined with the observation in the present study that virtually any sperm type is able to fertilize after ICSI, complements the suggestion by Yanagimachi (1994) that the function of the post-meiotic modification of sperm (spermiogenesis, maturation, activation of motility, acrosome reaction) is merely to enable the transfer of the male genome into the oocyte. These findings further advance the potential use of ICSI.

The results obtained in this study demonstrate that ICSI represents a significant advance in the management of severe male infertility. Fertilization is possible in spite of most types of sperm defect, even in cases previously thought to be irreversibly sterile. ICSI may be of limited use in some cases of extreme male infertility, although the true limits of this technology await further investigation.

Acknowledgments

We thank the clinical, laboratory and nursing staff of the Reproductive Biology Unit, Royal Women's Hospital and Melbourne IVF for their assistance in the management of these patients. In particular, we thank Michele McDonald, Felix Nieto and Anne Vassiliadis of the Royal Women's Hospital and Dr Gayle Jones,

Pam Matthews, and Linda Weiss of Melbourne IVF for performing the microinjection procedures, and Jessica Costa of the Royal Women's Hospital for the manufacture of pipettes for microinjection.

References

Baker, H. W. G., Liu, D.-Y., Bourne, H., and Lopata, A. (1993). Diagnosis of sperm defects in selecting patients for assisted fertilization. *Hum. Reprod. (Oxf.)* **8**, 1779–80.

Bongso, T. A., Sathananthan, A. H., Wong, P. C., Ratnam, S. S., Ng, S.-C., Anandakumar, C., and Ganatra, S. (1989). Human fertilization by micro-injection of immotile spermatozoa. *Hum. Reprod. (Oxf.)* **4**, 175–9.

Bourne, H., Liu, D.-Y., Clarke, G. N., and Baker, H. W. G. (1995). Normal fertilization and embryo development by intracytoplasmic sperm injection of round-headed acrosomeless sperm. *Fertil. Steril.* (In press.)

Cohen, J., Edwards, R., Fehilly, C., Fishel, S., Hewitt, J., Purdy, J., Rowland, C., Steptoe, P., and Webster, J. (1985). In vitro fertilization: a treatment for male infertility. *Fertil. Steril.* **43**, 422–32.

Cohen, J., Malter, H., Fehilly, C., Wright, G., Elsner, C., Kort, H., and Massey, J. (1988). Implantation of embryos after partial opening of oocyte zona pellucida to facilitate sperm penetration. *Lancet* **2**, 162.

Fishel, S., Jackson, P., Antinori, S., Johnson, J., Grossi, S., and Versaci, C. (1990). Subzonal insemination for the alleviation of infertility. *Fertil. Steril.* **54**, 828–35.

Fishel, S., Green, S., Dowell, K., Thornton, S., McDermott, H., Lisi, F., Rinaldi, L., Jacobson, M., and Gobetz, L. (1994). Fifty-nine cases of extreme male factor infertility — immotile spermatozoa, Kartagener syndrome, globozoospermia, spermatogenic arrest, testicular spermatozoa-treated by SUZI/ICSI. *Proc. 2nd Int. Meet. Br. Fertil. Soc.*, 5. [Abstr.]

Garrisi, J. G., Chin, A. J., Dolan, P. M., Nagler, H. M., Vasquez-Levin, M., Navot, D., and Gordon, J. W. (1993). Analysis of factors contributing to success in a program of micromanipulation-assisted fertilization. *Fertil. Steril.* **59**, 366–74.

Gordon, J. W., Grunfeld, L., Garrisi, G. J., Talansky, B. E., Richards, C., and Laufer, N. (1988). Fertilization of human oocytes by sperm from infertile males after zona pellucida drilling. *Fertil. Steril.* **50**, 68–73.

Harari, O., Bourne, H., Baker, G., Gronow, M., and Johnston, I. (1994). High fertilization rate with intracytoplasmic sperm injection in mosaic Klinefelter's syndrome. *Fertil. Steril.* **63**, 182–4.

Jeyendran, R. S., Van der Ven, H. H., Perez-Pelaez, M., Crabo, B. G., and Zaneveld, L. J. D. (1984). Development of an assay to assess the functional integrity of the human sperm membrane and its relationship to other semen characteristics. *J. Reprod. Fertil.* **70**, 219–28.

Lassalle, B., Testart, T., and Renard, J. P. (1985). Human embryo features that influence the success of cryopreservation with the use of 1, 2-propanediol. *Fertil. Steril.* **44**, 645–51.

Laws-King, A., Trounson, A., Sathananthan, H., and Kola, I. (1987). Fertilization of human oocytes by microinjection of a single spermatozoon under the zona pellucida. *Fertil. Steril.* **48**, 637–42.

Liu, D. Y., and Baker, H. W. G. (1994a). Disordered acrosome reaction of spermatozoa bound to the zona pellucida: a newly discovered sperm defect causing infertility with reduced sperm-zona pellucida penetration and reduced fertilization *in vitro*. *Hum. Reprod. (Oxf.)* **9**, 1694–700.

Liu, D. Y., and Baker, H. W. G. (1994b). Acrosome status and morphology of human spermatozoa bound to the zona pellucida and oolemma determined using oocytes that failed to fertilize *in vitro*. *Hum. Reprod. (Oxf.)* **9**, 673–9.

Lundin, K., Sjögren, A., Nilsson, L., and Hamberger, L. (1994). Fertilization and pregnancy after intracytoplasmic microinjection of acrosomeless spermatozoa. *Fertil. Steril.* **62**, 1266–7.

Lyon, M. F. (1974). Mechanisms and evolutionary origins of variable X-chromosome activity in mammals. *Proc. R. Soc. (Lond.) B* **187**, 243–68.

Mallidis, C., and Baker, H. W. G. (1994). Fine needle tissue aspiration biopsy of the testis. *Fertil. Steril.* **61**, 367–75.

Ng, S.-C., Bongso, A., Ratnam, S. S., Sathananthan, H., Chan, C. L. K., Wong, P. C., Hagglund, L., Anandakumar, C., Wong, Y. C., and Goh, V. H. H. (1988). Pregnancy after transfer of sperm under the zona. *Lancet* **2**, 790.

Oehninger, S., Acosta, A.A., Morshedi, M., Veeck, L., Swanson, R. J., Simmons, K. F., and Rosenwaks, Z. (1988). Corrective measures and pregnancy outcome in *in vitro* fertilization in patients with severe sperm morphology abnormalities. *Fertil. Steril.* **150**, 283–7.

Ogura, A., Matsuda, J., and Yanagimachi, R. (1994). Birth of normal young after electrofusion of mouse oocytes with round spermatids. *Proc. Natl Acad. Sci. USA* **91**, 7460–2.

Ord, T., Patrizio, P., Marello, E., Balmaceda, J. P., and Asch, R. H. (1990). Mini-Percoll: a new method of semen preparation for IVF in severe male factor infertility. *Hum. Reprod. (Oxf.)* **5**, 987–9.

Ord, T., Patrizio, P., Balmaceda, J. P., and Asch, R. H. (1993). Can severe male factor infertility be treated without micromanipulation? *Fertil. Steril.* **60**, 110–15.

Palermo, G., Joris, H., Devroey, P., and Van Steirteghem, A. C. (1992). Pregnancies after intracytoplasmic injection of single spermatozoon into an oocyte. *Lancet* **340**, 17–18.

Patrizio, P., and Asch, R. H. (1994a). The relationship between congenital absence of the vas deferens (CAVD), cystic fibrosis (CF) mutations and epididymal sperm. *Assist. Reprod. Rev.* **4**, 95–100.

Patrizio, P., Ord, T., Silber, S. J., and Asch, R. H. (1994b). Correlation between epididymal length and fertilization rate in men with congenital absence of the vas deferens. *Fertil. Steril.* **61**, 265–8.

Payne, D., McLaughlin, K. J., Depypere, H. T., Kirby, C. A., Warnes, G. M., and Matthews, C. D. (1991). Experience with zona drilling and zona cutting to improve fertilization rates of human oocytes *in vitro*. *Hum. Reprod. (Oxf.)* **6**, 423–31.

Payne, D., Flaherty, S. P., Newble, C. D., Swann, N. J., Wang, X.-J., and Matthews, C. D. (1994). The influence of sperm morphology and the acrosome reaction on fertilization outcome after sub-zonal injection (SZI) of human spermatozoa. *Hum. Reprod. (Oxf.)* **9**, 1281–8.

Schmutzler, A. G., Sushma, V., and Krebs, D. (1994). Treatment of teratozoospermia by cell surgery (micromanipulation). *Assist. Reprod. Rev.* **4**, 138–42.

Schoysman, R., Vanderzwalmen, P., Nijs, M., Segal, L., Segal-Bertin, G., Geerts, L., Van Roosendaal, E., and Schoysman, D. (1993). Pregnancy after fertilization with human testicular spermatozoa. *Lancet* **342**, 1237.

Silber, S. J., Ord, T., Balmaceda, J., Patrizio, P., and Asch, R. H. (1990). Congenital absence of the vas deferens. The fertilizing capacity of human epididymal sperm. *New Engl. J. Med.* **323**, 1788–92.

Silber, S. J. (1994). The use of epididymal sperm in assisted reproduction. In 'Frontiers in Endocrinology. Vol. 8. Male Factor in Human Infertility'. (Ed J. Tesarik.) pp. 335–68. (Ares-Serono Symposia: Rome.)

Silber, S. J., Nagy, Z. P., Liu, J., Godoy, H., Devroey, P., and Van Steirteghem, A. C. (1994). Conventional *in-vitro* fertilization versus intracytoplasmic sperm injection for patients requiring microsurgical epididymal sperm aspiration. *Hum. Reprod. (Oxf.)* **9**, 1705–9.

Tournaye, H., Devroey, P., Liu, J., Nagy, Z., Lissens, W., and Van Steirteghem, A. C. (1994). Microsurgical epididymal sperm aspiration and intracytoplasmic sperm injection: a new effective approach to infertility as a result of congenital bilateral absence of the vas deferens. *Fertil. Steril.* **61**, 1045–51.

Van Steirteghem, A. C., Liu, J., Joris, H., Nagy, Z., Janssenswillen, C., Tournaye, H., Derde M.-P., Van Assche, E., and Devroey, P. (1993a). Higher success rate by intracytoplasmic sperm injection than by subzonal insemination. Report of a second series of 300 consecutive treatment cycles. *Hum. Reprod. (Oxf.)* **8**, 1055–60.

Van Steirteghem, A. C., Nagy, Z., Joris, H., Liu, J., Staessen, C., Smitz, J., Wisanto, A., and Devroey, P. (1993b). High fertilization and implantation rates after intracytoplasmic sperm injection. *Hum. Reprod. (Oxf.)* **8**, 1061–6.

World Health Organization (1992). 'Laboratory Manual for the Examination of Human Semen and Sperm–Cervical Mucus Interaction'. 3rd Edn. (Cambridge University Press: Cambridge.)

Yanagimachi, R. (1994). Fertilization mechanisms in man and other mammals. In 'Frontiers in Endocrinology. Vol. 8. Male Factor in Human Infertility'. (Ed. J. Tesarik.) pp. 15–43. (Ares-Serono Symposia: Rome.)

Yovich, J. M., Edirisinghe, W. R., Cummins, J. M., and Yovich, J. L. (1990). Influence of pentoxifylline in severe male factor infertility. *Fertil. Steril.* **53**, 715–22.

Manuscript received 21 March 1995

Open Discussion

Sherman Silber (St Louis):

Your pregnancy rate was dramatically higher with testicular and epididymal sperm. Do you think it's simply a patient selection phenomenon, or with severe oligozoospermic patients, should we derive sperm from the testis?

Bourne:

Well, I think it comes back to David de Kretser's talk. With the obstruction patients you're likely to have normal spermatogenesis and good quality sperm, and therefore you'll have a good outcome when you collect sperm from the testis. But with some of the other cases there was no obstruction, but there were still poor quality sperm. The reason for the low sperm count is obscure, but it may relate to spermatogenesis.

Clinical Results From Intracytoplasmic Sperm Injection at Monash IVF

Robert I. McLachlan[A], Giuliana Fuscaldo,
Hwan Rho, Christine Poulos,
Julie Dalrymple, Peter Jackson and Carol A. Holden

Monash IVF, 185–187 Hoddle Street, Richmond, Vic. 3121, Australia.
[A] *To whom correspondence should be addressed.*

Abstract. The impact of a modification of the intracytoplasmic sperm injection (ICSI) technique on fertilization and pregnancy rates was examined in a retrospective analysis of 171 consecutive ICSI treatment cycles (156 patients). Patients were selected for ICSI on the basis of severe oligoasthenozoospermia (65 patients) or following conventional *in vitro* fertilization (IVF) with failed or poor fertilization (70 patients). Seven patients in which epididymal or testicular sperm was used, 10 patients with sperm antibodies and 4 patients with retrograde ejaculation or who required electro-ejaculation were also treated with ICSI. In the first 105 cycles (102 patients), single sperm, rendered immotile, were injected into the ooplasm of 979 metaphase II (M II) oocytes using an established technique (Method 1). In the following 66 cycles (513 M II oocytes injected), the ICSI procedure was modified by increased aspiration of the oolemma to ensure the intracytoplasmic deposition of sperm (Method 2). The patient groups did not differ between the two injection procedures. The normal (two pronuclear) fertilization rate increased significantly ($P < 0.001$) from 34.3% with Method 1 to 73.1% with Method 2, with no difference in the oocyte degeneration rate (4.3% v. 4.5% respectively). The incidence of failed fertilization was significantly ($P < 0.01$) reduced from 17.1% (18 cycles) to 1.6% (1 cycle) with the change in technique. As a consequence of the increased fertilization rates with Method 2, more embryos were available for assessment and transfer, and a pregnancy rate per oocyte retrieval of 21.2% was obtained for Method 2. Fertilization, embryo transfer and pregnancies were obtained in all patient groups treated with ICSI. To date, 8 normal children (including one set of twins) have been born. It is concluded that an optimal injection procedure is essential for the success of the ICSI technique.

Extra keywords: male infertility, ICSI, fertilization.

Introduction

The successful treatment of severe male factor infertility by microinjection techniques was first demonstrated clinically by placement of spermatozoa under the zona pellucida into the perivitelline space (Ng *et al.* 1988). This technique, sub-zonal injection (SUZI), has been successfully adopted by many clinics over the last 5 years. However, in common with other groups (Fishel *et al.* 1990; Lippi *et al.* 1993; Van Steirteghem *et al.* 1993a), we found that SUZI was limited by low normal fertilization rates, persistently high rates of polyspermic fertilization, poor success in certain subgroups (such as immotile or epididymal sperm) and clinical pregnancy rates that overall were lower than for patients having conventional *in vitro* fertilization (IVF).

In response to the impressive results with intracytoplasmic sperm injection (ICSI) reported by Van Steirteghem *et al.* (1994), we undertook to develop an ICSI programme for patients with severe defects of semen quality or who had previously failed to achieve fertilization *in vitro*. This technique also provided an opportunity to treat patients who demonstrated virtual azoospermia and those in whom only epididymal or testicular sperm could be retrieved. Our initial experience with the ICSI technique demonstrated improved fertilization rates compared with SUZI, and the latter procedure was subsequently abandoned. This report summarizes the retrospective analysis of our clinical results with ICSI and embryo transfer for 171 consecutive treatment cycles and demonstrates the significant impact of technical modifications of the ICSI injection procedure on fertilization and pregnancy rates.

Materials and Methods

Patient Selection

A total of 156 patients (171 cycles) were treated with ICSI between January and July 1994. Patients were directed to ICSI based on their likely or demonstrated need for microinjection in order to achieve reasonable (> 35%) fertilization rates. Patients with mild to moderate male factor or idiopathic infertility have so far not been treated.

Male factor patients in the following categories were included:

(1) Severe oligoasthenozoospermia ($n = 65$), which was defined as a total motile sperm count, following Percoll gradient centrifugation, of < 200 000. Such a yield rendered them unsuitable for other assisted reproductive technology (ART) techniques such as microdrop insemination. Virtual azoospermia (sometimes called cryptozoospermia) was defined as an initial sperm count of $<0 \cdot 2 \times 10^6$ mL^{-1} ($n = 13$).

(2) Previous poor fertilization (2-pronuclear fertilization rate < 35%) in one or more IVF or microdrop insemination cycle ($n = 70$).

(3) Sperm autoimmunity, with > 50% IgG- and/or IgA-binding to the sperm head ($n = 10$).

(4) Epididymal sperm retrieved at surgery (vasectomy reversal or congenital absence of the vas) were cryopreserved and later used for ICSI ($n = 5$). In two patients with intra-testicular obstruction to sperm outflow, sperm were retrieved from the testis by fine needle aspiration biopsy (Mallidis and Baker 1994). Sperm were dissected free from other cell types under a microscope; they were found to be immotile in both cases and were used immediately.

(5) Semen of poor quality obtained by electro-ejaculation ($n = 3$) or retrieved from urine after retrograde ejaculation ($n = 1$).

Semen Evaluation and Preparation

Patients proceeding with ICSI (excluding epididymal or testicular sperm patients) were required to have two semen analyses over a period of 6 months before treatment. Patients who demonstrated a sperm concentration of $<2 \times 10^6$ mL^{-1} were required to have an additional semen analysis approximately 2 weeks before the expected date of oocyte retrieval to determine if the sperm concentration had reduced further. Patients demonstrating virtual azoospermia were advised to have one or two ejaculates frozen in the event that no sperm could be retrieved from the sample produced on the day of oocyte collection. Sperm concentration, motility and morphology were assessed according to the guidelines set out by the World Health Organization (1992).

Progressively motile spermatozoa were selected from liquefied semen on discontinuous Percoll (Pharmacia, Uppsala, Sweden) density gradients (90%, 45%) by centrifugation at $200g$ for 20–30 min (Osborn et al. 1991).

Ovarian Stimulation

Ovarian stimulation was carried out using two protocols (down-regulation and BOOST). In both protocols, the gonadotrophin-releasing hormone-agonist (GnRHa) leuprorelin acetate (Lucrin; Abbott Australasia, Kurnell, NSW, Australia) was used in combination with purified urinary follicle-stimulating hormone (FSH) (Metrodin; Serono, Frenchs Forest, NSW). In the down-regulation protocol, Lucrin was administered subcutaneously from either the early follicular or mid-luteal phase until pituitary desensitization was achieved before the administration of FSH. In the short, or BOOST protocol, Lucrin was initiated on cycle Day 2, followed by FSH from Day 3. GnRHa and FSH were discontinued with the administration of human chorionic gonadotrophin (hCG) (Profasi; Serono) when adequate folliculogenesis was achieved. The luteal phase was supported in both protocols with hCG on Days 3, 6 and 9 post-egg pick-up (EPU).

Oocyte Preparation and Handling

Oocyte retrievals were performed 36 h after the administration of hCG by vaginal ultrasound-guided follicular puncture. The cumulus–oocyte complexes were collected and washed in human tubal fluid (HTF) medium (Quinn et al. 1985) supplemented with 10% maternal human serum (HS) and incubated at 37°C in 5% CO_2 in air for approximately 2 h before removal of the cumulus and corona radiata. Cumulus and corona cells were removed by incubation for approximately 30 s in HEPES-buffered HTF containing 80 I.U. mL^{-1} of hyaluronidase (Type VIII; Sigma, St Louis, MO, USA), followed by gentle aspiration in and out of hand-drawn glass pipettes. Oocytes were assessed for nuclear maturity by examination for the presence or absence of the first polar body and a germinal vesicle, and for cytoplasmic abnormalities. Oocytes were subsequently incubated in HTF containing 10% HS at 37°C in an atmosphere of 5% CO_2 in air for 3–4 h before microinjection. ICSI was performed on morphologically normal, mature oocytes in which the first polar body was clearly visible.

Microinjection Procedure

Unless otherwise indicated, the preparation of holding and injection pipettes and the ICSI procedure were performed as described by Van Steirteghem et al. (1993a, 1993b). Holding and injection pipettes were made from borosilicate glass capillary tubes (150 mm long, $0 \cdot 78$ mm inner diameter, $1 \cdot 0$ mm outer diameter; Clark Electromedical Instruments, Pangbourne, UK). The inner and outer diameters of the holding pipettes were 10–15 μm and 120–130 μm respectively. The injection pipettes were made with an outer diameter of approximately 7 μm, an inner diameter of 5 μm, and a bevelled angle of 50°. A sharp spike was made on the end of the injection pipettes in order to assist in the penetration of the zona pellucida and the oolemma.

Immediately before injection, sperm were washed in HEPES-buffered HTF, incubated at 37°C and then diluted 1:4 with a 10% solution of polyvinylpyrrolidone (PVP) (PVP-360, Sigma) which had been prepared in HEPES-buffered HTF (Van Steirteghem et al. 1993b).

Two microinjection techniques were applied in the present study. In both methods, single sperm were rendered immotile by touching the midpiece of the sperm tail with the tip of the injection pipette. The immobilized spermatozoon was then aspirated tail first into the microinjection pipette and positioned at the tip before puncturing the zona pellucida and passing the pipette through the ooplasm to a distance of approximately three-quarters of the egg diameter. In Method 1 (105 cycles), immobilized sperm were injected directly into the ooplasm of metaphase II (M II) oocytes based on our interpretation of the procedure reported by Van Steirteghem et al. (1993a, 1993b). The ooplasm was gently aspirated into the injection pipette to a point near the inner edge of the zona pellucida, the pipette was then pushed forward in an attempt to rupture the oolemma and the spermatozoon was injected into the oocyte. In Method 2 (66 cycles), the only modification to the ICSI injection procedure was an increased suction during aspiration of the oolemma into the injection pipette. The ooplasm was aspirated into the pipette until a sudden increase in the velocity of the ooplasm entering the pipette was observed. This was taken to indicate rupture of the oocyte membrane (D. Payne, personal communication). Aspiration was immediately ceased and the spermatozoon was placed directly into the ooplasm (Figs 1 and 2). Microinjection procedures were performed in an oil-filled chamber on an Olympus inverted microscope equipped with a heated stage (37°C).

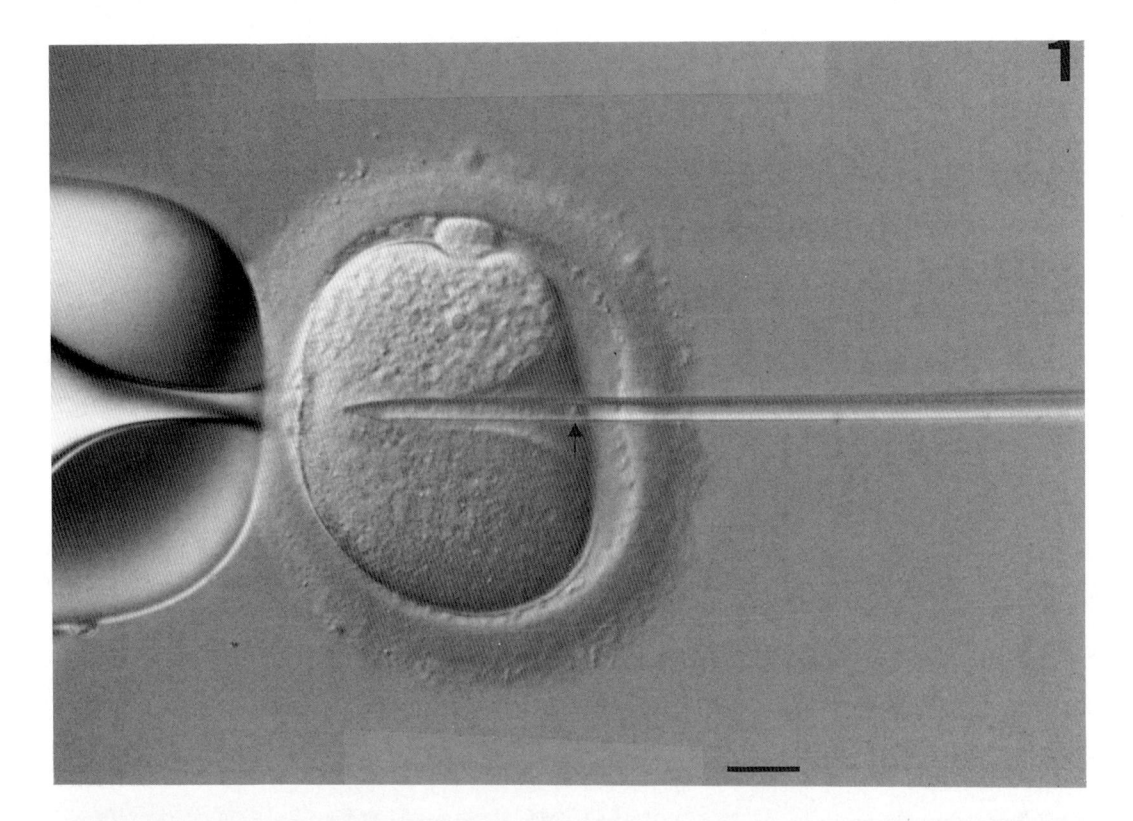

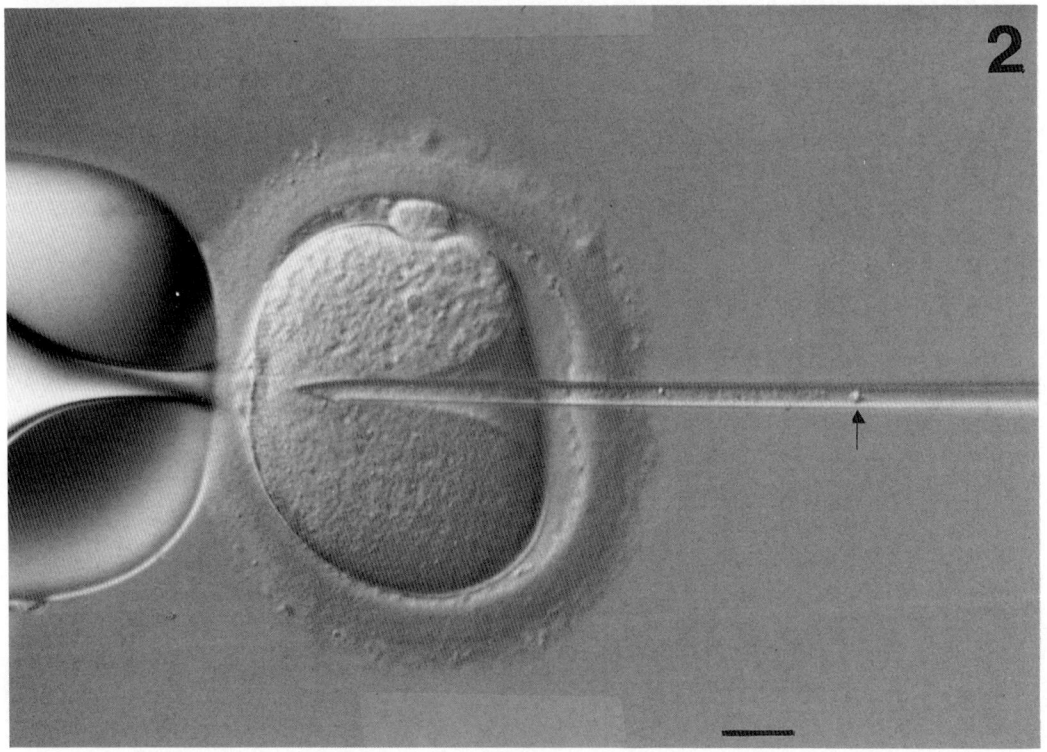

Figs 1 and 2. Modification of the injection technique. The placement of the sperm head and aspiration of oocyte cytoplasm is indicated with arrows. (**1**) Method 1: aspiration of cytoplasm to approximately the edge of the zona pellucida. (**2**) Method 2: aspiration of the cytoplasm is continued until the sperm head can be seen well past the level of the zona pellucida. Bars, 25 μm.

Table 1. Fertilization and pregnancy rates for the intracytoplasmic sperm injection (ICSI) programme at Monash IVF

Method 1 was the initial injection procedure whereas the injection procedure was altered in Method 2. EPU, egg pick up; ET, embryo transfer; M II, metaphase II; PN, pronuclei

	Overall	Method 1	Method 2
No. of patients	156	102	66
No. of cycles	171	105	66
No. of oocytes collected	1813	1172	641
No. of M II oocytes injected	1492	979	513
No. of 2 PN fertilized oocytes	711 (47·7%)	336 (34·3%)^A	375 (73·1%)^A
No. of 3 PN fertilized oocytes	21 (1·4%)	10 (1·0%)	11 (2·1%)
No. of degenerate eggs	65 (4·4%)	42 (4·3%)	23 (4·5%)
Day 2 cleavage rate	94·9%	93·5%	96·3%
No. of cycles with fertilization	152 (88·9%)	87 (82·9%)^A	65 (98·4%)^A
No. of ETs	148 (86·5%)	86 (81·9%)^B	62 (93·9%)^B
No. of cycles with frozen embryos	21 (12·2%)	9 (8·6%)	12 (18·2%)
No. of embryos frozen	61	29	32
No. of embryos transferred	370	207	163
Average no. embryos per ET	2·1	1·9	2·5
No. of pregnancies (clinical)	29 (26)	14 (12)	15 (14)
Pregnancy rate per EPU	17·0%	13·3%	22·7%
Pregnancy rate per cycle	19·6%	16·3%	24·2%
Clinical pregnancy rate per ET	17·6%	11·4%	21·2%
Implantation rate per embryo	8·1%	6·8%	9·8%

^{A} χ^2-test, Method 2 is significantly different from Method 1, $P < 0·01$.
^{B} χ^2-test, Method 2 is significantly different from Method 1, $P < 0·05$.

Table 2. Results for 11 patients who had a cycle before (Method 1) and after (Method 2) modification of the injection technique

EPU, egg pick up; ET, embryo transfer; M II, metaphase II; PN, pronuclei

	Method 1	Method 2
No. of cycles	11	11
No. of oocytes collected	105	113
No. of M II oocytes injected	82	86
No. of 2 PN fertilized oocytes	20 (24·4%)^A	65 (75·6%)^A
Cycles with fertilization	72·7%	100%
No. of embryos transferred	18	29
Average no. embryos per ET	1·6	2·6
Pregnancy rate per EPU	0	18·2%
No. of clinical pregnancies	0	1
Clinical pregnancy rate per ET	—	9·1%

^{A} χ^2-test, Method 2 is significantly different from Method 1, $P < 0·01$.

Injected oocytes were washed in a small volume of HTF containing 10% HS and then transferred to 25 μL drops of HTF containing 10% HS overlaid with mineral oil (Sigma) and incubated for a further 18–20 h at 37°C in an atmosphere of 5% CO_2, 5% O_2 and 90% N_2. Oocytes were examined for evidence of normal fertilization based on the presence of two pronuclei (PN) and the second polar body. Two pronuclear oocytes were subsequently evaluated for embryo cleavage after a further 24 h in culture. A maximum of 3 embryos which had cleaved and developed normally to 2–8 cells were selected for transfer to the uterine cavity, usually 48 h after microinjection. Supernumerary embryos which were morphologically normal were cryopreserved in propanediol by a slow freezing protocol (Lassalle et al. 1985).

Pregnancy Assessment

Pregnancy was confirmed by the detection of a positive serum hCG concentration (> 20 I.U. L^{-1}) on Day 16 after embryo transfer. Clinical pregnancies, defined by the presence of a gestational sac, were confirmed by ultrasound at 6 weeks gestation.

Statistical Analysis

Fertilization and pregnancy rates for method 1 and method 2 were compared by χ^2 analysis using the MINITAB statistical package 9·0 (Minitab, State College, Pennsylvania, USA). $P < 0·05$ was taken to indicate a significant difference.

Results

ICSI Results

The overall results of the programme, along with the separate results for Methods 1 and 2, are presented in Table 1. The impact of the methodological change is apparent from the significant increases in the normal (2 PN) fertilization rate ($P < 0·01$), the percentage of cycles in which fertilization occurred ($P < 0·01$) and

Table 3. Fertilization and pregnancy rates for patients with severe oligoasthenozoospermia

Method 1 was the initial injection procedure whereas the injection procedure was altered in Method 2. EPU, egg pick up; ET, embryo transfer; M II, metaphase II; PN, pronuclei

	Overall	Method 1	Method 2
No. of patients	65	49	20
No. of cycles	72	52	20
No. of oocytes collected	733	559	174
No. of M II oocytes injected	609	464	145
Fertilization (2 PN) rate	45.3%	36.2%[A]	74.5%[A]
No. of ETs	65 (90.3%)	45 (86.5%)	20 (100%)
No. of embryos transferred	161	107	54
Average no. embryos per ET	2.2	2.0	2.7
Pregnancy rate per EPU	20.8%	15.4%	35.0%
Pregnancy rate per ET	23.1%	17.8%	35.0%
No. of clinical pregnancies	13	7	6
Clinical pregnancy rate per ET	20.0%	15.6%	30.0%
Implantation rate per embryo	9.9%	7.5%	14.8%

[A] χ^2-test, Method 2 is significantly different from Method 1, $P < 0.01$.

Table 4. Intracytoplasmic sperm injection (ICSI) fertilization and pregnancy rates for patients who had previously experienced failed or poor fertilization in one or more conventional in vitro fertilization (IVF) cycles

Method 1 was the initial injection procedure whereas the injection procedure was altered in Method 2. EPU, egg pick up; ET, embryo transfer; M II, metaphase II; PN, pronuclei

	Overall	Method 1	Method 2
No. of patients	70	39	37
No. of cycles	76	39	37
No. of oocytes collected	816	434	382
No. of M II oocytes injected	653	355	298
Fertilization (2 PN) rate	51.2%	30.1%[A]	76.2%[A]
No. of ETs	63 (82.8%)	29 (74.4%)[B]	34 (91.9%)[B]
No. of embryos transferred	162	71	91
Average no. embryos per ET	2.1	1.7	2.4
Pregnancy rate per EPU	13.2%	7.7%	18.9%
Pregnancy rate per ET	15.9%	10.3%	20.6%
No. of clinical pregnancies	9	2	7
Clinical pregnancy rate per ET	14.3%	6.9%	20.6%
Implantation rate per embryo	5.5%	2.8%	7.7%

[A] χ^2-test, Method 2 is significantly different from Method 1, $P < 0.01$.
[B] χ^2-test, Method 2 is significantly different from Method 1, $P < 0.05$.

the embryo transfer rate ($P < 0.05$). The change in technique did not result in an increase in the oocyte degeneration rate. The apparent increases in the mean number of cycles with embryos frozen, the number of embryos transferred and the pregnancy rate did not reach statistical significance. The implantation rates of embryos produced using Methods 1 and 2 were similar.

Eleven patients underwent sequential ICSI treatment cycles using Methods 1 and 2 (Table 2) and a threefold improvement in the fertilization rate was observed ($P < 0.01$) with Method 2. Three of these patients initially failed to achieve fertilization with Method 1, but with a subsequent cycle using Method 2, fertilization and an embryo transfer was obtained. Pregnancies occurred in association with this improvement in fertilization rate.

Different patient subgroups also demonstrated significant improvements ($P < 0.01$) in their overall fertilization rates when the injection technique was modified. In the severe oligoasthenozoospermic group, fertilization rates using Method 2 were twice those of Method 1 (Table 3). In the group with a previous history of poor fertilization, significant improvements in fertilization ($P < 0.01$) and embryo transfer rates ($P < 0.05$) were achieved (Table 4).

Results from the oligoasthenozoospermic sub-group with virtual azoospermia, and from the other patient groups are shown in Table 5. The small number of treatment cycles in each group precludes division of the data according to the ICSI method employed. Fertilization and embryo transfer rates for these groups were similar to those in the total oligoasthenozoospermic and poor fertilization groups and pregnancies occurred in all groups except the testicular sperm group.

Table 5. Fertilization and pregnancy rates for different male factor infertility patient sub-groups

EPU, egg pick up; ET, embryo transfer; M II, metaphase II; PN, pronuclei

	Virtual azoospermia	Testicular sperm	Epididymal sperm	Sperm antibodies	Ejaculation problems[A]
No. of patients	13	2	5	10	4
No. of cycles	14	2	5	12	4
No. of oocytes collected	145	9	49	161	45
No. of M II oocytes injected	113	7	43	140	40
Fertilization (2 PN) rate	42·5%	28·6%	30·2%	46·4%	52·5%
Cycles with fertilization	92·9%	100%	100%	91·7%	100%
Cycles with ET	92·9%	100%	60%	91·7%	100%
No. of embryos transferred	32	2	7	28	10
Average no. embryos per ET	2·3	1·0	1·4	2·3	2·5
Pregnancy rate per EPU	14·3%	0	20·0%	16·7%	25·0%
Pregnancy rate per ET	15·4%	0	33·3%	18·2%	25·0%
Clinical pregnancy rate per ET	15·4%	—	33·3%	18·2%	25·0%
Implantation rate per embryo	6·3%	—	28·6%	7·1%	10·0%

[A] Retrograde ejaculation or electro-ejaculation cases.

The majority of supernumerary embryos did not meet the criteria for freezing (Table 1). The freezing rate was similar for embryos in the severely oligozoospermic (15%) and failed fertilization groups (23%). Embryos were available for cryopreservation in 21 patients, and to date, five patients have undergone transfer of 1–3 embryos with one pregnancy resulting. This pregnancy has been excluded from the pregnancy outcome data below.

Pregnancy Outcomes

In 26 of the 29 patients who showed a positive β-HCG at Day 16 post-EPU, clinical pregnancy was confirmed by ultrasound at 6 weeks gestation. A single gestational sac was seen in 21 (81%), 2 sacs were observed in 2 (8%) and three sacs was found in one (4%). There was one blighted ovum and one ectopic pregnancy. Pregnancy loss has subsequently occurred in the first trimester in two of the 24 patients with uterine pregnancies and in one patient at 20 weeks gestation. Chromosomal analysis of the products of conception was only obtained for the second trimester miscarriage and revealed trisomy 2. The spontaneous reduction of a twin to a singleton pregnancy occurred after the 12th week in one patient.

To date, 7 patients have delivered 6 singletons and 1 twin, comprising 4 girls and 4 boys, all of which were normal. Fourteen patients have ongoing pregnancies and are now beyond week 30. The overall pregnancy loss rate after the detection of β-HCG was 27·6%.

Discussion

We report the significant impact on our clinical ICSI results of a single technical modification, namely the modification of oocyte cytoplasm aspiration immediately before sperm injection. We attribute our recent improvement in ICSI results to the more vigorous aspiration of the oocyte cytoplasm. Although not proven, we deduce that the previous procedure (Method 1), although performed in a similar manner to the method of Van Steirteghem et al. (1993a, 1993b), was resulting in the frequent deposition of sperm within oolemmal fragments or outside the oolemma in the perivitelline space. In agreement with Van Steirteghem et al. (1993a, 1993b), we now find that ICSI has broad application to ejaculated sperm of any quality as well as to testicular and epididymal sperm.

In the current study, patients were initially managed with an ICSI technique which we thought closely followed that described by Palermo et al. (1993) and Van Steirteghem et al. (1993a, 1993b). This included the aspiration of a small amount of egg cytoplasm to ensure that the spermatozoon was released within the egg cytoplasm. In comparison with their published results, however, we were disappointed to achieve fertilization rates of only 34% but noted that our cleavage rates were similar (> 90%) and that our oocyte degeneration rates were not elevated. We interpreted this to indicate that our injection technique was not unduly traumatic on the oocytes and that the resultant embryos were of acceptable quality. However, the low fertilization rate suggested that sperm delivery into the oocyte was inadequate.

In discussions on our ICSI technique, it was suggested that aspiration of the oocyte cytoplasm immediately before sperm injection should be more vigorous to ensure that the spermatozoon was released into the cytoplasm (D. Payne, personal communication). Using this second procedure (Method 2), we observed immediate improvements in the fertilization rate, embryo yield and pregnancy rate in all groups. This conclusion was supported by the analysis of patients undergoing sequential treatments with the two methods. Since the only significant modification was the injection procedure, we attribute the improved results to a more certain delivery of the spermatozoon into the ooplasm.

An improvement in ICSI success was achieved in the two principal patient groups, severe oligoasthenozoospermia and poor fertilization. The small number of patients in the other categories limits any conclusions regarding success, however their overall fertilization rates were similar to the oligozoospermic and failed fertilization groups and pregnancies occurred in all groups except testicular sperm. We have since achieved a pregnancy using testicular sperm obtained by fine needle biopsy (data not shown). The ICSI technique is particularly applicable to cryopreserved epididymal sperm and permits multiple treatments from a single surgical sperm retrieval. The overall success of ICSI must take into account the impact of both freshly transferred and cryopreserved embryos. In our programme we initially transfer up to three of the best embryos and we have found that the majority of non-transferred embryos fail to meet our criteria for cryopreservation. As a result, the contribution of the cryopreserved embryos (18% of cycles) to our pregnancy rate is limited.

In terms of pregnancy outcomes, the pregnancy loss rate between the initial detection of hCG and the observation of a gestational sac at 6 weeks has been similar to that of our general IVF population. The loss of pregnancies after the detection of a gestational sac has also been similar to that expected for the general IVF population (Lancaster 1993). The validity of these conclusions will be tested when a larger data set is available. The rate of singleton and multiple pregnancies in our ICSI programme after the transfer of 2–3 embryos has also been similar to other IVF patient groups.

We observed one pregnancy loss associated with a trisomy 2 fetus. Although the Brussels group has reported a larger series of normal fetal karyotypes (Bonduelle et al. 1994), it seems prudent to continue to recommend amniocentesis or chorionic villous biopsy for the immediate future. It is of interest that, although all our patients are asked to consider these investigations, very few (< 5%) decided to undertake these procedures.

Since commencing ICSI in late 1993, we have had a total of 11 (10 singleton, 1 twin) live births from our ICSI programme, all of which have been normal. We believe that all aspects of the health and development of ICSI children should be closely monitored. Furthermore, we believe that this would be best achieved by national and international collaborative efforts.

In summary, we have found that the success of ICSI can be greatly enhanced by attention to the technique of ooplasm aspiration prior to sperm injection, thereby producing excellent fertilization rates. A greater knowledge of the less common male factor groups is required to determine whether differences in sperm characteristics have any bearing on ICSI success.

References

Bonduelle, M., Desmyttere, S., Buysse A., Van Assche, E., Schietecatte, J., Devroey, P., Van Steirteghem, A.C., and Liebaers, I. (1994). Prospective follow-up study of 55 children born after subzonal insemination and intracytoplasmic sperm injection. *Hum. Reprod. (Oxf.)* **9**, 1765–9.

Fishel, S., Jackson, P., Antinori, S., Johnson, J., Grossi, S., and Versaci, C. (1990). Subzonal insemination for the alleviation of infertility. *Fertil. Steril.* **54**, 828–35.

Lancaster, P. (1993). 'Assisted Conception Australia and New Zealand 1991'. (AIHW National Perinatal Statistics Unit, Fertility Society of Australia: Sydney.)

Lassalle, B., Testart, J., and Renard, J.-P. (1985). Human embryo features that influence the success of cryopreservation with the use of 1, 2 propanediol. *Fertil. Steril.* **44**, 645–51.

Lippi, J., Mortimer, D., and Jansen, R.P.S. (1993). Sub-zonal insemination for extreme male factor infertility. *Hum. Reprod. (Oxf.)* **8**, 908–15.

Mallidis, C., and Baker, H.W.G. (1994). Fine needle tissue aspiration biopsy of the testis. *Fertil. Steril.* **61**, 367–75.

Ng, S.-C., Bongso, A., Ratnam, S.S., Sathananthan, H., Chan, C.L.K., Wong, P.C., Hagglund, L., Anandakumar, C., Wong, Y.C., and Goh, V.H.H. (1988). Pregnancy after transfer of sperm under the zona. *Lancet* **2**, 790.

Osborn, J.C., Yates, C.A., Southwick G.J., Kovacs, G., Downing, B., Temple-Smith, P.D., and Wood, E.C. (1991). Pregnancy following intra-Fallopian insemination of spermatozoa from a male with obstructive azoospermia. *Hum. Reprod. (Oxf.)* **6**, 367–8.

Palermo, G., Joris, H., Derde, M.-P., Camus, M., Devroey, P., and Van Steirteghem, A. (1993). Sperm characteristics and outcome of human assisted fertilization by subzonal insemination and intracytoplasmic sperm injection. *Fertil. Steril.* **59**, 826–35.

Quinn, P., Kerin, J.F., and Warnes, G.M. (1985). Improved pregnancy rate in human *in vitro* fertilization with the use of a medium based on the composition of human tubal fluid. *Fertil. Steril.* **44**, 493–8.

Van Steirteghem, A.C., Liu, J., Joris, H., Nagy, Z., Janssenswillen, C., Tournaye, H., Derde, M.-P., Van Assche, E., and Devroey, P. (1993*a*). Higher success rate by intracytoplasmic sperm injection than by subzonal insemination. Report of a second series of 300 consecutive treatment cycles. *Hum. Reprod. (Oxf.)* **8**, 1055–60.

Van Steirteghem, A.C., Nagy, Z., Joris, H., Liu, J., Staessen, C., Smitz, J., Wisanto, A., and Devroey, P. (1993*b*). High fertilization and implantation rates after intracytoplasmic sperm injection. *Hum. Reprod. (Oxf.)* **8**, 1061–6.

Van Steirteghem, A., Liu, J., Joris, H., Nagy, Z., Staessen, C., Camus, M., Wisanto, A., Van Assche, E., and Devroey, P. (1994). Assisted fertilization by subzonal insemination and intracytoplasmic sperm injection. In 'The Infertile Male: Advanced Assisted Reproductive Technology'. *Reprod. Fertil. Dev.* **6**, 85–91.

World Health Organization (1992). 'Laboratory Manual for the Examination of Human Semen and Sperm–Cervical Mucus Interaction.' 3rd Edn. (Cambridge University Press: Cambridge.)

Manuscript received 20 February 1995

Clinical Intracytoplasmic Sperm Injection (ICSI) Results from Royal North Shore Hospital

James W. Catt[AB], John P. Ryan[A], Ian L. Pike[A], Chris O'Neill and Douglas M. Saunders

Human Reproduction Unit, Royal North Shore Hospital, St Leonards, NSW 2065, Australia.
[A] *Present address: North Shore ART, Clinic 20, Royal North Shore Hospital, St Leonards, NSW 2065, Australia.*
[B] *To whom correspondence should be addressed.*

Abstract. The technique of intracytoplasmic sperm injection (ICSI) was first introduced to the Royal North Shore Hospital in April 1993 as part of a controlled study of 100 patient cycles in which sibling oocytes were inseminated by either subzonal insemination (SUZI) or ICSI. This trial showed direct sperm injection to be superior in terms of fertilization. In that study, 58 embryo transfers of 101 ICSI-derived embryos resulted in 10 pregnancies. No miscarriages have occurred and a total of 10 fetal hearts (9·8% per embryo transferred) were detected on ultrasound. There have been 10 deliveries of 10 babies. Since the beginning of 1994, intracytoplasmic injection has been used exclusively for patients requiring micromanipulation to achieve fertilization. There have been 200 patient cycles with 1650 oocytes collected (8·8 oocytes per cycle). Of these oocytes, 1548 were mature (94%) and were subjected to ICSI, and normal fertilization occurred in 874 (56%) of the injected oocytes. The number of oocytes which cleaved and were suitable for fresh transfer or cryopreservation was 818 (94%). There have been 153 fresh embryo transfers of 326 embryos. Twenty-six pregnancies (17% per embryo transfer) have resulted, 22 of which proceeded to ultrasound examination in which 23 fetal hearts were detected (7% per embryo transferred). Three miscarriages have occurred, leaving 19 ongoing pregnancies. There have been 127 cryopreservation procedures involving 492 embryos. To date, there have been 47 embryo thaw cycles, and 93 of the 115 (81%) thawed embryos survived and were transferred. These 47 embryo transfers resulted in 10 pregnancies (21% per embryo transfer), one of which one has miscarried. All 9 ongoing pregnancies are singletons (9·7% fetal hearts per embryo transferred).

Extra keywords: fertilization, male infertility, SUZI.

Introduction

The idea and practicalities of injecting a single spermatozoon directly into the cytoplasm of a human oocyte, as a method of alleviating male factor infertility, has been investigated for a number of years (Lanzendorf *et al.* 1988; Ng *et al.* 1991). Palermo *et al.* (1992, 1993) and Van Steirteghem *et al.* (1993*a*, 1993*b*), showed that high fertilization rates could be achieved with intracytoplasmic sperm injection (ICSI) in the majority of cases and implantation rates were as high as conventional *in vitro* fertilization (IVF). Several other groups have used this methodology, one with equal success (Redgment *et al.* 1994), whereas others have achieved lower fertilization and implantation rates (Tucker *et al.* 1993; Fishel *et al.* 1994).

Against this background and the reported success rates with subzonal insemination (SUZI) (Cohen *et al.* 1991; Catt *et al.* 1994*a*), ICSI was first introduced to Royal North Shore Hospital in April 1993 as part of a controlled study comparing the fertilization and developmental potential of embryos generated by SUZI and ICSI. This study was completed in eight months and ICSI alone has been used since that time. During the past eighteen months, we have performed several investigations and refined our methodology and report these together with our overall results.

Materials and Methods

Patient Selection

Patients were categorized according to previous fertilization history or the results of semen analysis. Patients in one category had a history of failed or low (<15%) fertilization with conventional IVF (with a minimum of 10 oocytes). Patients in a second category had sperm parameters (after preparation for assisted reproductive techniques) of less than 1×10^6 motile, morphologically normal sperm (World Health Organization 1992). Our clinical experience has shown that these patients have a poor prognosis with IVF. A final group of patients were those from whom insufficient normal, motile sperm could be collected for any procedure. This group included severe oligozoospermic, complete asthenozoospermic, globozoospermic and testicular biopsy patients.

Ovarian Stimulation and Oocyte Recovery

All patients were given individualized, short gonadotrophin-releasing hormone agonist 'flare' stimulation protocols. Cumulus–oocyte complexes were recovered by transvaginal follicle aspiration and transferred to human tubal fluid (HTF) medium (Quinn et al. 1985), supplemented with 10% homologous serum (culture medium). The cumulus–oocyte complexes were treated with 300 I.U. mL^{-1} of hyaluronidase (Type VIII; Sigma, St Louis, MO, USA) about 3–5 h after recovery and aspirated through narrow pipettes to remove the cumulus cells. An oocyte was stripped of cumulus within 1 min. The denuded oocytes were kept in culture medium in an incubator (5% CO_2 in air).

Immature oocytes possessing a germinal vesicle were kept separate for further study, and those oocytes which did not exhibit a polar body (presumptive metaphase I oocytes) were injected last.

Sperm Preparation

After liquefaction, the sperm were separated on a two-step (45% and 87%) discontinuous Percoll density gradient. Sperm were harvested from the 87% fraction and were washed twice in culture medium by centrifugation (300g, 10 min). The final pellet was resuspended in a minimal volume of medium, and then underlaid beneath 0·2 mL of culture medium. The sperm were allowed to swim-up for 2 h. If the sperm concentration following this swim-up was $<5 \times 10^5$ mL^{-1} then the supernatant was centrifuged (3000g, 1 min) and the pellet was resuspended in 10 μL of HTF.

Polyvinylpyrrolidone (PVP) (PVP-360; Sigma) was used to retard sperm motility (Thadani 1980). A 10% (w/v) solution of PVP was extensively dialyzed against water to remove low molecular weight toxic components and the osmolarity of the dialysate was adjusted to 285±5 mOsm kg^{-1} using a 10×concentrated stock of HTF, and the concentrated PVP was adjusted to 8% with HTF. The sperm suspension was diluted 1:1 with this PVP solution.

Micromanipulation

A Nikon Diaphot inverted microscope (Nikon Instrument, Tokyo, Japan) equipped with Hoffman modulation contrast optics (Modulation Optics, Greenvale, NY, USA) was used for all manipulations. Injection pipettes were made from thin walled capillary glass (without a microfilament) which had an outer diameter (OD) of 1 mm and an inner diameter (ID) of 0·78 mm (GC100T-15; Clark Electromedical Instruments, Pangbourne, UK) using a P-87 pipette puller (Sutter Instrument, Novato, CA, USA). The two-stage programme pulled shallow tapered pipettes and these were cut to the correct diameter (6–7 μm OD, 5 μm ID) using a scalpel blade under a dissecting microscope. The pipettes were bevelled to 35–40° using an EG-9 wet grinding system (Narishige Instrument, Tokyo, Japan) and the tips were washed by aspirating boiling water. A bend was introduced 1–2 mm back from the bevel, to allow access to the manipulation droplets, and the pipettes were then dry heat sterilized before use.

Both the holding and injection pipettes were attached to Hamilton 0·5 mL screw-threaded plunger syringes via vinyl tubing which had previously been filled with light paraffin oil, to provide the necessary manipulating pressures. More recently, Fluorinert FC-40 (Sigma) has been used to completely fill the tubing and the tools, giving a more complete control over the operating pressures in the system. Manipulation was carried out in droplets (10–20 μL) of HTF on a 9 cm Petri dish lid, under heavy grade paraffin oil (BDH, Poole, UK). A central drop contained the sperm preparation and single oocytes were placed in peripheral drops. The paraffin oil had been pre-equilibrated for at least 5 days by incubating 40 mL of the oil over 10 mL of HTF in a CO_2 incubator.

Typically, a motile spermatozoon was selected, incised, aspirated into and then moved to the tip of the pipette. The incision of the sperm was carried out by lowering the injection pipette onto the sperm tail and swiping across it, causing it to bend at right angles to the longitudinal axis (see also the incision trial in the results section). This invariably immobilized the spermatozoon, enabling it to be aspirated into the injection pipette.

The oocyte was positioned on the holding pipette so that the polar body was orientated at 12 o'clock or 6 o'clock. This was so that the introduction of the injection pipette would be sufficiently distant from the metaphase II spindle to minimize any possible damage. To ensure cytoplasmic injection, back pressure was used to aspirate the oocyte cytoplasm into the injection pipette, until the cytoplasm moved freely past the sperm. This was found to be fundamental for successful injection. Intact cytoplasm could often be drawn >100 μm into the pipette before the oolemma ruptured. Up to 6 oocytes were injected in the same dish, usually in under 10 min, then returned to culture.

Fertilization Assessment and Zygote Culture

Injected oocytes were examined for second polar body abstriction and pronuclear formation using the Diaphot inverted microscope. Oocytes were examined at 16–18 h after insemination. After a further 24 h in culture, suitable cleaved embryos were either replaced by uterine transfer or cryopreserved. A maximum of two embryos were replaced in any one transfer, unless the patient had a history of at least three embryo transfer procedures without a pregnancy or the patient was over the age of 38.

Cryopreservation and Thawing

Cryopreservation of embryos was by a slow-freeze method based on that of Lassalle et al. (1985) using propanediol (PROH). Embryos were frozen two days post-insemination. Only those embryos with ≤30% fragmentation were cryopreserved. All media were supplemented with 10% homologous patient serum. Embryos were frozen individually in 0·25-mL straws (IMV, L'Aigle, France). Embryos were slow thawed individually and those with ≥50% intact blastomeres were transferred, on the same day as the thaw. The majority of embryos were transferred in natural, monitored cycles.

Patient Monitoring

In the absence of menses 18 days after embryo transfer, a urinary β-human chorionic gonadotrophin (hCG) pregnancy test was conducted. An ultrasound examination was conducted three weeks after a positive β-hCG test, to confirm the presence of a gestational sac and determine the number of fetal hearts.

Results

Clinical Results for the SUZI versus ICSI Sibling Oocyte Trial

The overall results of this trial are shown in Table 1. A detailed account of these results is given in Catt et al. (1995). There were four trials within this study, designed not only to compare SUZI with ICSI, but to define some of the injection parameters during the ICSI procedure. These are summarized in Fig. 1, where for ease of interpretation, some of the results from the trials have been combined. From this data it is clear that incision of the sperm tail resulted in an increase in the ICSI fertilization rate from 27% to 46% (χ^2-test, $P < 0.05$).

Table 1. Overall results for the subzonal insemination (SUZI) v. intracytoplasmic sperm injection (ICSI) sibling oocyte trial

Data from Catt et al. (1994b). PN, pronuclei; s.e.m., standard error of the mean

	SUZI	ICSI
No. of oocytes inseminated or injected	408	451
No. of normally fertilized oocytes (2 PN)	78 (19%)	183 (36%)
No. of embryos transferred or cryopreserved[A]	70 (89%)	166 (91%)
No. of embryo transfer procedures	27	58
Mean ±s.e.m. no. of embryos transferred	1·6±0·3	1·7±0·2
No. of pregnancies	4	10
Pregnancy rate per embryo transfer	15%	17·2%
No. of fetal hearts	4	10
Fetal heart rate per embryo transferred	9·3%	9·9%

[A] Values in parentheses are percentages of the normally fertilized oocytes.

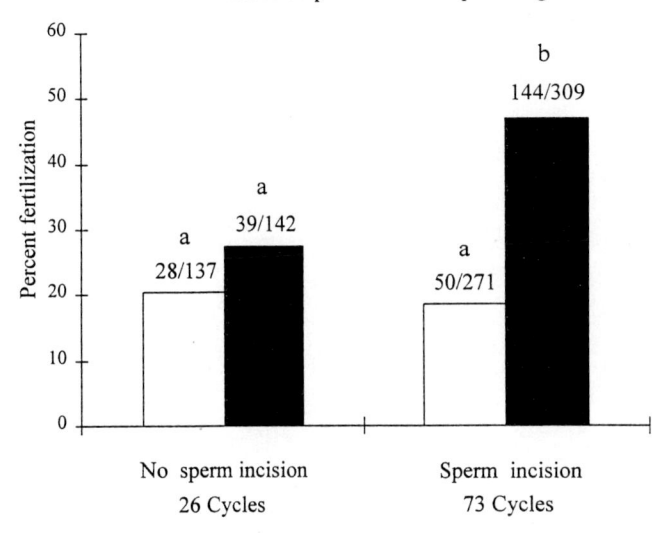

Fig. 1. Overall results of the SUZI trial (□) v. ICSI trial (■). Columns with different letters are significantly different. The numbers in the columns are the number of oocytes fertilized out of those injected.

The ten singleton ICSI pregnancies resulting from this trial (9·9% fetal hearts per embryo transferred) have all gone to term resulting in 6 female and 4 male babies. One male baby has a pansystolic heart murmur, a major congenital defect. All the others are normal and are part of an ongoing assessment programme.

Clinical Results for ICSI-only Cycles (from January 1994)

The results are presented in Tables 2, 3 and 4. The majority of oocytes recovered (94%) were mature (as judged by the first polar body abstriction) and these were inseminated 4–8 h after retrieval. Fertilization occurred in 188 of 200 patient cycles or 94% of the oocyte retrievals (OPU). The overall fertilization rate of injected oocytes was 56% (874/1548) and the overall degeneration rate was 13% (203/1548). The rate of normal fertilization did not increase over time but was variable, with lower fertilization rates and higher degeneration rates typically reflected in the training of new operators (Fig. 2).

Occasionally, immediate lysis was evident and tended to group around particular batches of oocytes. There may be cohorts of oocytes that are more susceptible to immediate lysis, despite precautions being taken such as the changing of microtools, manipulation media and personnel. Other cohorts inseminated on the same day showed no such degeneration. Underlying factors such as ovarian stimulation, the number of oocytes obtained and the percentage of mature oocytes did not correlate with degeneration (data not shown). Abnormal fertilization was a relatively rare occurrence (Table 2). Oocytes with one, three or more pronuclei comprised 3% of the injected oocytes.

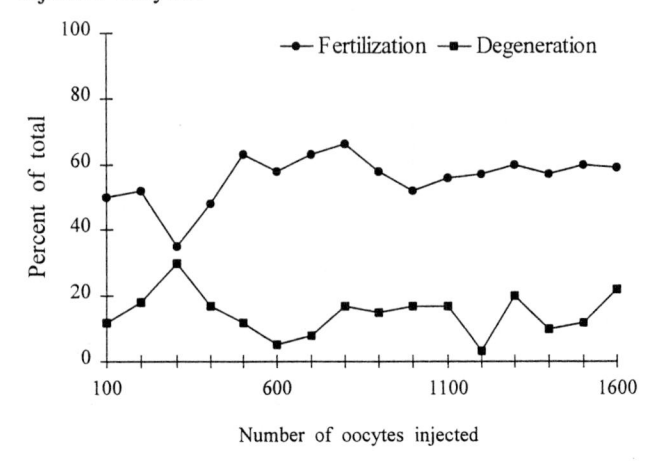

Fig. 2. Overall fertilization results (●) and degeneration results (■) after ICSI. The data are plotted for groups of 100 oocytes.

The cleavage rate for the normally fertilized zygotes was 97% (848/874) and 96% of these cleaved zygotes (818/848) were suitable for transfer or cryopreservation (Table 3). Transfer of fresh embryos occurred in 81% of patients (153/188) who had achieved fertilization. There were 153 transfer procedures utilizing 326 embryos, resulting in 26 elevated urinary β-hCG levels (biochemical pregnancy rate of 17% per embryo transfer). Ultrasound confirmed 22 of these pregnancies (with 23 fetal hearts) to give 7% fetal hearts per embryo transferred. A further

Table 2. Overall fertilization data for intracytoplasmic sperm injection (ICSI) at Royal North Shore Hospital

PN, pronuclei

No. of patients	152
No. of cycles	200
No. of oocytes collected	1650
No. of mature oocytes	1548 (94%)
No. of successfully injected oocytes[A]	1345 (87%)
Degeneration rate	13%
No. of normally fertilized oocytes (2 PN)	874
Normal fertilization rate per injected oocyte	56%
Normal fertilization rate per successfully injected oocyte	65%
No. of 'haploid' fertilized oocytes (1 PN)[A]	34 (2%)
No. of 'polyploid' fertilized oocytes ($\geq$3 PN)[A]	14 (1%)
No. of cycles with normally fertilized oocytes	188

[A] Values in parentheses are percentages of the mature oocytes.

Table 3. Fate of oocytes fertilized by intracytoplasmic sperm injection (ICSI)

hCG, human chorionic gonadotrophin

No. of cleaved zygotes[A]	848 (97%)
No. of embryos transferred or frozen[B]	818 (96%)
Useable embryos per injected oocyte	53%
No. of embryo transfer procedures	153
No. of embryos transferred	326
Mean no. of embryos transferred (range)	2·1 (1–3)
No. of pregnancies (positive β-hCG)	26
Pregnancy rate (β-hCG) per embryo transfer	17%
No. of fetal hearts detected by ultrasound	23 (1 set of twins)
No. of subsequent miscarriages	3
Fetal heart rate per embryo transferred	7%
No. of ongoing pregnancies	19

[A] Value in parentheses is the percentage of the fertilized oocytes.
[B] Value in parentheses is the percentage of the cleaved zygotes.

three of these pregnancies have since miscarried and there are 19 ongoing pregnancies from the fresh transfers.

Immature Oocytes

In a trial reported by Scuglia et al. (1994), injection of immature oocytes resulted in high rates of lysis and only occasional fertilization of presumptive metaphase I oocytes. No germinal vesicle stage oocytes were fertilized, although a small number (13% of those injected) did undergo apparent maturation and first polar body abstriction.

Cytological Examination of Abnormal Oocytes

A study was conducted to cytologically examine a series of oocytes that did not exhibit two pronuclei. Details of the experimental procedures have been presented elsewhere (Catt et al. 1994b). The results are shown in Fig. 3, and suggest that most oocytes failed to fertilize because the sperm was not correctly injected into the cytoplasm. Oocytes visually assessed as having one pronucleus were found to be haploid or they exhibited delayed male pronuclear formation and failed to develop further. Half of the oocytes assessed as polyploid were triploid and showed evidence of failure of second polar body abstriction (spindle fibres joining two of the pronuclei). Other polyploid oocytes showed multiple foci of decondensing chromatin, indicating metaphase spindle disruption and oocyte activation.

Sperm Incision Trial

The degree of sperm manipulation (incision) before injection was investigated in two trials of 8 and 11 patient cycles. For the first trial, half of the sibling oocytes (60) were injected using our standard conditions (swiping the sperm tail vigorously with the injection pipette) and the other oocytes (58) were injected with sperm that had not undergone any prior sperm manipulation. The second trial compared the standard method of tail swiping with minimal sperm manipulation (a light stroking of the tail along its longitudinal axis). The results are shown in Fig. 4. No differences in the fertilization rate were detected with sperm that had been manipulated before injection, but no manipulation resulted in a significant decrease in the fertilization rate (45% v. 64%, $P < 0.05$, χ^2-test).

the 492 embryos cryopreserved in 1994, 115 (23%) have been thawed and 93 (81%) survived. There were 47 embryo transfer procedures (mean 2·0±0·1 embryos per transfer). Ten pregnancies ensued, one miscarriage occurred and nine pregnancies are ongoing. These results give a pregnancy rate of 21% per embryo transfer and an implantation rate of 9·7% fetal hearts per embryo transferred.

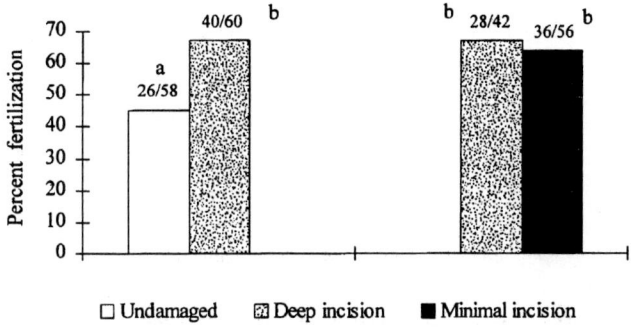

Fig. 4. Results of the sperm incision trial. Columns with different letters are significantly different. The numbers above the columns are the number of oocytes fertilized out of those injected.

Incidence of Failed Fertilization

Since the adoption of ICSI as our preferred method of manipulation, there have been 12 patient cycles with complete failure of normal fertilization. One cycle was abandoned because no sperm were found in three ejaculates on the day of oocyte collection. This patient had had a partially successful vasectomy reversal and his vas deferens had presumably occluded since the time of a previously successful ICSI attempt. Eight of the failed patient cycles had low numbers of oocytes collected, either 3 oocytes (2 cycles), 2 oocytes (3 cycles) or 1 oocyte (2 cycles), thus reducing the chances of successful injection. Another two patient cycles showed an abnormally high number of degenerate oocytes after injection. The reasons for this have been discussed above and may represent cohorts of susceptible oocytes. There was one other case of apparent fertilization failure in which 12 oocytes were inseminated, but at 16 and 24 h post-injection, there were no signs of pronuclear formation although most of the oocytes exhibited second polar body abstriction. After a further 24 h in culture, none of these oocytes showed any signs of fertilization or cleavage so they were fixed for cytological analysis. All the oocytes had 2 polar bodies with 2 internal areas of DNA condensation, reminiscent of early mitotic configurations. Our assumption was that the oocytes did not properly decondense the sperm heads and the meiotic plate on activation, but processed them through to two separate mitotic configurations. The sperm parameters for this patient were normal.

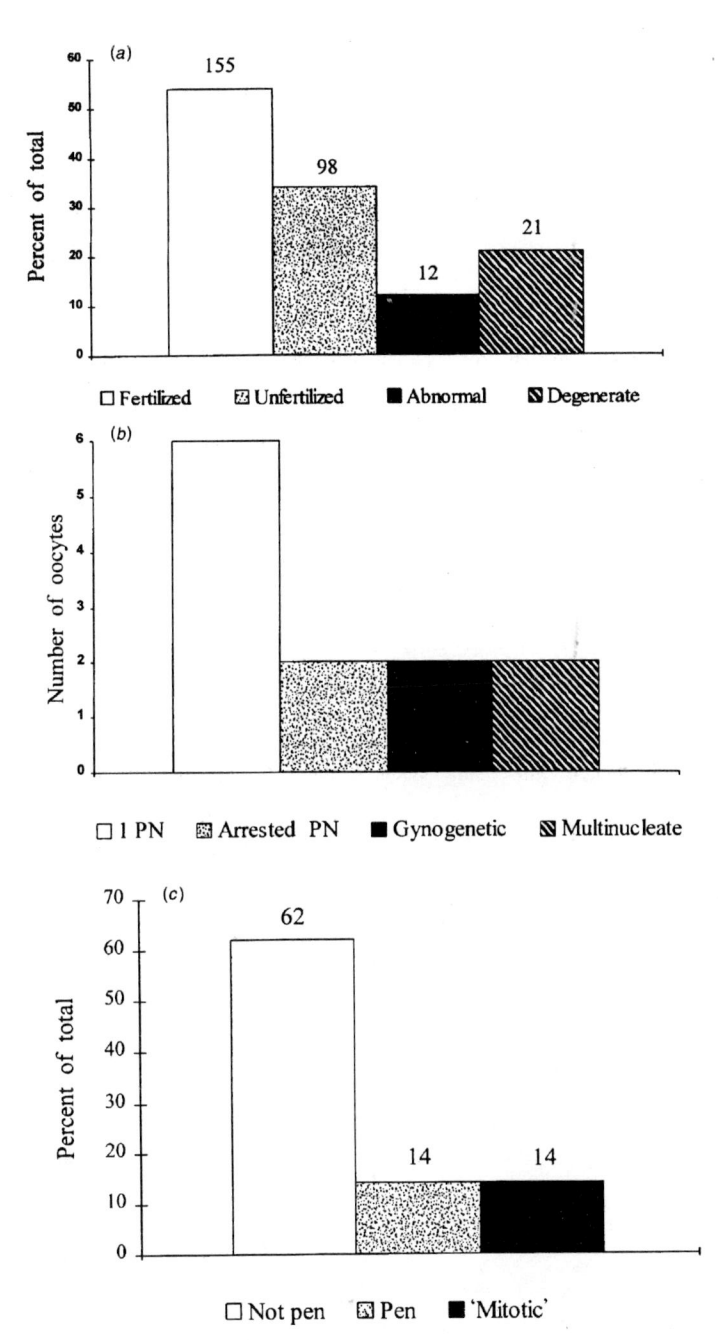

Fig. 3. (a) Fertilization data for 33 patient cycles (286 oocytes) in the failed or abnormal fertilization trial. (b) Cytology of 12 abnormally-fertilized oocytes. 1 PN, one pronucleus; arrested PN, normal female PN but retarded male PN; gynogenetic, failed second polar body abstriction giving 3 PN; multinucleate, multiple small PN-like structures. (c) Cytology of 90 oocytes which did not form 2 pronuclei. Not pen, no sperm penetration; Pen-not act, sperm found in cytoplasm but oocyte not activated; 'Mitotic', chromatin condensates in oocyte cytoplasm.

Cryopreservation and Thawing of ICSI Embryos

The results of embryo cryopreservation and thawing are shown in Table 4. To date there have been 127 cryopreservation procedures involving 492 embryos. Of

Table 4. Cryopreservation and frozen embryo transfer data
hCG, human chorionic gonadotrophin

No. of cryopreservation procedures	127
No. of embryos cryopreserved	492
No. of patients with all embryos frozen	35
No. of embryo thaws	47
No. of embryos thawed	115
No. of embryos surviving[A]	93 (81%)
No. of embryo transfers	47
No. of pregnancies (positive β-hCG)	10
Pregnancy rate (β-hCG) per embryo transfer	21%
No. of fetal hearts detected by ultrasound	9
Fetal heart rate per embryo thawed	7·8%
Fetal heart rate per embryo transferred	9·7%
No. of ongoing pregnancies	9

[A] Value in parentheses is the percentage of the thawed embryos.

Treatment of Specific Male Factor Groups

We have found no correlation between semen analysis results, fertilization and early embryonic development for those patients being referred to us for oligozoospermia, asthenozoospermia, teratozoospermia or poor results with IVF (data not shown), and pregnancies have been achieved in all groups of patients. We have observed a decreased fertilization rate for patients with globozoospermia, those requiring epididymal or testicular sperm recovery, or spinal injury patients requiring electro ejaculation. We have achieved pregnancies in almost all these patient types with the exception of testicular biopsy. The small number of cases in each group precludes meaningful analysis.

The Use of 'Live' and 'Dead' Immotile Sperm for ICSI

Fertilization is lower when immotile sperm are injected. We undertake to ensure that the sperm we inject have some degree of motility before incision and injection, but occasionally this is not possible. To date, we have had four cases in which the sperm were totally immotile and eosin red staining suggested less than 10% were viable. In all four of these cases, oocytes were injected with sperm selected on a morphology basis, as the hypo-osmotic swelling (HOS) test (World Health Organization 1992) did not yield any recognizable change in the sperm tail. The fertilization results from these patients were low (mean 26%, range 5–40%). Further work is needed to correlate the various parameters of sperm viability and the HOS test.

Discussion

The results presented here show that the Royal North Shore Hospital has a viable ICSI programme. Since the initiation of ICSI, our fertilization rate has steadily improved with continual monitoring and assessment of the programme. Micromanipulation programmes tend to be more fragile than conventional IVF programmes because of the increased handling and exposure to a greater variety of media, chemicals and temperature. Constant vigilance is therefore essential to keep the programme operational. A recent example of this was the identification of a batch of toxic paraffin oil used for covering media droplets, even though it had passed sperm longevity and mouse 2 cell culture tests. A more demanding mouse culture test (outbred pronucleate stage embryos grown in a glutamine and EDTA supplemented medium) indicated that the oil was toxic. Changing the batch of oil ended a sequence of 26 embryo transfers without a pregnancy.

The overall pregnancy rate of 17% per embryo transfer procedure may reflect our unit policy of transferring only two embryos. This policy has reduced the multiple pregnancy rate considerably, which is an obvious obstetric advantage. The success of the cryopreservation programme has increased our pregnancy rate per patient cycle and per patient treated. More time is needed to confirm this and ascertain the cumulative pregnancy rate per cycle.

We use a simple embryo grading system in the belief that pregnancies can ensue from most embryos, with the exception of those with >50% fragmentation. This grading system accounts for our high percentage of useable embryos (53% of oocytes injected) and may also explain our implantation rate of 7% per embryo transferred. Again, more time is needed for all the embryos to be transferred to give a true indication of the pregnancy potential of the embryos generated.

The manipulation of sperm before injection and the analysis of those oocytes which failed to fertilize suggest that a fertilization rate of 80% would be an achievable target in most cycles, with the exception of those in which immotile sperm were injected. The results obtained from ICSI around the world certainly justify its clinical use, but a more thorough understanding of the mechanisms whereby fertilization and competent development occur can only add to the overall success rate.

Acknowledgments

The authors thank the clinical, nursing and scientific staff of Clinic 20, Royal North Shore Hospital for providing the indispensable services to make these results possible.

References

Catt, J., Krzyminska, U., Tilia, L., Csehi, E., Ryan, J., Pike, I., and O'Neill, C. (1994a). Subzonal insertion of multiple sperm as a treatment for male factor infertility. *Fertil. Steril.* 61, 118–24.

Catt, J.W., Morton, M., and Saunders, D.M. (1994b). Should all oocytes fertilize after intracytoplasmic sperm injection? *Proc. Aust. Soc. Reprod. Biol.*, MP22 [Abstr.]

Catt, J.W., Ryan, J.P., Pike, I.L., and O'Neill, C. (1995). Intracytoplasmic sperm injection results in a higher fertilization rate than subzonal insemination, provided the sperm is incised prior to injection. *Fertil. Steril.* (In press.)

Cohen, J., Talansky, B.E., Malter, H., Alikani, M., Adler, A., Reing, A., Berkeley, A., Graf, M., Davis, O., Liu, H., Bedford, J.M., and Rosenwaks, Z. (1991). Microsurgical fertilization and teratozoospermia. *Hum. Reprod. (Oxf.)* 6, 118–23.

Fishel, S., Timson, J., Lisi, F., Jacobson, M., Rinaldi, L., and Gobetz, L. (1994). Micro-assisted fertilization in patients who have failed subzonal insemination. *Hum. Reprod. (Oxf.)* 9, 501–5.

Lanzendorf, S.E., Maloney, M.K., Veeck, L.L., Slusser, J., Hodgen, G.D., and Rosenwaks, Z. (1988). A preclinical evaluation of pronuclear formation by microinjection of human spermatozoa into human oocytes. *Fertil. Steril.* 49, 835–42.

Lassalle, B., Testart, J., and Renard, J.-P. (1985). Human embryo features that influence the success of cryopreservation with the use of 1,2-propanediol. *Fertil. Steril.* 44, 645–51.

Ng, S.-C., Bongso, A., and Ratnam, S.S. (1991). Microinjection of human oocytes: a technique for severe oligoasthenoteratozoospermia. *Fertil. Steril.* 56, 1117–23.

Palermo, G., Joris, H., Devroey, P., and Van Steirteghem, A.C. (1992). Pregnancies after intracytoplasmic injection of single spermatozoon into an oocyte. *Lancet* 340, 17–18.

Palermo, G., Joris, H., Derde, M.-P., Camus, M., Devroey, P., and Van Steirteghem, A. (1993). Sperm characteristics and outcome of human assisted fertilization by subzonal insemination and intracytoplasmic sperm injection. *Fertil. Steril.* 59, 826–35.

Quinn, P., Warnes, G.M., Kerin, J.F., and Kirby, C. (1985). Culture factors affecting the success rate of *in vitro* fertilization and embryo transfer. *Ann. N.Y. Acad. Sci.* 442, 195–204.

Redgment, C.J., Yang, D., Tsirigotis, M., Yazdani, N., Al Shawaf, T., and Craft, I.L. (1994). Experience with assisted fertilization in severe male factor infertility and unexplained failed fertilization *in vitro*. *Hum. Reprod. (Oxf.)* 9, 680–3.

Scuglia, P.M., Catt, J.W., Ryan, J.P., O'Neill, C., and Pike, I.L. (1994). The incidence of nuclear immaturity following ovarian stimulation and its influence on sperm microinjection procedures. *Proc. 13th Ann. Meet. Fert. Soc. Aust.*, MP113 [Abstr.]

Thadani, V.M. (1980). A study of hetero-specific sperm-egg interactions in the rat mouse and deer mouse using *in vitro* fertilization and sperm injection. *J. Exp. Zool.* 212, 435–53.

Tucker, M., Wiker, S., and Massey, J. (1993). Rational approach to assisted fertilization. *Hum. Reprod. (Oxf.)* 8, 1778.

Van Steirteghem, A.C., Liu, J., Joris, H., Nagy, Z., Janssenswillen, C., Tournaye, H., Derde, M.-P., Van Assche, E., and Devroey, P. (1993a). Higher success rate by intracytoplasmic sperm injection than by subzonal insemination. Report of a second series of 300 consecutive treatment cycles. *Hum. Reprod. (Oxf.)* 8, 1055–60.

Van Steirteghem, A.C., Nagy, Z., Joris, H., Liu, J., Staessen, C., Smitz, J., Wisanto, A., and Devroey, P. (1993b). High fertilization and implantation rates after intracytoplasmic injection. *Hum. Reprod. (Oxf.)* 8, 1061–6.

World Health Organization (1992). 'Laboratory Manual for the Examination of Human Semen and Sperm–Cervical Mucus Interaction'. 3rd Edn. (Cambridge University Press: Cambridge.)

Manuscript received 2 February 1995

Open Discussion

Harold Bourne (Melbourne):

You mentioned damaging the sperm tail before injection. Have you done any electron microscopy (EM) to determine the degree of damage?

Catt:

No, we haven't done any EM studies. There was a report at the 1994 ESHRE meeting by Dozortsev *et al.*; they included a vital stain in the PVP and they showed that swiping the injection pipette across the sperm tail allowed dye into the sperm. So there seems to be some form of membrane damage. It would be useful to examine this at the EM level.

Gianpiero Palermo (New York):

The sperm should be immobilized but not damaged, and they should be able to twitch or shake for a short while after touching the tail and then become immobilized. Only the membrane should be damaged, not the tail structure. I don't take sperm which have been damaged, only those which are immobilized.

Catt:

I think 'damage' is a misleading term, and that is why we prefer to use the term 'incision'. We're obviously doing something to the sperm to immobilize it, but we don't fully understand the extent of the damage.

Sean Flaherty (Adelaide):

When you stroke the sperm tail with the injection pipette, all you're doing is causing damage to the sperm plasma membrane. In doing so, you allow the cytosolic factors in the ooplasm which decondense the sperm head to enter the intracellular space of the sperm tail. It was previously thought that the nuclear ring at the base of the sperm head was impermeable, but there is evidence now that it's permeable. The factors which decondense the sperm head are small molecules and they probably enter through the damaged membrane in the midpiece of the sperm tail, and then permeate through the nuclear ring into the sperm head, and it swells as a result. So it doesn't matter whether or not the acrosome reaction has occurred. We shouldn't be too concerned about the significance of this immobilization step—it only needs to be done to permeabilize the membrane so that the oocyte decondensing factors can enter the sperm nucleus.

Catt:

That fits in with current thinking about how sperm activate oocytes.

Microfertilization Techniques — The Swedish Experience

Lars Hamberger [A,C], Anita Sjögren [A],
Kersti Lundin [A], Brita Söderlund [A],
Lars Nilsson [A], Christina Bergh [A],
Ulla-Britt Wennerholm [A], Matts Wikland [B],
Peter Svalander [B], Ann H. Jakobsson [B] and Ann-Sofie Forsberg [B]

[A] *Department of Obstetrics and Gynaecology, University of Göteborg, S-41345 Göteborg, Sweden.*
[B] *Fertility Centre Scandinavia, Box 5418, S-41255, Göteborg, Sweden.*
[C] *To whom correspondence should be addressed.*

Abstract. Intracytoplasmic sperm injection (ICSI) has been studied in this animal research programme since 1990. In 1993, the technique was first applied clinically and up to the present time (September 1994), a total of 456 couples have been studied in 538 cycles. The principal indication for the use of ICSI has been severe male sub-fertility as judged by a semen analysis. In addition, men with high titres of antisperm antibodies, blockage of the vas deferens and neurological disorders such as spinal cord lesions have been included in the programme. Men with genetic disorders such as cystic fibrosis and acrosome-deficient spermatozoa have also been treated successfully. The overall fertilization rate using ICSI was 59%, which is similar to the conventional *in vitro* fertilization (IVF) programme in Göteborg, however, the pregnancy rate per embryo transfer (29%) and the ongoing pregnancy rate per transfer (22%) were slightly lower. The total number of pregnancies was 144 with 111 of the pregnancies either ongoing or already delivered. To date, 36 healthy children have been born following 29 deliveries and no major malformations have been diagnosed. Being the first programme in Scandinavia to perform ICSI, this unit has experienced long waiting lists which indicates that severe male sub-fertility will be one of the major groups for treatment with assisted reproductive technologies in the future.

Extra keywords: male infertility, IVF, microinjection, ICSI.

Introduction

Ever since assisted reproduction was introduced as a clinical treatment, male sub-fertility has been one of the most important indications. However, it was soon recognized that conventional *in vitro* fertilization (IVF) was relatively ineffective for overcoming poor sperm quality and that more severe forms of male factor infertility could only be treated if the zona pellucida barrier could be overcome. A number of techniques, developed in different animal models, have been transferred to clinical application in the human over the last five years. Some methods which were initially presented with enthusiasm include zona drilling (ZD), partial zona dissection (PZD) and subzonal insemination (SUZI). However, with greater experience it was realized that the success rate for these techniques was disappointingly low. The most recent, and the most invasive of these new techniques, is intracytoplasmic sperm injection (ICSI). Several groups in the world with the technical knowledge and ability to perform ICSI hesitated to do so (Lanzendorf *et al.* 1988; Cohen *et al.* 1991) and the first successful application of ICSI in the human which resulted in viable term pregnancies was not reported until 1992 (Palermo *et al.* 1992). Since that first report, it has become evident from careful prenatal and postnatal investigations of the children that the risk of malformations or genetic defects from microfertilization techniques is not increased significantly (survey of clinical experience with ICSI until 31 December 1993; conducted by the European Society for Human Reproduction and Embryology).

Following a visit to the world's leading ICSI centre at the Free University of Brussels in 1992, we decided to apply the technique clinically to cases of severe male sub-fertility in which conventional IVF had already failed or in cases in which, for various other reasons, it was anticipated that IVF would fail. We now report our experience and results from the first 18 months of the clinical application of the ICSI technique in Göteborg.

Materials and Methods

Patients

A total of 456 couples have been treated during 538 cycles in the two collaborating units (Department of Obstetrics and Gynecology, University of Göteborg and Fertility Center Scandinavia, Göteborg). In the majority of the couples (~70%), the female partner was considered to be healthy according to standard infertility investigations which included hormonal profiles, a hysterosalpingogram and, in most cases, laparoscopic tubal assessment. In the remaining 30%, female infertility factors of varying degrees of severity were found including mild to moderate endometriosis which was a frequent finding in this group.

In a small group of our patients, ICSI has been tried successfully in men with undefined sperm disorders, including those men with seemingly normal spermiograms but repeated fertilization failure after conventional IVF.

Semen Analysis and Preparation

The male partners were evaluated with repeated semen analyses before treatment. We have followed the modified criteria set out by the World Health Organization (1992), but in the majority of cases included in this report, the strict criteria of Kruger *et al.* (1988) were utilized for sperm morphology evaluation. At the start of our ICSI study, the minimum criterion was set at 1×10^4 motile spermatozoa after preparation by swim-up or Percoll separation, but we now accept most men with a semen sample that contains any number of spermatozoa. Sperm preparation was either by a conventional swim-up when the sample had a high concentration of progressively motile sperm, or if not, by centrifugation through a four-step (45%, 70%, 80%, 90%) Percoll gradient (Hamberger *et al.* 1993a).

Preparation of Epididymal and Testicular Sperm

Microsurgical epididymal sperm aspiration (MESA) was performed for a variety of different indications in our programme. The caput epididymis was examined using microsurgical techniques under general anaesthesia, and fluid was gently aspirated from the tubules by use of a thin needle connected to a 1 mL syringe with constant slight negative pressure. Each sample was immediately checked under the microscope in the operating theatre and if possible, processed on a Percoll gradient to avoid long-term exposure of the sperm to red blood cells and debris. If epididymal sperm aspiration failed, the operation was concluded with a testicular biopsy, whereby a 3×3-mm tissue specimen was cut into very small pieces and the medium containing the dissociated tissue was centrifuged at 1800g for 5 min. Epididymal spermatozoa, not immediately utilized for ICSI, were cryopreserved for future use in small volumes (50–100 μL) in as many separate straws as possible.

Ovarian Hyperstimulation

Controlled ovarian hyperstimulation was performed in all cases utilizing long-term down-regulation with Buserelin (Suprefact; Hoechst AG, Frankfurt, Germany). This was followed by subcutaneous or intramuscular injections of follicle-stimulating hormone (FSH) (Fertinorm HP; Serono, Geneva, Switzerland) and/or human menopausal gonadotrophin (hMG) (Pergonal; Serono) until the leading follicles measured 18–22 mm in diameter (Wikland *et al.* 1994) and the endometrium was characterized using ultrasound as having a mature pattern, at which time human chorionic gonadotrophin (hCG) (Profasi; Serono) was administered. Follicle aspiration was performed 36–38 h after hCG using vaginal ultrasonography and follicle puncture (Wikland and Hamberger 1994).

The ICSI Procedure

Approximately 4 h after aspiration of the oocytes, the cumulus cells were removed by pipetting the oocytes in HEPES-buffered Earle's balanced salt solution (EBSS) (MediCult, Copenhagen, Denmark) containing 80 I.U. mL^{-1} hyaluronidase (Type VIII; Sigma, St Louis, MO, USA) for not more than 30 s. The oocytes were then rinsed three times in medium to remove the enzyme. The denuded oocytes were cultured in EBSS (MediCult) before sperm injection. The maturity of each oocyte was evaluated and only metaphase I and II oocytes were injected.

The microinjection procedure was performed on a heated stage attached to a Nikon Diaphot inverted microscope which was equipped with micromanipulators (Narishige, Tokyo, Japan). The pipettes were made from borosilicate glass capillary tubes. The holding pipettes had an internal diameter of 20 μm and the injection pipettes had an internal diameter of 5–7 μm with a 28° bevel. The injection procedure was carried out in a Petri dish with a central droplet of sperm suspension in culture medium diluted with 10% polyvinylpyrrolidone (PVP). Each oocyte was placed in a droplet of HEPES-buffered EBSS and the dish was covered with mineral oil. Following injection, the oocytes were placed in droplets of EBSS medium. About 18 h later, the injected oocytes were checked for fertilization. All fertilized oocytes were cultured for an additional 24–48 h depending on the cleavage rate, and 4–6-cell embryos of the highest possible grade were replaced. Additional, high quality embryos were cryopreserved using 1, 2-propanediol as described by Testart *et al.* 1987.

Table 1. Overall results of the intracytoplasmic sperm injection (ICSI) programme (March 1993–August 1994)

Biochemical pregnancies are not included. ET, embryo transfer; PN, pronuclei

No. of patients	456
No. of cycles	538
No. of oocytes injected	5231
No. of 2 PN fertilized oocytes	3018 (57·7%)
No. of 3 PN fertilized oocytes	60 (1·1%)
Patients who achieved fertilization	97%
Patients who had an embryo transfer	92%
Average no. of embryos transferred (range)	2·3 (1–3)
No. of clinical pregnancies	144
Implantation rate per embryo	13·6%
Pregnancy rate per ET	29%
Pregnancy rate per cycle	26·5%
Miscarriage rate	21%
No. of ongoing pregnancies and births	111
Ongoing pregnancy rate per ET	22·5%
No. of births	29
No. of children born	36

Results

Clinical ICSI Results

The results of all the ICSI cycles performed since the commencement of the programme, irrespective of the clinical indication, are summarized in Table 1. Fertilization was achieved in 97% of the treatment cycles. The slightly reduced percentage of cycles in which an embryo transfer occurred (92%) reflects the fact that some embryos were frozen for later transfer in cases where there was a risk of ovarian hyperstimulation syndrome (OHSS), or that ICSI and conventional IVF were sometimes performed in parallel for certain indications and embryos from conventional IVF were chosen for transfer. If these two reasons for exclusion are taken into account, embryo transfer could theoretically have been performed in 97% of the cycles in which oocytes were collected.

Currently, more than 2 embryos are seldom replaced in our IVF programme and we have adopted a similar philosophy for our ICSI programme. The pregnancy rate per embryo transfer (ET) of 29% does not include biochemical pregnancies, whereas the miscarriage rate of 21% corresponded exactly to that of our conventional IVF programme. Furthermore, there was a low ectopic pregnancy rate (1%). This could be partly due to the transfer technique which involved the replacement of embryos into the middle of the uterine cavity, as well as the fact that a majority of the women (~70%) had no uterine or tubal pathology.

Since only 2 embryos were usually replaced, a large number of high quality embryos were cryopreserved for 193 couples. As shown in Table 2, a pregnancy rate per ET of 16% was obtained after freezing and thawing of embryos fertilized by ICSI. This does not differ significantly from the pregnancy rate after freezing and thawing in our conventional IVF programme (18·5%). Most replacements were performed in natural cycles without hormone treatment.

Table 2. Freezing and thawing embryos generated by intracytoplasmic sperm injection (ICSI)

ET, embryo transfer

No. of patients with frozen embryos	193
No. of frozen embryos	765
No. of thaw cycles	106
No. of embryos surviving freezing and thawing	213/297 (72%)
No. of replacement cycles	82 (77%)
No. of embryos replaced	1–3
No. of clinical pregnancies	13
Pregnancy rate per ET	16%
Implantation rate per embryo	14%

Table 3. Pregnancies after microsurgical epididymal sperm aspiration (MESA) and intracytoplasmic sperm injection (ICSI)

ET, embryo transfer; PN, pronuclei

No. of patients	23
No. of cycles	29
No. of oocytes injected	359
No. of 2 PN fertilized oocytes	184 (51%)
No. of cycles with ET	27
No. of pregnancies	9
Pregnancy rate per ET	33%
No. of ongoing pregnancies (births)	5 (3)
Implantation rate per embryo	17%

The use of ICSI in combination with MESA has been performed on a limited scale, and the results are summarized in Table 3. Two children were born after this procedure was performed in men with cystic fibrosis (CF) and congenital absence of the vas deferens (Fogdestam et al. 1994). It should be stressed that both these men were young and in good physical condition and the female partners were free from the cystic fibrosis mutation on screening.

In another series of experiments, ICSI was performed with 24-h-old oocytes which had been exposed to spermatozoa in conventional IVF with low (< 20%) or no fertilization (Table 4). When 24-h-old spermatozoa were used for the ICSI procedure the fertilization rate was 36%, whereas freshly prepared spermatozoa from new ejaculates increased the fertilization rate to 56% (Table 4). When freshly prepared spermatozoa were used, 2 out of 9 embryo transfers resulted in ongoing clinical pregnancies. Where good quality embryos from both conventional IVF and ICSI were available in the same cycle, we preferred to replace IVF embryos.

Table 4. Intracytoplasmic sperm injection (ICSI) of one-day-old oocytes which failed to fertilize by conventional *in vitro* fertilization (IVF)

	Spermatozoa used for ICSI	
	24 h old	Fresh
No. of patients	16	17
Fertilization after IVF	13/190 (7%)	19/174 (11%)
Fertilization after ICSI	44/121 (36%)	63/122 (56%)
Cleavage after ICSI	40/44 (91%)	50/63 (83%)

	IVF	ICSI	IVF	ICSI
No. of embryo transfers	7[A]	2	3	9
No. of pregnancies	2	0	2	2[B]

[A] Three additional pregnancies were achieved with ICSI in the next cycle.
[B] One pregnancy was delivered in December 1994.

Special indications were present in a number of ICSI cycles and the results obtained thus far are summarized in Table 5. The use of acrosome-less, round-headed spermatozoa resulted in the term delivery of twins (Lundin et al. 1994a).

Table 5. Pregnancies achieved by intracytoplasmic sperm injection (ICSI) in specific patient subgroups

ASA, anti-sperm antibodies; Ig, immunoglobulin

	Cycles	Pregnancies
Spinal cord lesion	9	2
Frozen–thawed sperm injected	12	3
Acrosome-less spermatozoa	2	1
Severe ASA[A]	18	7

[A] IgA- and IgG-binding: 90–100%.

Children Born after ICSI

To date, 29 deliveries have resulted in 36 healthy children (Table 6). The incidence of premature delivery or low birth weight does not appear to differ from the normal population, but the results are as yet too small to allow any definite conclusions. The sex ratios (Table 6) also seem to be normal. No major malformations have been registered to date, although two minor malformations have been found by our expert team of paediatricians. One was a congenital hip subluxation and the other a discrete systolic heart murmur of no functional importance.

Table 6. Children born after intracytoplasmic sperm injection (ICSI) in Göteborg (1993–1994)

No. of births:	29
singletons	26 (83%)
twins	5 (17%)
No. of children born:	36
< 36 weeks	3 (8%)
< 37 weeks	4 (11%)
37–42 weeks	29 (81%)
Birth weights:	
< 2500 g	7 (19%)
2500–4000 g	29 (81%)
Sex ratio at birth:	
singleton births	12 male, 14 female
twin births	6 male, 4 female

Discussion

Intracytoplasmic injection of a single spermatozoon from men with severe sub-fertility into metaphase II oocytes, resulted in a surprisingly high fertilization rate. We now know that fertilization and pregnancy can be achieved in almost all cases of male infertility and sperm morphology also seems to be of less importance for ICSI. No marked differences in the fertilization and ongoing pregnancy rates have been found in our programme when sperm samples with < 10% or > 10% normal forms (strict criteria) were compared. In cases of azoospermia, MESA can be used and even spermatozoa isolated from testis biopsies can lead to fertilization, cleavage and clinical pregnancies (Schoysman et al. 1993).

Indeed, in our programme the overall fertilization rate was generally slightly higher than in our conventional IVF programme. The sperm used for ICSI were not exposed to any motility stimulants or acrosome reaction-inducing agents, and the majority of the injected sperm were therefore not acrosome reacted (Söderlund et al. 1994). Sperm preparative procedures may be important and have attracted our interest. The conventional use of 3–4 concentrations of Percoll in a discontinuous gradient may have negative consequences, not for fertilization, but for later cleavage stages and the incidence of fragmentation due to the putative presence of endotoxins (Hamberger et al. 1993b).

The use of PVP to decrease sperm motility is probably another factor of crucial importance for the outcome of ICSI. Different types of PVP are commercially available at present, and microinjection of these different types into fertilized mouse oocytes has led to significant differences in the cleavage rates and the morphology of mouse embryos (Bras et al. 1994).

It has been suggested that ICSI may completely replace conventional IVF in the future, as even better pregnancy rates might be expected if normal sperm were injected. This possibility has, to some extent, been explored in our IVF programme where a combination of IVF and ICSI were performed on a 1:1 basis in 42 cases of failed fertilization in earlier conventional IVF trials. In one-third of the cases (14/42), no fertilization occurred with conventional IVF in the second IVF cycle (Table 7), whereas in two-thirds (28/42), the fertilization and pregnancy rates were similar with both techniques (Table 8). Until more knowledge is gained concerning the outcome of the pregnancies, most centres have adopted the attitude that ICSI should only be applied when conventional IVF fails or is unlikely to be effective.

Table 7. Outcome of *in vitro* fertilization (IVF) and intracytoplasmic sperm injection (ICSI) in couples who had failed fertilization in a previous IVF cycle

ET, embryo transfer

	IVF	ICSI
No. of patients (cycles)	14	14
No. of oocytes	113	106
Fertilization rate	0%	49%
No. of ETs	—	14
No. of clinical pregnancies	—	5

Table 8. Outcome of *in vitro* fertilization (IVF) and intracytoplasmic sperm injection (ICSI) in couples who had failed fertilization in a previous IVF cycle

ET, embryo transfer

	IVF	ICSI
No. of patients	28	28
No. of oocytes	229	276
Fertilization rate	51%	69%
No. of ETs	9/22[A]	13/22[A]
No. of clinical pregnancies	3	3

[A] All embryos were frozen in 6 cycles.

Fortunately, no major malformations have been found in our ICSI children so far, and none of the amniocenteses performed on ongoing pregnancies have been abnormal. In this context, it is important to point out that all couples were offered and encouraged to have an amniocentesis in the case of a singleton pregnancy. Prior to treatment, the majority accepted our advice, but once pregnant, a relatively large number (about 40%) declined when informed that a small risk of miscarriage existed in connection with amniocentesis. This attitude has led us to karyotype all couples before ICSI and not to accept couples with a genetic disorder, especially those with translocations. It is, however, obvious that this only partially compensates for the risk that the fetus carries an abnormal karyotype.

The encouraging results with ICSI in men (7/18 cycles associated with pregnancy) with high antisperm antibodies (ASA) titres (Lundin et al. 1994b; Table 5) means that this infertility factor can now generally be treated. On the other hand, the application of conventional IVF can also be successful in some of these ASA cases, and in our view should be tried first. In our own programme, couples with ASA as the predominant infertility factor are treated with both IVF and ICSI on a 1:1 basis in the first cycle and then switched to either ICSI or IVF in subsequent treatment cycles as indicated.

In conclusion, the majority of severe male sub-fertility cases can now be successfully treated with ICSI and this rapid technical development has shifted andrology from a diagnostic discipline to a therapeutic one. Surgical procedures for varicocele or for vas deferens defects, as well as in most cases of hormonal treatments (e.g. gonadotrophins), have a much lower success rate than after ICSI (Palermo et al. 1993; Van Steirteghem et al. 1993). The next step in the development will most likely be a further simplification of the ICSI procedure. In our programme, much work has been devoted to the simplification of sperm preparation, the equipment used for microinjection and the culture conditions. Compared with conventional IVF, an ICSI procedure on 10–15 oocytes, adds approximately two hours of extra laboratory work which only increases the total technical cost moderately. However, because of the encouraging results with this technique on even the worst cases of male infertility, it is our belief that within a couple of years, ICSI will be adopted by all larger IVF centres and will be regarded as a routine procedure.

Acknowledgments

We thank Mrs Ann-Louise Dahl for skilful preparation of the manuscript and Dr Tom Bourne for revising the English language. Supported by a grant (no. 2873) from the Swedish Medical Research Council.

References

Bras, M., Dumoulin J.C.M., Pieters, M.H.E.C., Michiels, A.H.J.C., Geraedts, J.P.M., and Evers, J.L.H. (1994). The use of a mouse zygote quality control system for training purposes and toxicity determination in an ICSI programme. Hum. Reprod. (Oxf.) 9 (Suppl. 4), 23. [Abstr.]

Cohen, J., Talansky, B.E., Malter, H., Alikani, M., Adler, A., Reing, A., Berkeley, A., Graf, M., Davis, O., Liu, H., Bedford, J.M., and Rosenwaks, Z. (1991). Microsurgical fertilization and teratozoospermia. Hum. Reprod. (Oxf.) 6, 118–23.

Fogdestram, I., Hamberger, L., Lundin, K., Sjögren, A., Hjelte, L., and Strandvik, B. (1994). Successful pregnancies after IVF with sperm from men with cystic fibrosis. 19th Eur. Cystic Fibrosis Conf. [Abstr.]

Hamberger, L., Sjögren, A., Lundin, K., Svalander, P., Söderlund, B., Jacobsson, A.-H., Forsberg, A.S., and Wikland, M. (1993a). Fertilization of human oocytes by micromanipulation. In 'Frontiers in Gynecologic and Obstetric Investigation'. (Eds A.R. Genazzani, F. Petraglia and A.D. Genazzani.) pp. 489–501. (Parthenon Press: New York.)

Hamberger, L., Sjögren, A., Lundin, K., Söderlund, B., and Nilsson, L. (1993b). Microfertilization techniques — Scandinavian experience. Proc. Eur. Symp. Micromanipulation, 85–9.

Kruger, T.F., Acosta, A.A., Simmons, K.F., Swanson, R.J., Matta, J.F., and Oehninger, S. (1988). Predictive value of abnormal sperm morphology in in vitro fertilization. Fertil. Steril. 49, 112–17.

Lanzendorf, S.E., Maloney, M.K., Veeck, L.L., Slusser, J., Hodgen, G.D., and Rosenwaks, Z. (1988). A preclinical evaluation of pronuclear formation by microinjection of human spermatozoa into human oocytes. Fertil. Steril. 49, 835–42.

Lundin, K., Sjögren, A., Nilsson, L., and Hamberger, L. (1994a). Fertilization and pregnancy after ICSI of acrosomeless spermatozoa. Fertil. Steril. 62, 1266–7.

Lundin, K., Sjögren, A., Nilsson, L., and Hamberger, L. (1994b). Antisperm antibodies: IVF or microinjection? Hum. Reprod. (Oxf.) 9 (Suppl. 4), 72. [Abstr.]

Palermo, G., Joris, H., Devroey, P., and Van Steirteghem, A.C. (1992). Pregnancies after intracytoplasmic injection of single spermatozoon into an oocyte. Lancet 340, 17–18.

Palermo, G., Joris, H., Derde, M.-P., Camus, M., Devroey, P., and Van Steirteghem, A. (1993). Sperm characteristics and outcome of human assisted fertilization by subzonal insemination and intracytoplasmic sperm injection. Fertil. Steril. 59, 826–35.

Schoysman, R., Vanderzwalmen, P., Nijs, M., Segal, L., Segal-Bertin, G., Geerts, L., Van Roosendaal, E., and Schoysman, D. (1993). Pregnancy after fertilization with human testicular spermatozoa. Lancet 342, 1237.

Söderlund, B., Lundin, K., and Hamberger, L. (1994). Results from IVF and ICSI correlated to sperm morphology. Hum. Reprod. (Oxf.) 9 (suppl. 4), 46. [Abstr.]

Testart, J., Lasalle, B., Belaisch-Allart, J., Forman, R., Hazout, A., Volante, M., and Frydman, R. (1987). Human embryo viability related to freezing and thawing procedures. Am. J. Obstet. Gynecol. 157, 168–71.

Van Steirteghem, A.C., Nagy, Z., Joris, H., Liu, J., Staessen, C., Smitz, J., Wisanto, A., and Devroey, P. (1993). High fertilization and implantation rates after intracytoplasmic sperm injection. Hum. Reprod. (Oxf.) 8, 1061–6.

Wikland, M., and Hamberger, L. (1994). The role of ultrasonography in oocyte retrieval for in vitro fertilization and other assisted reproductive technologies. In 'Imaging in Infertility and Reproductive Endocrinology'. (Eds R. Jaffe and J.B. Pierson.) pp. 191–9. (Lippincott: Washington.)

Wikland, M., Borg, J., Hamberger, L., and Svalander, P. (1994). Simplification of IVF: minimal monitoring and the use of subcutaneous highly purified FSH administration for ovulation induction. Hum. Reprod. (Oxf.) 9, 1430–6.

World Health Organization (1992). 'Laboratory Manual for the Examination of Human Semen and Semen–Cervical Mucus Interaction'. 3rd Edn. (Cambridge University Press: Cambridge.)

Manuscript received 3 April 1995

Open Discussion

Robert McLachlan (Melbourne):

After one cycle of failed conventional IVF, you recommend that a second cycle be performed because you couldn't tell if they would achieve fertilization in the next cycle. Do you use any tests of sperm function such as zona binding or acrosome reactions to decide whether it's worth trying IVF or ICSI in the second cycle?

Hamberger:

Of course there is a group in whom you can go directly to ICSI. I am talking about totally unexpected fertilization failures and the conclusion I want to draw from this is that just because you get fertilization failure in one IVF cycle, you shouldn't switch immediately to ICSI. If you do, then you are frequently successful with ICSI in the second cycle, but it doesn't mean that ICSI was necessary.

Alan Trounson (Melbourne):

You mentioned that you injected metaphase I eggs. What you injected were eggs that had undergone germinal vesicle breakdown (GVBD). If you injected them prior to metaphase I (and you wouldn't know that), they would have to form a diploid female nucleus and the outcome wouldn't be normal. But if they were at metaphase I or later, then they would possibly form the two normal pronuclei and two polar bodies. What proportion of eggs were in that category?

Hamberger:

About 9·5%.

Trounson:

So if you took that data out, I suspect your fertilization rate would improve.

Hamberger:

Yes, by almost 10% to about 68%. If we see a germinal vesicle (GV), we try to mature that egg for scientific purposes but we never use it for clinical purposes. If we don't see a GV or a polar body, we inject it. Since we don't completely denude the eggs, we sometimes fail to see the polar body and we classify the egg as metaphase I, when it may well have been a metaphase II egg.

Intracytoplasmic Sperm Injection (ICSI): the Brussels Experience

Herman Tournaye[AD], Jian Liu[A], Zsolt Nagy[A], Hubert Joris[A],
Ari Wisanto[A], Maryse Bonduelle[B], Josiane Van der Elst[A],
Catherine Staessen[A], Johan Smitz[A], Sherman Silber[C],
Paul Devroey[A], Inge Liebaers[B] and André Van Steirteghem[A]

[A] *Centre for Reproductive Medicine and* [B] *Centre for Medical Genetics,*
University Hospital and Medical School, Dutch-speaking Brussels Free University,
Laarbeeklaan 101, Brussels B-1090, Belgium.
[C] *Department of Urology, St Luke's Hospital, St Louis, MO 63017, USA.*
[D] *To whom correspondence should be addressed.*

Abstract. The present report covers the results of a 26-month period in which 1275 consecutive treatment cycles by intracytoplasmic sperm injection (ICSI) were performed in 919 couples. These couples were afflicted with male factor infertility and had had at least one previous failed conventional *in vitro* fertilization (IVF) treatment cycle. In other couples, the husband had semen parameters incompatible with conventional IVF or suffered from excretory azoospermia which required microsurgical epididymal sperm aspiration or testicular sperm retrieval. Overall, the 2 pronuclear (PN) fertilization rate was 47·7% per retrieved oocyte–cumulus complex and 66·4% per successfully injected metaphase II oocyte. Embryo transfer was performed in 90·8% of started cycles and 362 clinical pregnancies were recorded, giving a clinical pregnancy rate of 28·4% per started cycle or 31·3% per transfer. In addition, updated results on the outcome of pregnancies after microassisted fertilization are presented. As of 30 August 1994, 416 children have been born. Although 16 major congenital malformations have been observed (3·9%), there appears to be no reason for serious concern as regards the occurrence of major congenital anomalies after ICSI.

Extra keywords: fertilization failure, epididymal sperm, testicular sperm, cryptozoospermia, cryopreservation, congenital malformations.

Introduction

In contrast to female factor infertility, the treatment of male factor infertility has generally been disappointing and, since most patients suffer from a non-specific male factor, the specific therapeutic choices are limited. For years, most patients with male factor infertility were treated empirically, for example by gonadotrophins, anti-oestrogens, androgens or antibiotics, in an attempt to optimize the patient's semen profile. However, retrospective studies have only provided inconsistent results and controlled trials have not demonstrated any real benefit from such empirical treatments (O'Donovan *et al.* 1993). New hopes have recently been raised by the introduction of the technique of *in vitro* fertilization (IVF) and embryo transfer. This technique has allowed non-specific male factor infertility to be treated with greater efficiency (Mahadevan *et al.* 1983; Marrs *et al.* 1983).

Although one of the most successful treatments for male factor infertility, IVF tends to be less successful than in treating female factor infertility (Mahadevan and Trounson 1984; Yovich and Stanger 1984). This is because IVF relies on several conditions, among them an adequate number of selected functional spermatozoa and normal cleavage of the fertilized oocytes, which tends to be reduced when there are sperm disorders. Innovative techniques of gamete and/or embryo replacement, such as gamete intra-Fallopian transfer (GIFT) or zygote intra-Fallopian transfer (ZIFT) failed to render the treatment more successful in cases of male factor infertility (Tournaye *et al.* 1991*a*, 1992*b*). Many corrective measures have been proposed in order to improve the fertilization rate *in vitro*, which is assumed to be the major bottleneck for success in IVF. The use of higher numbers of spermatozoa for *in vitro* insemination has been suggested (Oehninger *et al.* 1988; Ord *et al.* 1993). Modifications of the insemination procedures have been proposed (Van der Ven *et al.* 1989; Hammitt *et al.* 1991; Ord *et al.* 1993) and various methods to improve the fertilizing potential of the spermatozoa used for insemination have been reported. Glass–wool column filtration of semen has proven beneficial in cases of poor quality semen

(Van der Ven *et al.* 1988) and discontinuous Percoll gradient centrifugation has also been shown to improve fertilization rates *in vitro* (Ord *et al.* 1990; Sapienza *et al.* 1993). Methods for improving the fertilizing potential of the spermatozoa also include metabolic stimulation *in vitro* of the recovered spermatozoa (Yovich *et al.* 1988, 1990). Finally, the use of micromanipulation was introduced (Laws-King *et al.* 1987).

In our centre, IVF results for male factor patients were markedly reduced (Tournaye *et al.* 1992a) and methods of improving the fertilizing potential such as stimulation of sperm function *in vitro*, failed to improve the results (Tournaye *et al.* 1993, 1994a, 1994b). The introduction of micromanipulation in our centre led to hopes for greater success, but the technique of sub-zonal insemination (SUZI) failed to increase success rates substantially in cases with severe male factor infertility (Palermo *et al.* 1992a, 1992b). The most dramatic improvement was achieved only by the development of the technique of intracytoplasmic sperm injection (ICSI) (Palermo *et al.* 1992b, 1992c, 1993; Van Steirteghem *et al.* 1993a, 1993b, 1993c). The present paper reviews the results after ICSI, which has now become the preferred method for treating severe male factor infertility in our centre.

Materials and Methods

The present survey reviews the results of 1275 consecutive ICSI treatment cycles from October 1991 until December 1993 and also presents updated results on the outcome of pregnancies after micro-assisted fertilization.

Patient Selection

Initially, ICSI was proposed to those couples suffering from severe male factor infertility in whom no fertilization had occurred in at least two conventional IVF cycles. Later, the technique was also used for couples in whom the husband showed sperm parameters incompatible with success by conventional IVF and, from the start of our microsurgical epididymal sperm aspiration (MESA) programme in 1992, ICSI was performed using epididymal sperm and, from 1993 onwards, testicular sperm.

In the cycles included in this survey, ICSI was performed using freshly ejaculated sperm ($n = 1189$), frozen–thawed ejaculated sperm ($n = 5$), frozen–thawed deferential sperm ($n = 2$), fresh epididymal sperm ($n = 49$), frozen–thawed epididymal sperm ($n = 10$) and testicular sperm ($n = 17$). Ejaculated sperm samples were obtained after a 3 day abstinence period and were considered normal if the sample contained $\geq 40 \times 10^6$ motile spermatozoa (World Health Organization 1987) and if $\geq 14\%$ of the spermatozoa showed a normal morphology according to strict criteria (Kruger *et al.* 1986). The methodologies for sperm cryopreservation and retrieval of epididymal and testicular sperm have been reported elsewhere (Tournaye *et al.* 1991b, 1994c; Devroey *et al.* 1994; Silber *et al.* 1994).

Clinical and Laboratory Procedures

All the female partners were superovulated using a gonadotrophin-releasing hormone analogue (GnRHa) suppression protocol combining Buserelin (Suprefact nasal spray; Hoechst, Frankfurt, Germany) with human menopausal gonadotrophin (hMG) (Humegon; Organon, Oss, The Netherlands or Pergonal; Serono, Brussels, Belgium) (Smitz *et al.* 1988, 1992). Oocytes were recovered by transvaginal ultrasound-guided pick-up, 36 h after administration of 10 000 I.U. of human chorionic gonadotrophin (hCG).

Cumulus–oocyte complexes were maintained at 37°C and transported to the microinjection laboratory in modified Earle's medium, equilibrated with 5% O_2, 5% CO_2 and 90% N_2. In the microinjection laboratory, cumulus cells were removed before performing the ICSI procedure. The full description of oocyte preparation, sperm preparation and the sperm injection procedure has been described in detail elsewhere (Van Steirteghem *et al.* 1993a; Liu *et al.* 1994a). Briefly, after removing the surrounding cumulus and corona cells, the nuclear maturation of the oocytes was assessed using an inverted microscope. Oocytes which had extruded their first polar body (metaphase-II oocytes), were then injected with a single spermatozoon, directly into the ooplasm. Further culture of injected oocytes was performed in 25-μL drops of B2 medium under lightweight paraffin oil. Fertilization was confirmed after 18 h if 2 distinct pronuclei (PN) were observed under an inverted microscope. Cleavage was assessed 24 h later and cleaved embryos with <50% of their volume filled with anucleate fragments were considered for transfer. Two to three, or in exceptional cases four, embryos were replaced into the uterine cavity 48 h after the sperm injection procedure. If the patient was <37 years old and we obtained >6 embryos with <20% of fragmentation, we electively only replaced 2 embryos in the patient's first three treatment cycles (Staessen *et al.* 1993). Supernumerary embryos with <20% fragmentation were frozen using dimethylsulfoxide as a cryoprotectant (Camus *et al.* 1989). Luteal supplementation was given by daily intravaginal administration of 3×200 mg natural micronized progesterone (Utrogestan; Piette, Brussels) (Smitz *et al.* 1992).

Pregnancy Assessment and Follow-up

A rise in serum hCG concentration on two consecutive occasions from 11 days after transfer was taken as an indication of pregnancy. Clinical pregnancies were defined by the presence of a gestational sac on ultrasound examination about 5 weeks after transfer. In cases in which no pregnancy occurred, cryopreserved embryos were replaced in a subsequent cycle as described previously (Camus *et al.* 1989).

Since the evaluation of the safety of this novel technique is of utmost importance, pregnancy follow-up and the follow-up of the children born have been organized in a prospective manner (Bonduelle *et al.* 1994; Buysse *et al.* 1994). Most couples agreed to participate in this prospective follow-up study. The pregnant patients and their referring gynaecologists were contacted during the pregnancy and after the eventual delivery. Patients were advised to undergo prenatal diagnosis by means of chorionic villous sampling (CVS) at 9–10 weeks or amniocentesis at 16 weeks of gestation. If possible, children born after ICSI were examined about 2 months after birth. Otherwise a detailed report was obtained from the paediatrician or house officer looking after the child.

Results

Overall Clinical Results

In the 26-month period surveyed, a total of 1275 ICSI cycles were started in 919 couples. ICSI could not be performed in only 5 treatment cycles (0·4%) because either no sperm ($n = 3$) or no oocytes ($n = 2$) were available for injection.

Overall, 16 109 oocyte–cumulus complexes (OCC) were retrieved (average = 12·6 per cycle). After removal of the surrounding cumulus cells, 95% of the OCC contained an oocyte with an intact zona pellucida and clear cytoplasm

Table 1. Characteristics of freshly ejaculated semen samples used in 1189 intracytoplasmic sperm injection (ICSI) procedures

Sperm concentration and motility were scored according to the World Health Organization (1987) criteria. Sperm morphology was scored according to the Tygerberg strict criteria (Kruger et al. 1986)

	No. of cycles		% of cycles
Normal semen	77		6·5
Single sperm defect:	177		14·9
oligozoospermia		49	
asthenozoospermia		64	
teratozoospermia		64	
Double sperm defects:	345		29·0
oligoteratozoospermia		145	
asthenoteratozoospermia		92	
oligoasthenozoospermia		108	
Triple sperm defect: Oligoasthenoteratozoospermia	590		49·6

Table 2. Semen parameters of epididymal and testicular sperm used in 76 intracytoplasmic sperm injection (ICSI) procedures

Values are mean (range). Sperm concentration and motility were scored according to the World Health Organization (1987) criteria. Sperm morphology was scored according to the Tygerberg strict criteria (Kruger et al. 1986). n.a., not assessed

	Fresh epididymal sperm	Frozen–thawed epididymal sperm	Testicular sperm
Total sperm count ($\times 10^6$)	46·2 (0–248)	0·15 (0–4·4)	0·54 (0·3–3·4)
Total motility (%)	12 (0–49)	0 (0–5)	0 (0–15)
Progressive motility (%)	2 (0–20)	0 (0–5)	0
Normal morphology (%)	9 (0–33)	0 (0–15)	n.a.

Table 3. Oocyte recovery and fertilization after 1270 intracytoplasmic sperm injection (ICSI) procedures

M II, metaphase II; OCC, oocyte–cumulus complex; PN, pronuclei

	Number	Percentage of:		
		OCC	M II oocytes	intact oocytes
OCC recovered	16 109			
M II oocytes injected	13 047	81·0		
Intact oocytes	11 565	71·8	88·6	
Fertilized oocytes: 2 PN	7683	47·7	58·9	66·4
3 PN	492	3·1	3·8	4·3
1 PN	438	2·7	3·4	3·8

Table 4. Fertilization rates after intracytoplasmic sperm injection (ICSI) in relation to sperm origin

Values in parentheses are percentages. M II, metaphase II; PN, pronuclei

	Source of sperm:		
	ejaculate	epididymis	testis
No. of cycles	1189	59	17
No. of M II oocytes injected	12 017	759	242
No. of intact oocytes after ICSI[A]	10 655 (88·6)	683 (90·0)	217 (89·7)
No. of fertilized (2 PN) oocytes[B]	7228 (67·9)[C]	331 (48·5)[C]	108 (49·8)[C]

[A] Values in parentheses are percentages of the injected oocytes.
[B] Values in parentheses are percentages of the intact eggs.
[C] χ^2-test, $P < 0.001$.

Table 5. Intracytoplasmic sperm injection using sperm from extremely impaired semen

Values in parentheses are percentages. M II, metaphase II; PN, pronuclei

	Cryptozoospermia	100% immotile sperm	100% teratozoospermia
No. of cycles	57	66	48
No. of M II oocytes injected	601	678	488
No. of intact oocytes	516 (85·9)	611 (90·1)	436 (89·3)
No. of fertilized (2PN) oocytes[A]	320 (62·0)[B]	316 (51·7)[B]	295 (67·7)[B]
No. of embryos transferred or frozen[C]	236 (73·8)	197 (62·3)	198 (67·1)
No. of clinical pregnancies	15 (26·3)	8 (12·2)	13 (27·1)

[A] Values in parentheses are percentages of the intact oocytes.
[B] χ^2-test, $P < 0·05$.
[C] Values in parentheses are percentages of the 2 PN fertilized eggs.

Table 6. Causes of fertilization failure in 1124 intracytoplasmic sperm injection (ICSI) cycles

	No. of cycles	No. of patients
Only one oocyte available	8	8
Only 100% immotile sperm available	8	7
Gross abnormalities in oocytes	5	4
Round-headed sperm used	4	3
Unexplained fertilization failure	4	4
No intact oocytes after injection	2	2
Testicular sperm used	2	2

Table 7. Embryo development after intracytoplasmic sperm injection (ICSI) in relation to the semen category (ejaculated sperm)

Values in parentheses are percentages. PN, pronuclei

	Sperm defect:			
	none	single	double	triple
No. of cycles	77	177	345	590
No. of fertilized (2PN) oocytes	489	1126	2164	3424
Type A embryos (0% fragmentation)	42	93	216	305
	(8·6)	(8·3)	(10·0)	(8·9)
Type B embryos (1–20% fragmentation)	238	599	1210	1828
	(48·7)	(53·2)	(55·9)	(53·4)
Type C embryos (21–50% fragmentation)	62	142	224	391
	(12·7)	(12·6)	(10·4)	(11·4)

($n = 15\,387$). Nuclear maturation was assessed using an inverted microscope at 200×, and 85% of the oocytes were at metaphase II, 4% were at metaphase I and 11% were still at the germinal vesicle stage.

Tables 1 and 2 show the characteristics of the sperm used for injection. ICSI was performed on 13 047 metaphase II oocytes, of which 1482 were damaged (destruction rate = 11·3%). Overall, 7683 zygotes showed 2 distinct PN 18 h after ICSI (66·4% of intact oocytes), whereas 438 (3·8%) zygotes showed only one pronucleus and three pronuclei were recorded in 492 (4·3%) zygotes (Table 3). Table 4 shows the fertilization rates after ICSI in relation to the origin of the sperm used (Nagy et al. 1995). The fertilization rate was significantly reduced after ICSI with epididymal or testicular sperm.

The ICSI results for freshly ejaculated sperm in selected subgroups are presented in Table 5 (Nagy et al. 1994). These subgroups included patients with virtual azoospermia (cryptozoospermia), patients with 100% immotile sperm and those with 100% morphologically abnormal sperm. The fertilization, cleavage and clinical pregnancy rates were lower in patients with 100% immotile sperm but the difference was statistically significant only for the fertilization rate. We also reviewed a subgroup of 1124 ICSI cycles from January 1992 to December 1993 (Liu et al. 1994b) and found that complete failure of fertilization only occurred in 33 of the cycles (2·9%) in 30 patients. Table 6 shows the causes of these failures. It is interesting to note that in 10 of the 30 patients, fertilization occurred in a subsequent ICSI cycle.

Of the 7683 normally fertilized oocytes, 5129 (66·8%) developed into good quality embryos suitable for transfer ($n = 2915$) or cryopreservation ($n = 2214$). Table 7 shows the embryo quality after ICSI using freshly ejaculated sperm in relation to the semen category, in which no significant differences were observed. Table 8 compares

Table 8. Embryo development after intracytoplasmic sperm injection (ICSI) in relation to sperm origin

Values are percentages

	Source of sperm		
	ejaculate	epididymis	testis
Type A embryos (0% fragmentation)	9.1	6.7	4.6
Type B embryos (1–20% fragmentation)	53.8	45.3	50.0
Type C embryos (21–50% fragmentation)	11.4	13.3	7.4
Embryos transferred or frozen	67.2[A]	60.7[A]	61.1[A]
Cycles with embryo freezing	43.5[B]	27.1[B]	29.4[B]

[A] χ^2-test, $P < 0.03$. [B] χ^2-test, $P < 0.03$.

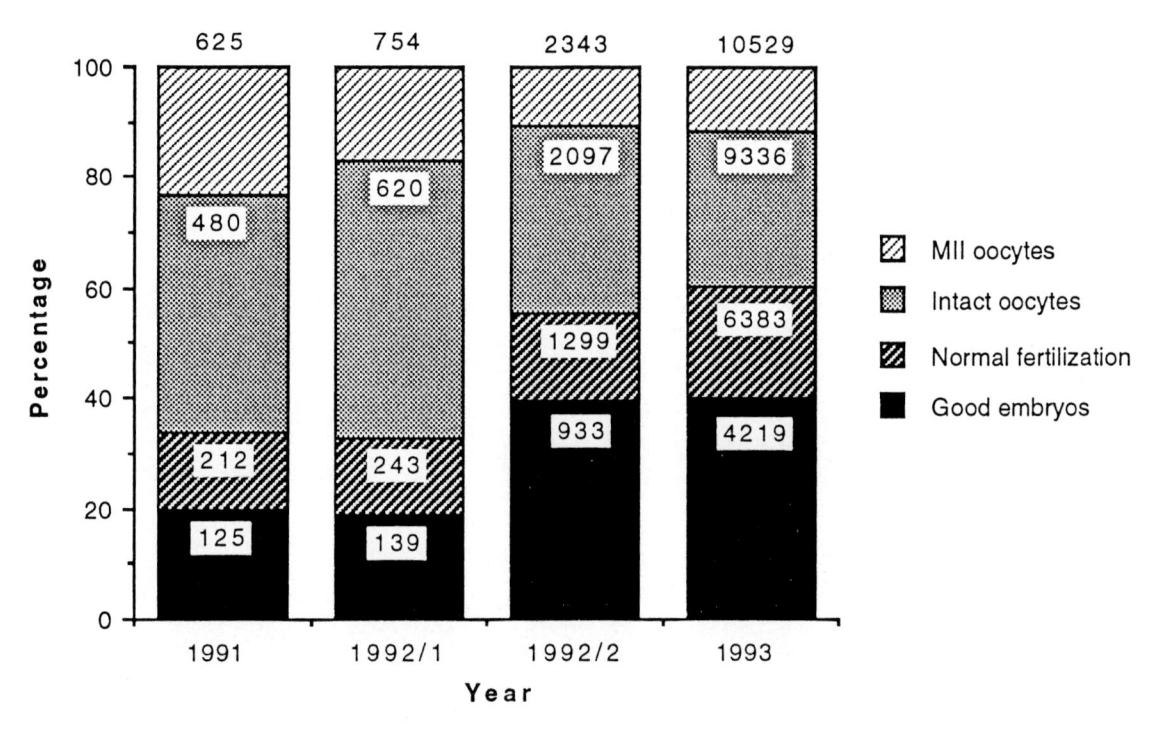

Fig. 1. Evolution of the overall ICSI results from October 1991 to December 1993.

Table 9. Number of embryos transferred in relation to semen characteristics

Values in parentheses are percentages

	Sperm defect:			
	none	single	double	triple
No. of cycles	77	177	345	590
No. of transfers	70 (90.9)	164 (92.7)	322 (93.3)	529 (89.7)
Embryos transferred:				
1	5 (7.1)	13 (7.9)	26 (8.1)	51 (9.6)
2	21 (30.0)	53 (32.3)	127 (39.4)	187 (35.3)
3	41 (58.6)	93 (56.7)	166 (51.6)	277 (52.4)
>3	3 (4.3)	5 (3.0)	3 (0.9)	14 (2.7)

embryo quality and the proportion of embryos acceptable for transfer or cryopreservation in relation to the sperm origin. When epididymal or testicular sperm were used for ICSI, fewer good quality embryos were obtained for transfer or cryopreservation.

Fig. 1 shows the evolution of the overall ICSI results during the period reviewed here. Although there was a continuous decrease in the damage rate, the fertilization rate increased markedly from the second-half of 1992. Embryo development followed the evolution of the fertilization rate over this period.

A total of 2915 embryos were replaced in 1158 transfers (90.8% of started cycles) and 2214 supernumerary embryos were cryopreserved. An average of 2.5 embryos were transferred per fresh transfer. There were no significant differences in the number of embryos replaced in relation to the semen category (Table 9).

Overall, 460 pregnancies were recorded, of which 362 were clinical (78·7%). The total (hCG positive) pregnancy rate and the clinical pregnancy rate per started ICSI treatment cycle were 36·1% and 28·4% respectively (Table 10). There were no significant differences between the clinical pregnancy rates per transfer after ICSI with ejaculated (30·7%), epididymal (34·0%) or testicular (38·5%) sperm. The pregnancy rate per transfer was 39·0% for ICSI cycles using ejaculated sperm. Table 11 shows the impact of our transfer policy on the total pregnancy rate (hCG positive); transfer of 2 embryos in selected cases resulted in a pregnancy rate comparable to that obtained when 3 embryos were replaced. However, when the patient requested the replacement of 3 good quality embryos, the total pregnancy rate increased to 49·1%.

Table 10. Transfer and pregnancy rates after 1275 intracytoplasmic sperm injection (ICSI) procedures

	Number	Percentage of: cycles	transfers	pregnancies
Cycles started	1275			
Transfers	1158	90·8		
Pregnancies (total)	460	36·1	39·7	
Clinical pregnancies	362	28·4	31·3	78·7

In addition to the 460 pregnancies obtained after the ICSI cycles in this series, of which some originated from the use of epididymal sperm ($n = 26$) and testicular sperm ($n = 6$), a further 26 pregnancies were obtained from cycles in which both SUZI and ICSI were performed at random but only ICSI embryos were transferred (51 transfers). Table 12 shows the obstetric outcome of these 486 ICSI pregnancies. Twin pregnancies occurred in 22·3% of cycles, triplet pregnancies in 5·9% of cycles and only one pregnancy was a quadruplet (0·2%). At the time of analysis, 189 patients had delivered 231 children. There were 118 boys (51·7%) and 110 girls (48·3%), giving a sex ratio at birth of 1·07. The sex of the children was unavailable for 3 deliveries. Table 13 presents an overview of the obstetric complications in those ongoing pregnancies in which follow-up has been completed.

Table 12. Outcome of 486 pregnancies after intracytoplasmic sperm injection (ICSI)

	Number	Percentage
Subclinical abortions	55	11·3
Clinical abortions	60	12·3
Ectopic pregnancies	2	0·4
Late abortions	3	0·6
Ongoing pregnancies	150	30·9
Deliveries	189	38·9
Unknown outcome	27	5·5

Table 13. Pregnancy complications observed in ongoing pregnancies after intracytoplasmic sperm injection (ICSI)

IUGR, intrauterine growth retardation; HELLP, hypertension, elevated liver enzymes and low platelets; PROM, premature rupture of the membranes

	Singleton $n = 119$	Twin $n = 48$	Triplet $n = 4$
Bleeding	23	8	1
Pre-term labour	13	10	3
Cerclage	1	2	—
PROM	2	7	2
Pre-term delivery	13	20	4
Hypertension	5	7	—
IUGR	4	3	—
HELLP syndrome	—	1	1
Oligohydramnios	2	—	—
Death *in utero*	1	—	—
Perinatal loss	—	1	1

Table 11. Embryo transfers and total pregnancy rate after intracytoplasmic sperm injection (ICSI) in relation to numbers of embryos replaced in cycles using ejaculated sperm

hCG, human chorionic gonadotrophin

	Number	Percentage
Cycles	1194	
Cycles with cryopreservation	519	43·5[A]
Embryo transfers	1090	91·3[A]
Pregnancy rate (hCG positive) per transfer:		
overall	425/1090	39·0
1 embryo	10/95	10·5
2 embryos	41/154	26·6
2 embryos (elective)[B]	96/235	40·9
3 embryos	133/305	43·6
3 embryos (elective)[C]	135/275	49·1
>3 embryos	10/26	38·5

[A] Percentage of cycles.
[B] Two excellent embryos were replaced, although others were available.
[C] Three excellent embryos were replaced at the patient's request.

Table 14. Pregnancies after transfer of frozen-thawed embryos
hCG, human chorionic gonadotrophin

	Number	Percentage of embryos:		
		thawed	survived	replaced
Embryos thawed	1165			
Embryos surviving	673	57·8		
Embryos replaced	646	55·4	96·0	
Pregnancies (hCG positive)	43	3·7	6·4	6·7

Table 15. Cases of major congenital malformations in 439 children born after intracytoplasmic sperm injection (ICSI)

Number	Malformation
1	Holoprosencephaly
2–3	Palatochisis (twin)
4	Femur–fibula–ulna syndrome
5	Malformation of the left hip and left leg
6	Hypospadias
7	Diaphragma eventration
8	Down's syndrome
9	Tetralogy of Fallot
10	Situs inversus
11	Pre-axial polydactylia
12	Pseudo-arthrogryposis plus Pierre Robin syndrome
13	Hypospadias plus unilateral cryptorchidia
14	Cheilopalatochisis plus malformation of the foot
15	Hypospadias
16	Polymalformative syndrome (gastrochisis, body stalk, malformations of the foot and leg)

Frozen–Thaw Embryo Transfer Cycles

In 329 cycles, a total of 1171 supernumerary ICSI embryos were frozen. At the last update (Van der Elst et al. 1994), 1165 embryos had been thawed in 310 thaw cycles. As shown in Table 14, 673 embryos had at least 50% of their blastomeres intact, giving a survival rate of 57·8%. After replacing these embryos in 260 transfers, 43 pregnancies occurred (16·5% per transfer). However, the pregnancy wastage in the first trimester was remarkably high, with 14 biochemical pregnancies (32·5%), 10 miscarriages (23·3%), 2 ectopic pregnancies (4·7%) and one patient had her pregnancy interrupted. Seven patients have given birth and 9 pregnancies are still ongoing.

Pregnancy Outcomes

As of 30 August 1994, a total of 794 ICSI pregnancies have been established in our centre, including 47 pregnancies after the replacement of frozen–thawed embryos. Prenatal karyotypes were obtained in 371 pregnancies and 366 (98·6%) were found to be normal, including 7 which showed transmitted 'benign' structural aberrations. Five (1·4%) karyotypes were abnormal: 47XXY ($n = 2$), 47XXX, 47XYY and 47XX+20. The number of ICSI children born was 413, and 16 (3·9%) major congenital malformations have been recorded. These are listed in Table 15. The obstetric outcome of ICSI pregnancies has been reported by Wisanto et al. (1995).

Discussion

Although the introduction of IVF represented a major breakthrough in the treatment of male factor infertility, many couples could not be helped because this treatment failed or their sperm parameters were too low for IVF to be even considered. In other cases, for example congenital bilateral absence of the vas deferens, the results after conventional IVF were unacceptably low (Silber et al. 1994). ICSI uses only one single spermatozoon in order to inseminate the oocyte and bypasses gamete interaction at the level of the zona pellucida and the vitelline membrane. For this reason, patients with quantitative sperm disorders such as those with surgically uncorrectable excretory azoospermia or cryptozoospermia, as well as patients with qualitative sperm disorders such as globozoospermia or 100% immotile sperm, may benefit from this technique.

The results of the current survey corroborate the initial reports on ICSI from this centre (Van Steirteghem et al. 1993a, 1993b). Furthermore, high fertilization rates were achieved after ICSI and the 2 PN fertilization rate per retrieved OCC was comparable to conventional IVF in non-male factor cases (Tournaye et al. 1992). The patients included in this series, however, had severe male factor infertility for which conventional IVF was not indicated, even using improved insemination conditions. Analysis of the damage rates in our centre over the 26-month period indicates that the ICSI technique followed a learning curve. The sharp increase in the fertilization rate observed from the second-half of 1992 onwards may coincide with changes in the sperm preparation and injection protocols (Liu et al. 1994a).

From the moment a single viable spermatozoon could be successfully injected into a metaphase II oocyte, the fertilization rate was invariably the same, regardless of the extent of sperm defects in the semen sample. Even in patients with virtual azoospermia, in which no sperm were observed by standard microscopic examination but only after centrifugation and further preparation, the fertilization rate was similar to cases in which the sperm parameters were normal. In cases with 100% teratozoospermia, high fertilization rates were also observed after ICSI using morphologically abnormal sperm. Only in cases in which immotile sperm had to be injected did the fertilization rate appear to be reduced. This can be explained by the presence of ultrastructural abnormalities at the axonemal level which might have interfered with the events of fertilization after sperm injection. On the other hand, the use of completely immotile sperm also makes it more difficult to be certain that a vital spermatozoon has been selected for injection. Nevertheless, it is important to stress that complete fertilization failure occurred in only 2·9% of the ICSI cycles, and in one-quarter of these, failure was associated with the injection of immotile sperm. Attempts have been made to improve the selection of vital sperm from samples with 100% immotile sperm by using the hypo-osmotic swelling (HOS) test (Desmet et al. 1994). In a research set-up, 50 one-day-old unfertilized oocytes were injected with immotile sperm which showed a positive HOS test and 30% of the oocytes underwent normal (2 PN) fertilization. Since to date these experiments have not been repeated using fresh oocytes, it remains to be proven whether or not the HOS test represents a useful tool to improve fertilization when using 100% immotile spermatozoa. On the other hand, this problem might be overcome in selected cases such as necrozoospermia by using sperm recovered from a testicular biopsy. The second main cause of ICSI failure was a low number of oocytes available for injection. In contrast to conventional IVF in which the OCC are inseminated, ICSI requires injection of metaphase II oocytes without damage. Since only about 72% of the OCC contained a metaphase II oocyte which could be successfully injected, it is not surprising to find fertilization failures in the subgroup of patients who only had a few eggs. Injection of round-headed sperm was also associated with ICSI failure, although in our present experience, fertilization failure is merely a patient-related phenomenon. Unexplained fertilization failure occurred in only 0·3% of the ICSI cycles.

Although fertilization rates after ICSI with epididymal sperm were reduced in comparison to those obtained using ejaculated sperm, they were still remarkably high compared with those achieved after conventional IVF (Silber et al. 1994). The lower fertilization rate using epididymal sperm may be explained by the fact that in some of the patients undergoing MESA, only immotile, and therefore possibly senescent, sperm were available for injection. The use of testicular sperm for conventional IVF has been reported, but as for epididymal sperm, fertilization after IVF with testicular sperm will certainly be lower than after ICSI. This would be expected from the low number of motile sperm which can be obtained from a testicular biopsy. In cases involving the use of epididymal and testicular sperm, embryo development was found to be reduced and fewer supernumerary embryos were available for cryopreservation.

In this series, about 91% of the patients had an embryo transfer, and in approximately 80% of these cases, 2 or 3 embryos were electively replaced. The number of embryos replaced after ICSI depends on the number requested by the patient or the number proposed as a result of the transfer policy of our centre (Staessen et al. 1993), rather than on the availability of good quality embryos. When using ejaculated sperm, supernumerary embryos with <20% fragmentation were available for transfer in 43% of the cycles. Neither the number of embryos available for transfer nor the quality of these embryos was affected by the sperm quality.

The clinical pregnancy rate was 28·4% per started cycle. This figure corresponds with the pregnancy rate for tubal factor patients in our conventional IVF programme, but exceeds the IVF pregnancy rate for patients with moderate male factor infertility (Tournaye et al. 1992a). The obstetric outcome of pregnancies after microassisted fertilization was comparable to that of pregnancies after conventional IVF for male factor infertility (Tournaye et al. 1992a).

So far, no substantial increase in chromosomal abnormalities has been observed in the prenatal karyotypes. The incidence and types of major congenital malformations have been comparable to that of our general population. To date, we have therefore been unable to find reasons for any great concern as regards the occurrence of major congenital anomalies after ICSI. However, the size of the sample studied here is limited and data collection is still ongoing. The European Society for Human Reproduction and Embryology (ESHRE) is currently constructing a multi-centre database on the outcome of pregnancies after ICSI.

Acknowledgments

Geertrui Bocken, An Vankelecom, Heidi Van Ranst and Bart Desmet are specially acknowledged for their technical skills in the assisted fertilization technique. The authors also gratefully acknowledge the assistance of Frank Winter, M.A. in correcting this manuscript. Thanks are also extended to all our clinical, scientific and paramedical colleagues in the Centre for Reproductive Medicine.

References

Bonduelle, M., Desmyttere, S., Buysse, A., Van Assche, E., Schietecatte, J., Devroey, P., Van Steirteghem, A. C, and Liebaers, I. (1994). Prospective follow-up study of 55 children born after subzonal insemination and intracytoplasmic sperm injection. *Hum. Reprod (Oxf.).* **9**, 1765–9.

Buysse, A., Magnus, M., Schiettecatte, J., Bonduelle, M., Liebaers, I., Joris, H., Tournaye, H., Wisanto, A., Devroey, P., and Van Steirteghem, A.C. (1994). A paramedical approach to the follow-up of pregnancies and babies born after assisted fertilization. *Hum. Reprod. (Oxf.)* **9** (Suppl 4), 79. [Abstr.]

Camus, M., Van den Abbeel, E., Van Waesberghe, L., Wisanto, A., Devroey, P., and Van Steirteghem, A. C. (1989). Human embryo viability after freezing with dimethylsulfoxide as a cryoprotectant. *Fertil. Steril.* **51**, 460–5.

Desmet, B., Joris, H., Nagy, Z., Liu, J., Bocken, G., Vankelecom, A., Van Ranst, H., Devroey, P., and Van Steirteghem, A. C. (1994). Selection of vital immotile spermatozoa for intracytoplasmic sperm injection by the hypo-osmotic swelling test. *Hum. Reprod. (Oxf.)* **9** (Suppl. 4), 24. [Abstr.]

Devroey, P., Liu, J., Nagy, Z., Tournaye, H., Silber, S. J., and Van Steirteghem, A. C. (1994). Normal fertilization of human oocytes after testicular sperm extraction and intracytoplasmic sperm injection. *Fertil. Steril.* **62**, 639–41.

Hammitt, D. G., Walker, D. L., Syrop, C. H., Miller, T. M., and Bennett, M. R. (1991). Treatment of severe male-factor infertility with high concentrations of motile sperm by microinsemination in embryo cryopreservation straws. *J. In Vitro Fertil. Embryo Transfer* **8**, 101–10.

Kruger, T. F., Menkveld, R., Stander, F. S., Lombard, C. J., Van der Merwe, J. P., van Zyl, J. A., and Smith, K. (1986). Sperm morphologic features as a prognostic factor in *in vitro* fertilization. *Fertil. Steril.* **46**, 1118–23.

Laws-King, A., Trounson, A., Sathananthan, H., and Kola, I. (1987). Fertilization of human oocytes by microinjection of a single spermatozoon under the zona pellucida. *Fertil. Steril.* **48**, 637–42.

Liu, J., Nagy, Z., Joris, H., Tournaye, H., Devroey, P., and Van Steirteghem, A. C. (1994a). Intracytoplasmic sperm injection does not require special treatment of the spermatozoa. *Hum. Reprod. (Oxf.)* **9**, 1127–30.

Liu, J., Joris, H., Nagy, Z., Devroey, P., and Van Steirteghem, A. C. (1994b). Analysis of 33 fertilization failures in 1124 intracytoplasmic sperm injection cycles. *Hum. Reprod. (Oxf.)* **9** (Suppl. 4), 26–7. [Abstr.]

Mahadevan, M. M., Trounson, A. O., and Leeton, J. F. (1983). The relationship of tubal blockage, infertility of unknown cause, suspected male infertility, and endometriosis to success of *in vitro* fertilization and embryo transfer. *Fertil. Steril.* **40**, 755–62.

Mahadevan, M. M., and Trounson, A. O. (1984). The influence of seminal characteristics on the success rate of human *in vitro* fertilization. *Fertil. Steril.* **42**, 400–5.

Marrs, R. P., Vargyas, J. M., Saito, H., Gibbons, W. E., Berger, T., and Mishell, D. R. (1983). Clinical applications of techniques used in human *in vitro* fertilization research. *Am. J. Obstet. Gynecol.* **146**, 477–81.

Nagy, Z. P., Liu, J., Joris, H., Bocken, G., Tournaye, H., Devroey, P., and Van Steirteghem, A. C. (1994). Extremely impaired semen parameters and the outcome of the intracytoplasmic sperm injection. *Hum. Reprod. (Oxf.)* **9** (Suppl. 4), 20. [Abstr.]

Nagy, Z., Liu, J., Janssenswillen, C., Silber, S., Devroey, P., and Van Steirteghem, A. (1995). Using ejaculated, fresh and frozen–thawed epididymal and testicular spermatozoa gives rise to comparable results after intracytoplasmic sperm injection. *Fertil. Steril.* **63**, 808–15.

O'Donovan, P. A., Vandekerckhove, P., Lilford, R. J., and Hughes, E. (1993). Treatment of male infertility: is it effective? Review and meta-analyses of published randomized controlled trials. *Hum. Reprod. (Oxf.)* **8**, 1209–22.

Oehninger, S., Acosta, A. A., Morshedi, M., Veeck, L., Swanson, R. J., Simmons, K. F., and Rosenwaks, Z. (1988). Corrective measures and pregnancy outcome in *in vitro* fertilization in patients with severe sperm morphology abnormalities. *Fertil. Steril.* **50**, 283–7.

Ord, T., Patrizio, P., Marello, E., Balmaceda, J. P., and Asch, R. H. (1990). Mini-Percoll: a new method of semen preparation for IVF in severe male factor infertility. *Hum. Reprod. (Oxf.)* **5**, 987–9.

Ord, T., Patrizio, P., Balmaceda, J. P., and Asch, R. H. (1993). Can severe male factor infertility be treated without micromanipulation? *Fertil. Steril.* **60**, 110–15.

Palermo, G., Joris, H., Devroey, P., and Van Steirteghem, A. C. (1992a). Induction of acrosome reaction in human spermatozoa used for subzonal insemination. *Hum. Reprod. (Oxf.).* **7**, 248–54.

Palermo, G., Joris, H., Devroey, P., and Van Steirteghem, A. C. (1992b). Pregnancies after intracytoplasmic injection of single spermatozoon into an oocyte. *Lancet* **340**, 17–18.

Palermo, G., Joris, H., Derde, M.-P., Camus, M., Devroey, P., and Van Steirteghem, A. (1993). Sperm characteristics and outcome of human assisted fertilization by subzonal insemination and intracytoplasmic sperm injection. *Fertil. Steril.* **59**, 826–35.

Sapienza, F., Verheyen, G., Tournaye, H., Janssens, R., Pletincx, I., Derde, M., and Van Steirteghem, A. C. (1993). An auto-controlled study in *in-vitro* fertilization reveals the benefit of Percoll centrifugation to swim-up in the preparation of poor-quality semen. *Hum. Reprod. (Oxf.)* **8**, 1856–62.

Silber, S. J., Nagy, Z. P., Liu, J., Godoy, H., Devroey, P., and Van Steirteghem, A. C. (1994). Conventional *in-vitro* fertilization *versus* intracytoplasmic sperm injection for patients requiring microsurgical epididymal sperm aspiration. *Hum. Reprod. (Oxf.)* **9**, 1705–9.

Smitz, J., Devroey, P., Camus, M., Khan, I., Staessen, C., Van Waesberghe, L., Wisanto, A., and Van Steirteghem, A. C. (1988). Addition of Buserelin to human menopausal gonadotrophins in patients with failed stimulations for IVF or GIFT. *Hum. Reprod. (Oxf.)* **3**, (Suppl. 2), 35–8.

Smitz, J., Devroey, P., Faguer, B., Bourgain, C., Camus, M., and Van Steirteghem, A. C. (1992). A prospective randomized comparison of intramuscular or intravaginal natural progesterone as a luteal phase and early pregnancy supplement. *Hum. Reprod (Oxf.).* **7**, 168–75.

Staessen, C., Janssenswillen, C., Van Den Abbeel, E., Devroey, P., and Van Steirteghem, A. C. (1993). Avoidance of triplet pregnancies by elective transfer of two good quality embryos. *Hum. Reprod. (Oxf.)* **8**, 1650–3.

Tournaye, H., Camus, M., Bollen, N., Wisanto, A., Van Steirteghem, A. C., and Devroey, P. (1991a). *In vitro* fertilization with frozen–thawed sperm: a method for preserving the progenitive potential of Hodgkin patients. *Fertil. Steril.* **55**, 443–5.

Tournaye, H., Camus, M., Kahn, I., Staessen, C., Van Steirteghem, A. C., and Devroey, P. (1991b). *In-vitro* fertilization, gamete- or zygote intra-Fallopian transfer for the treatment of male infertility. *Hum. Reprod. (Oxf.)* **6**, 263–6.

Tournaye, H., Devroey, P., Camus, M., Staessen, C., Bollen, N., Smitz, J., and Van Steirteghem, A. C. (1992a). Comparison of in-vitro fertilization in male and tubal infertility: a 3 year survey. *Hum. Reprod. (Oxf.)* **7**, 218–22.

Tournaye, H., Devroey, P., Camus, M., Valkenburg, M., Bollen, N., and Van Steirteghem, A. C. (1992b). Zygote intrafallopian transfer or *in vitro* fertilization and embryo transfer for the treatment of male-factor infertility: a prospective randomized trial. *Fertil. Steril.* **58**, 344–50.

Tournaye, H., Janssens, R., Camus, M., Staessen, C., Devroey, P., and Van Steirteghem, A. C. (1993). Pentoxifylline is not useful in enhancing sperm function in cases with previous *in vitro* fertilization failure. *Fertil. Steril.* **59**, 210–15.

Tournaye, H., Janssens, R., Verheyen, G., Camus, M., Devroey, P., and Van Steirteghem, A. (1994a). An indiscriminate use of pentoxifylline does not improve *in-vitro* fertilization in poor fertilizers. *Hum. Reprod. (Oxf.)* **9**, 1289–92.

Tournaye, H., Janssens, R., Verheyen, G., Devroey, P., and Van Steirteghem, A. (1994b). *In vitro* fertilization in couples with previous fertilization failure using sperm incubated with pentoxifylline and 2-deoxyadenosine. *Fertil. Steril.* **62**, 574–9.

Tournaye, H., Devroey, P., Liu, J., Nagy, Z., Lissens, W., and Van Steirteghem, A. (1994c). Microsurgical epididymal sperm aspiration and intracytoplasmic sperm injection: a new effective approach to infertility as a result of congenital bilateral absence of the vas deferens. *Fertil. Steril.* **61**, 1045–51.

Van der Elst, J., Van den Abbeel, E., Joris, H., Camus, M., Devroey, P., and Van Steirteghem, A. C. (1994). Cryopreservation of supernumerary multicellular human embryos obtained after intracytoplasmic sperm injection. *Hum. Reprod. (Oxf.)* **9** (Suppl. 4), 55. [Abstr.]

Van der Ven, H. H., Jeyendran, R. S., Al-Hasani, S., Tünnerhoff, A., Hoebbel, K., Diedrich, K., Krebs, D., and Perez-Pelaez, M. (1988). Glass wool column filtration of human semen: relation to swim-up procedure and outcome of IVF. *Hum. Reprod. (Oxf.)* **3**, 85–8.

Van der Ven, H. H., Hoebbel, K., Al-Hasani, S., Diedrich, K., and Krebs, D. (1989). Fertilization of human oocytes in capillary tubes using very low number of spermatozoa. A new treatment of severe oligozoospermia? *Ann. Urol.* **23**, 317–21.

Van Steirteghem, A. C., Liu, J., Joris, H., Nagy, Z., Janssenswillen, C., Tournaye, H., Derde, M.-P., Van Assche, E., and Devroey, P. (1993a). Higher success rate by intracytoplasmic sperm injection than by subzonal insemination. Report of a second series of 300 consecutive treatment cycles. *Hum. Reprod. (Oxf.)* **8**, 1055–60.

Van Steirteghem, A. C., Nagy, Z., Joris, H., Liu, J., Staessen, C., Smitz, J., Wisanto, A., and Devroey, P. (1993b). High fertilization and implantation rates after intracytoplasmic sperm injection. *Hum. Reprod. (Oxf.)* **8**, 1061–66.

Van Steirteghem, A. C., Nagy, Z., Liu, J., Joris, H., Janssenswillen, C., Smitz, J., Tournaye, H., Bonduelle, M., and Devroey, P. (1993c). Intracytoplasmic sperm Injection. *Assist. Reprod. Rev. (Oxf.)* **3**, 160–3.

Wisanto, A., Bonduelle, M., Liu, J., Liebars, I., Magnus, M., Van Steirteghem, A., and Devroey, P. (1995). Obstetric outcome of 424 pregnancies after intracytoplasmic single sperm injection (ICSI). *Hum. Reprod. (Oxf.)* (In press).

World Health Organization (1987). 'Laboratory Manual for the Examination of Human Semen and Semen–Cervical Mucus Interaction'. 2nd Edn. (Cambridge University Press: Cambridge.)

Yovich, J. L., and Stanger, J. D. (1984). The limitations of *in vitro* fertilization from males with severe oligospermia and abnormal sperm morphology. *J. In Vitro Fertil. Embryo Transfer* **1**, 172–9.

Yovich, J. M., Edirisinghe, W. R., Cummins, J. M., and Yovich, J. L. (1988). Preliminary results using pentoxifylline in a pronuclear stage tubal transfer (PROST) program for severe male factor infertility. *Fertil. Steril.* **50**, 179–81.

Yovich, J. M., Edirisinghe, W. R., Cummins, J. M., and Yovich, J. L. (1990). Influence of pentoxifylline in severe male factor infertility. *Fertil. Steril.* **53**, 715–22.

Manuscript received 21 March 1995

Open Discussion

Robert Edwards (Cambridge):

Can you associate any of the abnormalities in the children with any aspect of ICSI, especially sperm morphology? I noticed that many of your trisomies involved the Y chromosome, so presumably most of them were generated through the sperm.

Tournaye:

Yes, that's possible but we haven't seen a clear relationship. I think the series is still too limited to draw any valid conclusions. This research must continue and I think every unit must do these follow-ups.

David de Kretser (Melbourne):

What percentage of patients refuse prenatal diagnosis?

Tournaye:

In the beginning, we were pushing them to get the results of prenatal assessments as a requirement of institutional approval and most patients agreed, but now there is less pressure and only about one in three will have prenatal diagnosis.

Simon Fishel (Nottingham):

What is your unit's long-term paediatric follow-up plan?

Tournaye:

There are several people involved. One paramedical nurse is looking after the pregnancies in relation to the obstetrical outcome, phoning people etc., while another is looking at the children. There are two doctors from the Department of Genetics who are looking closely at the children. The way we do the follow-up is that normally once we know that the patient is pregnant, we send an extensive questionnaire to the patient and to the referring doctor, even if they are patients from abroad. The first questionnaire is sent after the first trimester in order to record miscarriages and, if it is an ongoing pregnancy, we send another questionnaire to both the patient and the referring doctor after the expected time of delivery. In 9 out of 10 cases we receive one or both of the questionnaires, so it's a good system.

Lars Hamberger (Göteborg):

ESHRE has a study group on the follow-up of ICSI children, so you can report data to me, André Van Steirteghem or Basil Tarlatzis.

Sean Flaherty (Adelaide):

At the 1994 ESHRE meeting, your unit presented the minor malformation rate as well, and I recall a total malformation rate including minor abnormalities of about 13%. Here you have only presented the major malformations?

Tournaye:

I might not notice a minor malformation in a child whereas someone who has been trained to find them would. I think there is a major bias in that 13% figure, because now we get patients from all around the world and the follow-up is mainly by questionnaires. In the early years, which was the data presented at ESHRE, many patients brought their 3 month old children to the hospital and they also recorded all the minor details about the children themselves. So I suspect that the minor malformation rate will decrease, because now we are really reliant on what information the referring doctor sends us.

Sherman Silber (St Louis):

Do you have a control study of the children born from conventional IVF *versus* ICSI?

Tournaye:

That was also presented at the 1994 ESHRE meeting. There were no differences in the frequency of abnormalities in the two groups.

Fertilizing Capacity of Epididymal and Testicular Sperm using Intracytoplasmic Sperm Injection (ICSI)

Sherman J. Silber [AC], Paul Devroey [B], Herman Tournaye [B] and André C. Van Steirteghem [B]

[A] St Luke's Hospital, 224 South Woods Mill Road, Suite 730, St Louis, Missouri 63017, USA.
[B] Centre for Reproductive Medicine, University Hospital and Medical School, Dutch-Speaking Brussels Free University, Laarbeeklaan 101, B-1090 Brussels, Belgium.
[C] To whom correspondence should be addressed.

Abstract. For men with uncorrectable obstructive azoospermia, their only hope of fathering a child is microsurgical epididymal sperm aspiration (MESA) combined with *in vitro* fertilization (IVF). In 1988, proximal epididymal sperm were demonstrated to have better motility than senescent sperm in the distal epididymis, and it was thought that retrieval of motile sperm from the proximal epididymis would yield reliable fertilization and pregnancy rates after conventional IVF. However, the results to date have been poor, and although a minority of patients achieved good fertilization rates with IVF, the vast majority (81%) had consistently poor or no fertilization and the pregnancy rate averaged only 9%. Recently, intracytoplasmic sperm injection (ICSI) has been successfully used to achieve fertilization and pregnancies for patients with extreme oligoasthenozoospermia. ICSI has therefore been applied to cases of obstructive azoospermia and, in this report, 67 MESA–IVF cases are compared with 72 MESA–ICSI cases. The principle that motile sperm from the proximal segments of the epididymis should be used for ICSI was followed, although in the most severe cases in which there was an absence of the epididymis (or absence of sperm in the epididymis), testicular sperm were obtained from macerated testicular biopsies. These sperm only exhibited a weak, twitching motion. In 72 consecutive MESA cases, ICSI resulted in fertilization and normal embryos for transfer in 90% of the cases, with an overall fertilization rate of 46%, a cleavage rate of 68%, and ongoing or delivered pregnancy rates of 46% per transfer and 42% per cycle. The pregnancy and take-home baby rates increased from 9% and 4·5% with IVF to 53% and 42% with ICSI. There were no differences between the results for fresh epididymal, frozen epididymal or testicular sperm, and the number of eggs collected did not affect the outcome. The results were also unaffected by the aetiology of the obstruction such as congenital absence of the vas deferens or failed vasoepididymostomy. The only significant factor which affected the pregnancy rate was female age. It is concluded that although complex mechanisms involving epididymal transport may be beneficial for conventional fertilization of human oocytes (*in vivo* or *in vitro*), none of these mechanisms are required for fertilization after ICSI. Given the excellent results with epididymal and testicular sperm, ICSI is obligatory for all future MESA patients. Finally, the use of ICSI with testicular sperm from men with non-obstructive azoospermia is also discussed.

Extra keywords: IVF, congenital absence of the vas, MESA, TESE, cystic fibrosis.

Introduction

Congenital absence of the vas deferens (CAV) and irreparable obstructive azoospermia due to failed vaso-epididymostomy (V-E), are the cause of male infertility in a large and frustrating group of patients who have normal spermatogenesis, and from whom large numbers of sperm are surgically retrievable for *in vitro* fertilization (IVF) (Temple-Smith *et al.* 1985; Silber *et al.* 1990). A treatment protocol consisting of microsurgical epididymal sperm aspiration (MESA) from the proximal region of the epididymis and IVF was developed to solve this problem. The first successful fertilization and pregnancies using this approach were achieved in CAV patients (Silber *et al.* 1988, 1990) and this technique was applied to all cases of obstructive azoospermia including failed vasectomy reversal and epididymal blockage. In some men, successful V-E was also performed at the time of the MESA. The two major achievements from

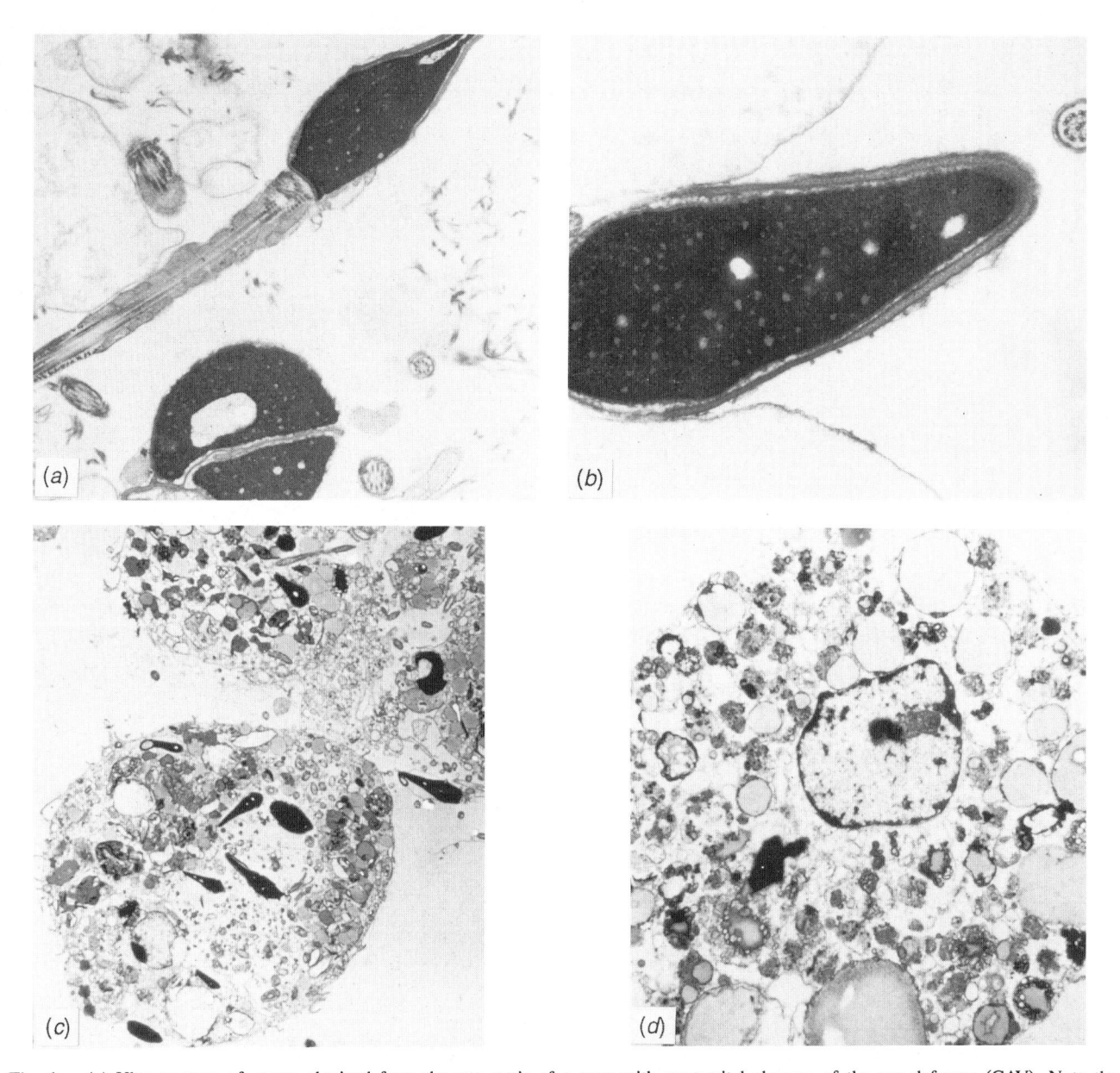

Fig. 1. (a) Ultrastructure of sperm obtained from the rete testis of a man with congenital absence of the vas deferens (CAV). Note the normal organization of the nucleus, acrosome and flagella. (b) Ultrastructure of a spermatozoon obtained from the vasa efferentia of a man with CAV. The organization of the nucleus, acrosome and flagella is similar to that of normal ejaculated sperm. (c) Ultrastructure of macrophages obtained from the corpus epididymis in a man with CAV. The cytoplasm of the macrophages contains large amounts of sperm remnants at different stages of degradation and digestion. (d) Ultrastructure of a macrophage obtained from the cauda epididymis of a man with CAV. Note the presence of prominent whorls of membranes and numerous lipid droplets indicating advanced stages of sperm degradation.

this work were: *(1)* the establishment of a successful treatment for male infertility caused by a condition that had previously been untreatable; and *(2)* a demonstration that in the human, sperm passage through the epididymis was not always required for fertilization and the live birth of normal children.

However, subsequent to the initial enthusiasm for using IVF with aspirated epididymal sperm, it soon became apparent that these sperm often failed to fertilize. The reason for this was not readily apparent and there were no recognizable differences between the quality of epididymal sperm that did or did not fertilize after IVF (Silber 1994). Most centres have obtained very low ($\leq$10%) fertilization rates and pregnancy rates of $\leq$9% (Anon. 1994).

Epididymal Sperm Motility and Conventional IVF

Sperm with the greatest motility are always found in the most proximal portion of the obstructed epididymis (Silber *et al.* 1990). Although the percent motility is usually low (1–30%), the greatest motility is always found, paradoxically, in the most proximal region. The most distal site from which progressively motile sperm are usually recovered is the proximal corpus epididymis, and this only occurs in about 10% of cases. Incubation of proximal epididymal sperm usually results in a dramatic improvement in progressive motility, whereas incubation of distal epididymal sperm does not improve their motility.

The fertilizing capacity of sperm which have not traversed the entire epididymis can ideally be studied with the human clinical model. In every mammal that has been studied, spermatozoa from the caput epididymis are only capable of weak circular motion at most and are not able to fertilize (Orgebin-Crist 1969), whereas sperm from the corpus epididymis can occasionally fertilize but the pregnancy rate is low. However, few of these animal studies allowed the sperm time to mature *in vivo* and thereby potentially develop the capacity for fertilization. In our clinical procedures, sperm are aspirated from specific regions of the obstructed epididymis, which allows them time to mature in the epididymis despite the absence of epididymal transit. In animal studies in which the epididymis was experimentally ligated to determine if time alone could mature sperm, the obstructed environment was so pathological that no firm conclusion about fertility could be reached, and the initial increase in motility was followed subsequently by sperm senescence and poor motility associated with obstruction (Gaddum and Glover 1965; Bedford 1966; Gaddum 1969; Glover 1969).

Thus, the most striking finding in the retrieval of sperm from the chronically-obstructed epididymis is the inversion of the usual pattern of motility one would expect in a non-obstructed epididymis. Sperm in the distal regions of an obstructed epididymis have poor or no motility because of senescence, and sperm in the proximal regions have the best motility. Therefore, the poor fertilization rate obtained using distal epididymal sperm is probably due to aging as well as immaturity (Krylov and Borovikov 1984). There is experimental support for this concept. Young (1931) ligated the guinea-pig epididymis at various levels and examined the proximal sperm that had been trapped for varying periods of time. Contrary to expectation, the more distal sperm had the poorest motility and the proximal sperm had the best. Young (1931) concluded that in the obstructed epididymis the more distal sperm are senescent, whereas the more proximal sperm have had time to mature despite having not passed through the epididymis. Thus, sperm maturation (development of progressive motility) appears to be intrinsic in nature, and may not require epididymal transit.

Clinical studies of V-E in humans have demonstrated equivalent pregnancy rates irrespective of whether the sperm had passed through a long or short length of the corpus epididymis, and even when sperm had only passed through a portion of the caput, there were reasonable pregnancy rates (Silber 1989a, 1989b). Two pregnancies have been documented (with proven paternity) after end-to-end anastomosis of the vas deferens to the vasa efferentia, with normal motile sperm found in the post-operative ejaculate. Thus sperm do not require transit through the epididymis in order to fertilize oocytes (Silber 1980, 1988; Weiske 1994). However, despite good motility, sperm collected from the proximal regions of the obstructed epididymis by MESA often do not fertilize oocytes by conventional IVF (Silber 1994).

We demonstrated with electron microscopy (EM) that after vasectomy, sperm which are proximal to the site of occlusion undergo senescence and degeneration into what appears by light microscopy to be debris and dead sperm, but is in fact globules of broken-down sperm heads and tails (Friend *et al.* 1976). The debris and dead sperm are initially seen in the ejaculate after vasovasostomy, however, if there is no secondary epididymal occlusion, the ejaculate eventually contains normal sperm. More recent studies have demonstrated that the reason for poor sperm motility in the distal epididymis of MESA patients is exactly the same senescent phenomenon. The quality and integrity of sperm aspirated from the rete testis, vasa efferentia, and caput is always markedly superior to the sperm aspirated from the corpus and cauda of the obstructed epididymis. The distal epididymis contains mostly degenerating and necrotic sperm along with large numbers of giant sperm-engulfing macrophages. This is similar to the senescence changes in sperm proximal to a vas occlusion. Sperm aspirated from the vasa efferentia, rete testis, and caput epididymis are usually similar to ejaculated sperm in normospermic subjects (Fig. 1). The only difference is that some of the proximal epididymal sperm possess a cytoplasmic droplet around the posterior portion of the head and the initial segment of the flagellum. With that exception and regardless of IVF success or failure, all of the proximal epididymal sperm we examined had a normal ultrastructure.

Nevertheless, it is still difficult to predict the fertilizing capacity of epididymal sperm from the sperm characteristics. Some samples with good motility yield no fertilization, whereas a small number of samples with poor motility yield good fertilization rates.

Intracytoplasmic Sperm Injection and MESA

Intracytoplasmic sperm injection (ICSI) has been successfully used to treat extreme oligoasthenozoospermia (Palermo *et al.* 1992, 1993; Van Steirteghem *et al.* 1993a, 1993b). We have therefore examined the proposal that ICSI could be used to improve the poor fertilization and pregnancy rates obtained with MESA–IVF. The present collaborative studies confirm that ICSI using epididymal or testicular sperm in men with CAV or any other cause of obstructive azoospermia gives reliable, and much higher, fertilization and pregnancy rates than conventional IVF with MESA (Tournaye et al. 1994; Silber et al. 1994, 1995).

The purpose of this paper is to: *(1)* document the first large-scale, systematic use of ICSI to treat obstructive azoospermia due to CAV, failed V-E or irreparable obstruction; *(2)* document the first systematic use of ICSI with testicular sperm; *(3)* predict the use of testicular sperm and ICSI for the treatment of non-obstructive azoospermia due to Sertoli cell-only syndrome and maturation arrest; and *(4)* review what the ICSI technique reveals about epididymal and testicular physiology.

Materials and Methods

Induction of Follicular Development and Oocyte Retrieval

The female partners underwent routine induction of multiple follicular development. Briefly, the protocol involved the daily subcutaneous administration (1 mg) of leuprolide acetate (Lupron; TAP Pharmaceuticals, North Chicago, IL, USA) until the day of follicular aspiration. After desensitization, patients received human follicle-stimulating hormone (FSH) (Metrodin; Serono, Randolph, MA, USA) and/or human menopausal gonadotrophin (hMG) (Pergonal; Serono) until multiple follicles 2·0 cm in diameter were noted by ultrasound. At that time, 10 000 I.U. of human chorionic gonadotrophin (hCG) (Profasi; Serono) was administered intramuscularly and, 35 h later, patients underwent transvaginal follicle aspiration.

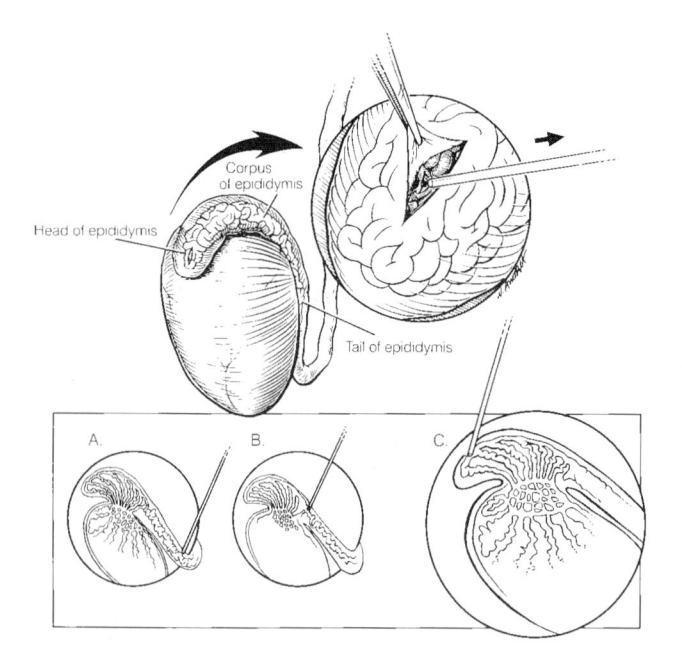

Fig. 2. Sperm were microsurgically aspirated from distal and proximal regions of the epididymis. The samples with the best motility were used for IVF. From Silber (1994).

Microsurgical Epididymal Sperm Aspiration

The male partners underwent scrotal exploration and MESA to obtain sufficient numbers of motile sperm for IVF or ICSI. The surgical technique was as follows. The scrotal contents were extruded through a small incision, the tunica vaginalis was opened and the epididymis was exposed. Under 10–40× magnification with an operating microscope, a tiny incision was made with micro-scissors in the epididymal tunic to expose the tubules in the proximal portion of the obstructed epididymis. Sperm were aspirated directly from the opening in the tubule with a plastic micropipette (Medicuts 22G, 0·7 mm/22 mm; Cook Urological, Spencer, IN, USA). The epididymal fluid was immediately diluted in HEPES-buffered Earle's medium and an aliquot was examined for motility and quality of progression. If sperm exhibited poor motility or no motility, another aspiration was made more proximally (Figs 2 and 3). Motile sperm were usually not obtained until the proximal caput epididymis or vasa efferentia were reached (Silber et al. 1988, 1990). The rationale for proceeding proximally to find the most motile sperm for ICSI was based on the following presumptions: *(1)* ICSI with ejaculated sperm is most efficient when there is some motility, no matter how poor, as a verification of 'vitality'; and *(2)* the most proximal sperm are least likely to have undergone degenerative changes in the sperm head due to senescence.

Testicular Sperm Extraction

When there was no epididymis, the entire scrotum was massively scarred, or there simply were no sperm in the epididymis, testicular sperm extraction (TESE) was performed to recover sperm for ICSI. The surgical technique for testicular biopsy was extremely simple. A small 1-cm horizontal incision was made in the scrotal skin and carried through the peritoneal tunica vaginalis. Then a 0·5-cm incision was made in the tunica albuginea and a small piece of extruded testicular tissue was excised and placed in a small Petri dish with 3 mL of HEPES-buffered Earle's medium. The tunica albuginea was closed with several 3–0 vicryl intracuticular stitches. When the retrieval of testicular tissue was performed as a last resort after unsuccessful MESA, the incision was more extensive because it was known that only testicular sperm would be available.

The testicular tissue was finely minced in HEPES-buffered Earle's medium and the suspension was placed in a 5-mL tube and centrifuged for 5 min at 300*g*. The supernatant was removed with a Pasteur pipette, and after adding 0·1–0·2 mL of Earle's medium, the pellet was gently resuspended. The sperm suspension was kept at 37°C in an incubator gassed with 5% O_2, 5% CO_2 and 90% N_2 until the injection procedure was performed. The number of sperm in the resulting droplet was few, so individual sperm had to be selected for ICSI from among the debris, red blood cells, and spermatid-laden Sertoli cells. The barely motile testicular sperm were placed in a PVP droplet which resulted in immediate and complete immotility.

In the 72 cases reported here, our first choice was to obtain epididymal sperm. The reason was that we could freeze and save the majority of the epididymal sperm for subsequent ICSI cycles without the need for further surgery. Freezing of testicular sperm was not considered because of the small numbers of sperm and their extremely poor motility.

MESA and Conventional IVF

Epididymal sperm were first diluted and examined in a 5-mL volume and then concentrated into a volume of 0·3 mL, layered onto a discontinuous mini-Percoll gradient (Ord et al. 1990), and centrifuged for 30 min. The entire 95% Percoll fraction was then washed twice and added to the entire cohort of eggs in a tube in 1 mL of HTF culture media (Quinn et al. 1985). After incubation at

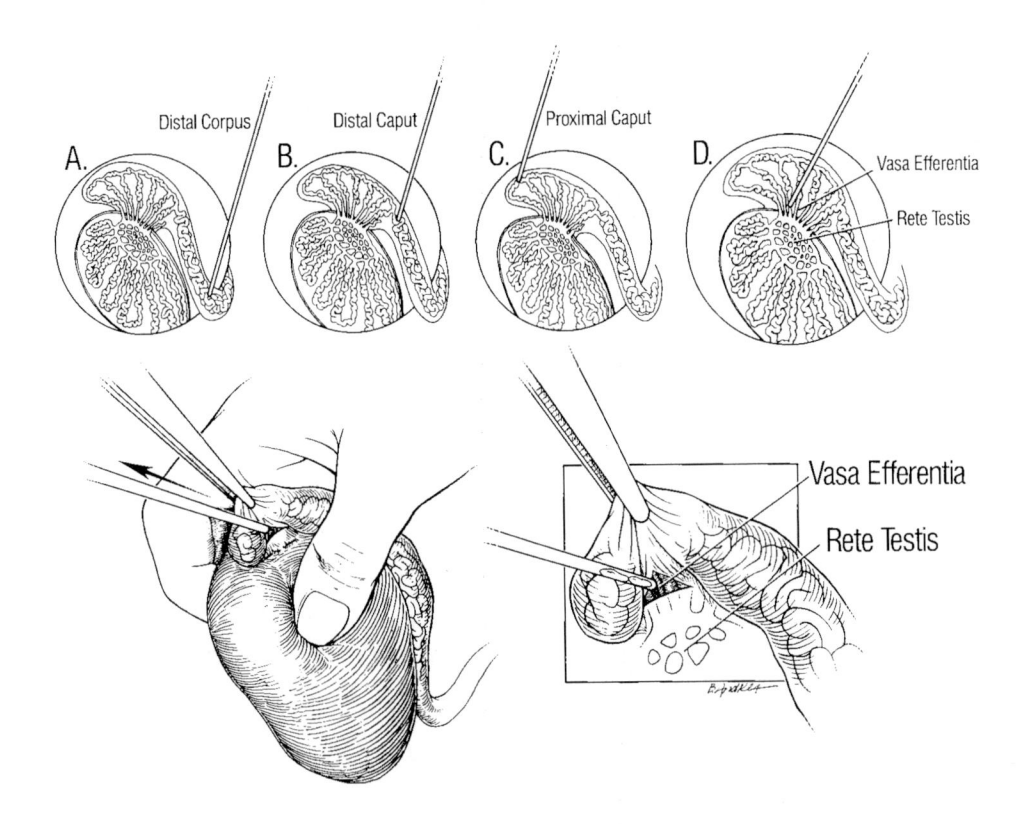

Fig. 3. Sperm in the distal and sometimes proximal epididymis were often immotile or poorly motile, and in these cases, vasa efferentia fluid was collected and usually contained the most motile sperm. From Silber (1994).

37°C and 5% CO_2 in air for two days, the embryos were transferred to the Fallopian tubes or to the uterus. The female partners received 50 mg day^{-1} progesterone in oil (intramuscularly), beginning on the day of oocyte collection.

MESA and ICSI

The procedures for sperm and oocyte preparation, microinjection and culture were essentially as described by Van Steirteghem et al. (1993a, 1993b). Details are provided below. A slightly different approach was used for MESA–ICSI. Since only very small numbers of sperm with weak motility (vitality) were required for ICSI, the unused epididymal fluid was diluted 1:1 with sperm freezing medium, drawn into 0·25-mL straws, frozen in liquid nitrogen vapour then plunged into liquid nitrogen.

Oocyte Preparation for ICSI

After oocyte retrieval, up to 8 cumulus–oocyte complexes were transferred into a tube containing Earle's medium. The tubes were gassed, tightly closed and then transported in a thermobox (37°C) to the microinjection laboratory which was about 500 m away. The cells of the cumulus and corona radiata were removed by incubation for about 30 s in HEPES-buffered Earle's medium containing 80 I.U. mL^{-1} of hyaluronidase (Type VIII; specific activity 320 I.U. mg^{-1}; Sigma, St Louis, MO, USA). Removal of the cumulus and coronal cells was enhanced by aspiration of the complexes in and out of hand-drawn glass pipettes with an opening of about 200 μm. The oocytes were rinsed several times in HEPES-buffered Earle's and B_2 media and then assessed at 200× magnification for nuclear maturity (germinal vesicle, polar body) and cytoplasmic abnormalities.

Oocytes were then incubated in 25-μL microdrops of B_2 medium covered by lightweight paraffin oil (BDH, Brussels, Belgium) at 37°C in an atmosphere of 5% CO_2, 5% O_2 and 90% N_2. About 3–4 h later, the immature oocytes were checked to determine if any of them had extruded the first polar body. Intracytoplasmic sperm injection was carried out on all morphologically intact oocytes that had extruded the first polar body (metaphase II stage).

Preparation of ICSI Pipettes

The holding and injection pipettes were made from 30-μL borosilicate glass capillary tubes which were 78 mm long and had an inner diameter (ID) of 0·69 mm and an outer diameter (OD) of 0·97 mm (Drummond Scientific Company, Broomall, PA, USA). The capillaries were sonicated for 30 min in Milli RO or Milli Q water (Millipore, Brussels, Belgium) containing 2% (v/v) detergent (7X-PF O-MATIC; Flow Laboratories, Irvine, Scotland), then rinsed in running Milli Q water for 30 min. This cleaning procedure was repeated before the capillary tubes were finally dried and sterilized at 100°C for 6 h in a ULE 500 oven (Memmert, Schwabach, Germany). The second sonication was done in water without detergent.

The pipettes were made using a Type 753 horizontal micro-electrode puller (Campden Instruments, Loughborough, Leicestershire, UK). The holding pipettes were cut and fire-polished on a MF-9 microforge (Narishige, Tokyo, Japan) to obtain an OD of 50 μm and an ID of 20 μm. To prepare the injection pipettes, the pulled capillaries were opened on an EG-4 microgrinder (Narishige) to an OD of 7 μm, an ID of 5 μm and a bevel angle of 50°. The microforge was used to make a sharp spike on each injection pipette and to bend the edge of the holding and injection pipettes to an angle of about 45° in order to facilitate injection in a Petri dish.

ICSI Procedure

A 3–5-μL sperm droplet was placed in the centre of a Petri dish (Falcon 1006; Becton Dickinson, Lincoln Park, NJ, USA), surrounded by eight 5-μL droplets of HEPES-buffered Earle's medium which contained 0·5% crystalline bovine serum albumin (BSA). The droplets were covered with about 3·5 mL of lightweight paraffin oil. The ICSI procedure was carried out at 37°C on a Diaphot inverted microscope (Nikon, Tokyo, Japan) at 400× magnification using Hoffman modulation contrast optics (Modulation Optics, Greenvale, NY, USA) and a THN-60/16 heated stage (Linkam Scientific Instruments, London, UK). The microscope was equipped with a F-601M camera (Nikon) for still pictures and a DXC-755P video camera (Sony, Brussels, Belgium) that allowed the procedure to be followed on a PVM-1443MD Trinitron colour video monitor (Sony). The microscope was equipped with two coarse positioning manipulators (3D Motor Driven Coarse Control Manipulator MM-188; Narishige) and two three-dimensional hydraulic remote-control micromanipulators (Joystick Hydraulic Micromanipulator MO-188; Narishige). The holding and injection pipettes were fitted to tool holders and were connected by Teflon tubing (CT-1; Narishige) to IM-6 microinjectors (Narishige). Fluid delivery was controlled by a 1-μL resolution vernier micrometer.

A single, almost immotile spermatozoon was selected from the central droplet and aspirated tail-first into the tip of the injection pipette. The Petri dish was then moved in order to visualize an oocyte in one of the droplets surrounding the sperm suspension. The oocyte was immobilized against the holding pipette by slight negative pressure. The oocyte was positioned so that the polar body was at 12 o'clock or 6 o'clock and the injection pipette was pushed through the zona pellucida and the oolemma into the ooplasm at 3 o'clock. The spermatozoon was injected into the ooplasm with about 1–2 pL of medium. The injection pipette was withdrawn gently and the injected oocyte was released from the holding pipette. This was repeated until all the metaphase II oocytes had been injected. The injected oocytes were then washed in B_2 medium, transferred to 25-μL droplets of B_2 medium in Petri dishes covered by lightweight paraffin oil and incubated in a B5060 EK/O_2 incubator (Heraeus, Brussels, Belgium) at 37°C in an atmosphere of 5% CO_2, 5% O_2 and 90% N_2.

Assessment of Fertilization and Embryo Cleavage

Further handling of the injected oocytes followed our standard IVF procedures. About 16–18 h after microinjection, the oocytes were observed under an inverted microscope at 200× or 400× magnification for any sign of damage and for the presence of pronuclei (PN) and polar bodies. Fertilization was considered to be normal when two distinct PN containing nucleoli were observed. The presence of one PN or three PN was noted together with the presence of one, two or fragmented polar bodies. If a single PN was observed, a second evaluation was carried out about 4 h later to see if another PN appeared. Cleavage of the 2 PN oocytes was evaluated after a further 24 h in culture and embryos were scored according to the equality of size of the blastomeres and the number of anucleate fragments. Cleaved embryos with < 50% of their volume filled with anucleate fragments were eligible for transfer. Up to three embryos, and occasionally more (depending on female age and embryo quality), were loaded into a Frydman catheter (LG 4·5; Prodimed, Neuilly-en-Thelle, France) in a small volume of Earle's medium and transferred to the uterine cavity. Embryo replacement was usually done about 48 h after microinjection. If supernumerary embryos with < 20% anucleate fragments were available, they were cryopreserved on Day 2 or Day 3 by a slow-freezing protocol using dimethylsulfoxide (DMSO).

Establishment and Follow-up of Pregnancies

Pregnancy was confirmed by detection of increasing serum hCG concentrations on at least two occasions, at least 10 days after embryo replacement. Clinical pregnancy was determined by observing a gestational sac by means of ultrasound screening at 7 weeks of pregnancy. Prenatal diagnosis was carried out by chorionic villus sampling at 9–10 weeks of gestation or by amniocentesis at 16 weeks of gestation. Genetic counselling was given in view of the prenatal diagnosis and for planning a prospective follow-up study of the children born after ICSI. The referring gynaecologist and the patients were asked to provide detailed information on the outcome of the pregnancy and the delivery.

Results and Discussion

Comparison of MESA–ICSI and MESA–IVF

The objective of our first study of 17 patients with CAV or irreparable obstructive azoospermia who had consistently failed to achieve fertilization in previous cycles with MESA–IVF was to determine whether ICSI could produce better results than MESA–IVF (Silber *et al.* 1994). When ICSI was used with epididymal or testicular sperm, we achieved good fertilization rates and normal embryos in 82% of the cases, compared with only 19% with conventional IVF. Table 1 summarizes the results and also demonstrates that 11 of the 15 patients (70%) with CAV had common cystic fibrosis (CF) carrier genotypes and 8 had the ΔF508 mutation. The CF carrier status had no adverse effect on the fertilization or pregnancy rates after ICSI. The overall ICSI fertilization rate was 45% (85% cleaved normally), compared with a 7% fertilization rate for conventional IVF. The pregnancy rate with MESA–ICSI was 47% per cycle (normal delivery rate of 30%) compared with 4·5% for MESA–IVF.

We concluded from this first series of 17 MESA–ICSI cycles that complex mechanisms facilitated by epididymal passage are required by sperm for conventional fertilization of human oocytes (whether *in vivo* or *in vitro*), but these mechanisms are not required for fertilization after ICSI. Because of the consistently good results using epididymal sperm with ICSI in comparison to conventional IVF, and also the good results in extreme cases requiring testicular tissue sperm, we concluded that ICSI would be essential for all future MESA patients with CAV or irreparable obstructive azoospermia.

This has been fully validated by the results of an additional 72 consecutive cycles of MESA–ICSI which were compared with 67 previous consecutive cycles of MESA–IVF. Fifty-three of the MESA–ICSI cycles were performed for CAV, 18 were for failed V-E, and one was for irreparable blockage. Since the results were equivalent for CAV and failed V-E, all the data were analysed as one group of 72 patients. Table 2 compares

Table 1. Results for the 17 patients in the first MESA–ICSI series based on cystic fibrosis genotype

CAV, congenital absence of the vas deferens; FR, fertilization rate; ICSI, intracytoplasmic sperm injection; MESA, microsurgical epididymal sperm aspiration; M II, metaphase II; N, normal genotype; PN, pronuclei. From Silber et al. (1994)

No.	Genotype if CAV	No. of M II eggs	No. of 2 PN eggs	No. embryos transferred	FR(%)	Female: age	Pregnant
1	ΔF508, N	9	3	3	33	42	No
2	N, N	14	5	5	36	39	No
3	ΔF508, N	22	11	6	50	31	No
4	ΔF508, N	10	5	5	50	33	No
5	R117H, R117H	14	6	4	43	31	Yes
6	ΔF508, N	18	6	4	33	28	Yes
7	W1282X, N	16	5	3	31	36	Yes
8	ΔF508, N	3	2	2	67	25	No
9	N, N	3	0	0	0	40	No
10	N, N	7	3	3	43	28	Yes
11	N, N	10	8	3	80	38	No
12	ΔF508, N	8	1	1	13	35	Yes
13	ΔF508, N	12	5	3	42	36	Yes
14	ΔF508, N	10	0	0	0	35	No
15	R117H, N	11	5	3	45	29	Yes
16	N, N	22	10	3	45	32	No
17	N, N	8	5	2	63	42	Yes
Totals		197	89	50	41%		8/17(47%)

Table 2. Comparison of MESA–ICSI and MESA–IVF in a similar patient population

ICSI, intracytoplasmic sperm injection; IVF, in vitro fertilization; MESA, microsurgical epididymal sperm aspiration; PN, pronuclei; PR, pregnancy rate. Adapted from Silber et al. (1994)

	MESA–IVF	MESA–ICSI
No. of cycles	67	72
No. of mature eggs	1427	962
No. of 2 PN eggs	98	443
Fertilization rate	7%	46%
No. (%) of embryo transfers	13 (19%)	65 (90%)
PR (ongoing or delivered PR)	9% (4·5%)	53% (42%)

Table 3. Fertilization, cleavage and pregnancy rates after ICSI with fresh epididymal sperm, frozen epididymal sperm and testicular sperm

ET, embryo transfer; ICSI, intracytoplasmic sperm injection; MESA, microsurgical epididymal sperm aspiration; M II, metaphase II; PN, pronuclei; PR, pregnancy rate; TESE, testicular sperm extraction

	Fresh epididymal sperm (MESA)	Frozen epididymal sperm	Testicular sperm (TESE)	Combined totals
No. of cycles	33	7	32	72
No. of M II eggs injected	431	95	436	962
No. of 2 PN eggs	201	27	215	443
Fertilization rate	47%	28%	49%	46%
No. (%) of cleaved embryos	127 (63%)	20 (74%)	155 (72%)	302 (68%)
No. (%) of ETs	31 (94%)	7 (100%)	27 (84%)	65 (90%)
No. of clinical pregnancies	20	4	14	38
Clinical PR per ET	65%	57%	52%	58%
No. of ongoing[A] pregnancies	15	3	12	30
Ongoing[A] PR per ET	48%	43%	44%	46%
Ongoing[A] PR per cycle	45%	43%	38%	42%

[A] Ongoing or delivered pregnancies.

the results of these 72 MESA–ICSI cycles with the 67 MESA–IVF cycles. The overall fertilization rate with MESA–IVF was 7% and only 19% of the patients had an embryo transfer. With ICSI, using epididymal or testicular sperm, the fertilization rate was 46% and 90% of the patients had an embryo transfer. The ongoing or delivered pregnancy rate per stimulated cycle was 4·5% after MESA–IVF compared with 42% after MESA–ICSI. This represents a 7–10-fold improvement in the results with ICSI, and is all the more impressive because the 72 ICSI cycles included 32 patients who had no epididymal sperm and thus required the use of testicular sperm.

Overall Results with TESE–ICSI and MESA–ICSI

After establishing that ICSI was preferable to conventional IVF for MESA, we compared the results among the different groups of patients (Table 3). The standard MESA procedure was the preferred approach because large numbers of sperm could be obtained from the epididymis and frozen for use in subsequent cycles without the need for further surgery. However, in many of the men who had undergone MESA on several earlier occasions, epididymal sperm could not be retrieved, and in these cases we often used testicular sperm. The patients in each of the three groups did not represent mixtures of clinical conditions or techniques. For example, if fresh epididymal sperm were used, then no eggs in that patient were injected with frozen epididymal sperm or testicular sperm. Similarly, if testicular sperm were used, then none of the eggs were injected with epididymal sperm.

The 2 PN fertilization rates were remarkably similar with fresh epididymal (MESA) sperm (47%) and testicular sperm (49%), whereas frozen epididymal sperm yielded a lower fertilization rate (28%). The cleavage rates were similar in all three groups: 63% for MESA, 74% for frozen epididymal sperm and 72% for testicular sperm (Table 3). Despite the lower 2PN fertilization rate with frozen–thawed epididymal sperm, all of these patients had embryo transfers after ICSI. Fresh MESA yielded a 94% transfer rate, whereas the transfer rate was 84% with testicular sperm. The ongoing or delivered pregnancy rates per transfer were 48% (MESA), 43% (frozen–thawed epididymal sperm) and 44% (TESE). The ongoing or delivered pregnancy rates per cycle were 45% (MESA) and 43% (frozen–thawed epididymal sperm). The pregnancy rate per cycle was lower (38%) for testicular sperm because of the lower transfer rate. A significant number (16%) of TESE–ICSI cases resulted in no fertilization, whereas there were very few fresh or frozen epididymal sperm cases with no fertilization. Nevertheless, the pregnancy rate per transfer was similar in all three groups.

MESA–ICSI for Irreparable Obstructive Azoospermia

Table 4 summarizes the results in 18 of the 72 patients whose indication for MESA was irreparable, failed V-E. The results for these patients were not different from those with CAV or from the combined results for the 72 patients. The 2PN fertilization rate was 50%, the cleavage rate was 79%, and 94% of the patients had embryos for transfer. Forty-four percent of the couples achieved a clinical pregnancy, which indicates that the aetiology of obstructive azoospermia had no influence on the results.

Table 4. The use of MESA–ICSI for failed vasoepididymostomy

ET, embryo transfer; ICSI, intracytoplasmic sperm injection; MESA, microsurgical epididymal sperm aspiration; M II, metaphase II; PN, pronuclei; PR, pregnancy rate

No. of patients	18
No. of M II eggs	249
No. of 2 PN eggs	124
Fertilization rate	50%
No. (%) of cleaved embryos	98 (79%)
No. (%) of patients with ET	17 (94%)
No. of clinical pregnancies	8
Clinical PR per cycle	44%

Virtually all the couples preferred to have a concurrent V-E or vasectomy reversal because we could assure them of an 88% chance of surgical success (Silber 1989a, 1989b, 1989c). As such, the couple could consider having more children in the future without the need for further ICSI. Since our normal policy was not to perform MESA–ICSI on reconstructable cases, this means that the 18 patients in Table 4 were a selected group who had no chance for pregnancy without MESA–ICSI. The results in this seemingly dismal group were still quite acceptable.

Results of MESA–ICSI or TESE–ICSI in Relation to Female Factors

Clearly, it was unimportant whether the sperm were derived from the epididymis (frozen or fresh) or the testis, or whether the male had CAV or irreparable obstruction. The CF genotype, sperm morphology and quality of motility also had no impact. The only factor in the 72 couples which affected success was the female age. The only female selection criteria were a normal uterus based on a hysterosalpingogram and a normal menstrual cycle. Several patients had tubal disease, polycystic ovary disease (PCO), some degree of endometriosis, or non-intraluminal uterine fibroids.

Table 5 summarizes the fertilization and pregnancy rates for MESA–ICSI in relation to the number of metaphase II oocytes that were retrieved. The 2 PN fertilization rate was not related to the number of mature

Table 5. Fertilization and pregnancy rates after MESA–ICSI in relation to the number of mature eggs

ET, embryo transfer; ICSI, intracytoplasmic sperm injection; MESA, microsurgical epididymal sperm aspiration; PN, pronuclei; PR, pregnancy rate

	No. of metaphase II eggs:			Totals
	< 10	10–19	≥20	
No. of patients	24	30	18	72
2 PN fertilization rate	48%	48%	43%	46%
Cleavage rate	83%	77%	65%	68%
Average no. of embryos per ET	2·3	3·5	3·5	2·9
No. of pregnancies	8	20	10	38
PR per cycle	33%	67%	56%	53%

Table 6. Fertilization and pregnancy rates after MESA–ICSI in relation to female age

ET, embryo transfer; ICSI, intracytoplasmic sperm injection; MESA, microsurgical epididymal sperm aspiration; M II, metaphase II; PN, pronuclei; PR, pregnancy rate

	Female age (years):			Combined totals
	< 30	30–37	> 37	
No. of patients	20	35	17	72
No. of M II eggs	293	479	190	962
No. of 2 PN eggs	138	220	85	443
Fertilization rate	47%	46%	45%	46%
No. (%) of cleaved embryos	91 (66%)	160 (73%)	51 (60%)	302 (68%)
Total no. of embryos transferred	54	104	51	209
Average no. of embryos per ET	2·7	3·0	3·0	2·9
No. of pregnancies	15	19	4	38
PR per cycle	75%	54%	24%	53%

Table 7. Ongoing implantation rates per embryo after ICSI with epididymal and testicular sperm

ICSI, intracytoplasmic sperm injection; MESA, microsurgical epididymal sperm aspiration; TESE, testicular sperm extraction

	Epididymal (MESA)	Testicular (TESE)
No. of patients	16	12
No. of embryo transfers	16	9
No. of embryos transferred	47	30
No. of foetal hearts	12[A]	7[B]
Ongoing implantation rate	25·5%	23·3%

[A] Includes 2 sets of triplets. [B] Includes 2 sets of twins.

eggs but the cleavage rate was higher when fewer eggs were retrieved. Fewer embryos were transferred when fewer eggs were obtained, however, the implantation rates per embryo were similar (16–20%) regardless of whether there was a high or low number of mature eggs. The pregnancy rate was reduced (33% v. 53%) in women with < 10 eggs, but this was due to the lower number of embryos transferred (2·3 v. 3·5). In the 72 cycles, there were 962 metaphase II eggs and 302 cleaved embryos (Table 3), which is an average of 4·2 embryos per patient. An average of only 2·9 embryos were transferred per patient because only the best quality embryos were selected for fresh transfer.

Table 6 demonstrates the effect of female age. The 2 PN fertilization rate (45–47%) and the cleavage rate was unrelated to female age. However, increased female age dramatically reduced the implantation and pregnancy rates. When the female partner was < 30 years of age, 75% of the MESA–ICSI cycles resulted in pregnancy. When the female was 30–37 years of age, 54% became pregnant, but when the woman was > 37 years of age, only 24% became pregnant. Thus, of all the factors which might have been predicted to affect the treatment of obstructive azoospermia by ICSI, only the age of the female had an impact, and this was not on the fertilization rate but on the implantation and pregnancy rates.

Implantation Rates after MESA–ICSI and TESE–ICSI

Although embryo transfer rates were high with both MESA–ICSI and TESE–ICSI, a significant percentage (16%) of the TESE–ICSI cycles resulted in no fertilization. This was rare with MESA–ICSI. Hence, we performed a prospective study in a series of 16 MESA cases and 12 TESE cases to determine if the implantation rate was different for embryos derived from ICSI using epididymal (MESA) and testicular sperm (TESE). The results are summarized in Table 7. There was complete failure of fertilization in 3 (25%) of the TESE cycles, whereas fertilization and an embryo transfer occurred in all of the MESA cycles. However, the ongoing implantation rates per embryo were not different (25·5% v. 23·3%) for epididymal and testicular sperm. Thus, for reasons we do not yet understand, testicular sperm do not always fertilize eggs after ICSI, but if fertilization does occur, the cleavage and implantation rates are not different from epididymal sperm.

Clinical Approach to Managing the CF Issue in CAV Patients Undergoing MESA

Virtually all patients with clinical CF, the most common genetic disorder in humans, also have CAV. Until recently, most CF patients did not survive long enough to consider fatherhood. None of the CAV patients we have treated thus far have had clinical CF. Until recently (Silber *et al.* 1991; Anguiano *et al* 1992; Patrizio *et al.* 1993), it was not recognized that infertile males with CAV had an isolated genital form of CF that was inherited via a mutation of the CF gene.

We routinely screen all CAV patients for the 36 most common CF mutations. About 70% of otherwise normal CAV patients have one of these CF mutations, despite a normal chloride sweat test and no clinical symptoms of CF. Our studies of the parents of these CAV patients, as well as their offspring, have revealed that: *(1)* one of the parents of the CF-positive, CAV male always has the same heterozygous mutation as their son; *(2)* male siblings of a CAV male have a 1 in 4 chance of also having CAV; *(3)* offspring of CAV males (after successful MESA) have in theory a 50% chance of having the same CF heterozygous mutation as the CAV father; *(4)* the CF heterozygous male offspring do not themselves have CAV, and indeed have normal bilateral vasa deferentia; *(5)* the presumption is that CF carrier status alone does not cause CAV; the child must acquire a mutation (perhaps undetectable with current methods) from both parents to develop CAV (Mercier *et al.* 1995); and *(6)* 10% of CAV patients have two different CF mutations, either two weak ones, or a weak and a strong one. These compound heterozygous carriers do not have clinical CF nor a positive sweat chloride test, yet compound heterozygosity can cause CF.

It is crucial to screen for CF in men with CAV and in their partners. If the female partner is negative for the 36 common CF mutations, we feel it is quite safe to perform MESA–ICSI since the chances of any male offspring having CAV are remote, and the chances of the child having CF is probably less than in a normal, unscreened population. However, if she turns out to be a CF carrier (4% incidence in the general population), the couple can still undergo MESA–ICSI, but pre-implantation embryo diagnosis or prenatal diagnosis should be performed.

We have published the first report of successful pre-implantation embryo diagnosis after MESA–ICSI in a couple in which the man had CAV and both partners were carriers of the ΔF508 CF mutation (Liu *et al.* 1994). Both were 35 years of age and they had given up hope many years earlier of ever having a child because of the low success rate of MESA–IVF. With the introduction of ICSI, they finally decided to attempt MESA, but the woman was also found to have the ΔF508 mutation on routine pre-MESA screening. This couple thus reflected a major question for those who are CF carriers, as both were heterozygous for ΔF508. Twelve metaphase II oocytes were retrieved and microinjected. One degenerated, 5 fertilized and cleaved to 4–8-cells by Day 3 post-oocyte recovery. One or 2 blastomeres were then removed with a micropipette, and underwent PCR and genetic analysis. Two of the 5 embryos were found to be homozygous for ΔF508 and therefore were not transferred. The other three embryos were all heterozygous-positive for ΔF508. The couple accepted the possibility of a child who was a CF carrier since they were both CF carriers themselves and 3 heterozygous embryos were replaced. The dilemma was that if the ΔF508 mutation in the embryo originated from the mother, then some unknown CF mutation from the father might be transmitted to the child along with the mother's ΔF508 mutation. Thus, any male child would not be a true heterozygote but would be similar to his father and would therefore most likely have CAV. Since the father had no phenotypic expression of CF other than CAV, it was felt there would be little or no risk of the child having CF. If the ΔF508 mutation in the embryo originated from the father, then there would be no undue concern. The woman became pregnant and delivered a normal baby boy who was confirmed to be a heterozygous ΔF508 carrier. The child's chloride sweat test was normal and both vasa deferentia were present and normal, indicating that the ΔF508 deletion probably originated from the father.

A more serious problem arises when the woman is discovered to have a CF mutation different from the man. In that case, unless both mutations can be tested for in the embryo, 50% of embryos (i.e. all embryos presenting with just one of the detectable mutations) would have to be discarded, even though only 25% would be expected to be potentially dangerous compound heterozygotes.

In summary, the issue of CF in the offspring from CAV males must be addressed seriously in any MESA–ICSI programme. Nonetheless, with routine, inexpensive CF genetic screening of the prospective parents and the availability of pre-implantation diagnosis, we are not aware of any children born with a CF phenotype or CAV despite transmission to the offspring of the father's CF gene mutation. But only with proper attention to these details can this potential risk to the offspring remain remote.

TESE–ICSI for Non-obstructive Azoospermia and Other Conditions

To date, our major effort with MESA–ICSI and TESE–ICSI has been concentrated on obstructive azoospermia. The results presented here indicate that all cases of obstructive azoospermia have the potential to be treated successfully and the only limitations appear to be the age and egg quality of the female partner. For ICSI, it is the vitality of the sperm and not their motility which is important, therefore retrieval of testicular sperm for ICSI enables injection of non-senescent, viable sperm when the ejaculated sperm are completely immotile.

No matter what the cause of total asthenozoospermia, the key to success with ICSI is to inject viable sperm. Selection of viable sperm is difficult when they are all immotile, so one solution to this problem is to retrieve sperm from the testis for ICSI. Although the motility of testicular sperm is always poor, the percentage of viable sperm should be high. This approach has been successful in a case of maturation arrest and in a case of Kartagener's syndrome. In addition, we have reviewed the slides of many of our azoospermic patients with diagnoses of Sertoli cell only syndrome or maturation arrest, and we found very small numbers of mature spermatids in these samples, indicating that TESE–ICSI could be used successfully in many of these non-obstructive azoospermic cases. Therefore, whenever the ejaculate fails to contain the few motile sperm that are required for ICSI, testicular sperm extraction provides a simple back-up solution.

Conclusions

Three years ago, ICSI provided a major breakthrough in the treatment of severe male factor infertility. Initial efforts were directed at severe oligozoospermia or oligoasthenozoospermia, and the only serious limitation was if there were no sperm in the ejaculate or if they were all immotile. This review documents the solution to the problem of obstructive azoospermia. If microsurgery is impractical or unsuccessful, MESA–ICSI or TESE–ICSI provide the most successful treatment. In fact, when we perform vasectomy reversals or V-E, we now always freeze a sample of motile epididymal sperm in case the microsurgery is unsuccessful. Thus, almost every case of obstructive azoospermia is now amenable to microsurgery and ICSI. The next step is to utilize TESE–ICSI to treat cases of non-obstructive azoospermia, and this will be the direction of our future research.

Acknowledgments

The authors thank the many staff in the Centre for Reproductive Medicine at the Dutch-Speaking Brussels Free University for their scientific altruism, the administrative staff in Brussels, namely Gi De Mesmaeker and Marlene Magnus, and S.J.S.'s office staff for the complex job of coordinating this collaboration. We also thank the organizers of the ICSI Symposium at Kooralbyn for their help in making ICSI a universally understood procedure.

References

Anguiano, A., Oates, R.D., Amos, J.A., Dean, M., Gerrard, B., Stewart, C., Maher, T.A., White, M.B., and Milunsky, A. (1992). Congenital bilateral absence of the vas deferens. A primarily genital form of cystic fibrosis. *J. Am. Med. Assoc.* **267**, 1794–7.

Anon. (1994). The sperm microaspiration retrieval techniques study group. Results in the United States with sperm microaspiration retrieval techniques and assisted reproductive technologies. *J. Urol.* **151**, 1255–9.

Bedford, J.M. (1966). Development of the fertilizing capacity of spermatozoa in the epididymis of the rabbit. *J. Exp. Zool.* **162**, 319–20.

Friend, D.S., Galle, J., and Silber, S.J. (1976). Fine structure of human sperm, vas deferens, epithelium, and testicle biopsy specimens at the time of vasectomy reversal. *Anat. Rec.* **184**, 584.

Gaddum, P. (1969). Sperm maturation in the male reproductive tract; development of motility. *Anat. Rec.* **161**, 471–2.

Gaddum, P., and Glover, T.D. (1965). Some reactions of rabbit spermatozoa to ligation of the epididymis. *J. Reprod. Fertil.* **9**, 119–30.

Glover, T.D. (1969). Some aspects of function in the epididymis; experimental occlusion of the epididymis in the rabbit. *Int. J. Fertil.* **14**, 216–21.

Krylov, V.S., and Borovikov, A.M. (1984). Microsurgical method of reuniting ductus epididymis. *Fertil. Steril.* **41**, 418–23.

Liu, J., Lissens, Silber, S.J., Devroey, P., Liebaers, I., and Van Steirteghem, A.C. (1994). Birth after preimplantation diagnosis of the cystic fibrosis ΔF508 mutation by polymerase chain reaction in human embryos resulting from intracytoplasmic sperm injection with epididymal sperm. *J. Am. Med. Assoc.* **23**,1858–60.

Mercier, B., Verlingue, C., Lissens, W., Silber, S.J., Novelli, G., Bonduelle, M., Raguenes, O., Quere, I., Audrezet, M.P., and Ferec, C. (1995). Is congenital bilateral absence of vas deferens primarily a form of cystic fibrosis? Results of a large study of the CFTR gene in CBAVD patients. *Am. J. Hum. Genet.* **56**, 272–7.

Ord, T., Patrizio, P., Marello, E., Balmaceda, J.P., and Asch, R.H. (1990). Mini-Percoll: a new method of semen preparation for IVF in severe male factor infertility. *Hum. Reprod. (Oxf.)* **5**, 987–9.

Orgebin-Crist, M.-C. (1969). Studies of the function of the epididymis. *Biol. Reprod.* **1** (Suppl. 1), 155–75.

Palermo, G., Joris, H., Devroey, P., and Van Steirteghem, A.C. (1992). Pregnancies after intracytoplasmic injection of single spermatozoon into an oocyte. *Lancet* **340**, 17–18.

Palermo, G., Joris, H., Derde, M.-P., Camus, M., Devroey, P., and Van Steirteghem, A. (1993). Sperm characteristics and outcome of human assisted fertilization by subzonal insemination and intracytoplasmic sperm injection. *Fertil. Steril.* **59**, 826–35.

Patrizio, P., Asch, R.H., Handelin, B., and Silber, S.J. (1993). Aetiology of congenital absence of the vas deferens: genetic study of three generations. *Hum. Reprod. (Oxf.)* **8**, 215–20.

Quinn P., Kerin, J.F., and Warnes, G.M. (1985). Improved pregnancy rate in human in vitro fertilization with the use of a medium based on the composition of human tubal fluid. *Fertil. Steril.* **44**, 493–8.

Silber, S.J. (1980). Vasoepididymostomy to head of epididymis: recovery of normal spermatozoal motility. *Fertil. Steril.* **34**, 149–53.

Silber, S.J. (1988). Pregnancy caused by sperm from vasa efferentia. *Fertil. Steril.* **49**, 373–5.

Silber, S.J. (1989a). Apparent fertility of human spermatozoa from the caput epididymis. *J. Androl.* **10**, 263–9.

Silber, S.J. (1989b). Pregnancy after vasovasostomy for vasectomy reversal: a study of factors affecting long-term return of fertility in 282 patients followed for 10 years. *Hum. Reprod. (Oxf.)* **4**, 318–22.

Silber, S.J. (1989c). Results of microsurgical vasoepididymostomy: role of epididymis in sperm maturation. *Hum. Reprod. (Oxf.)* **4**, 298–303.

Silber, S.J. (1994). A modern view of male infertility. In 'The Infertile Male: Advanced Assisted Reproductive Technology.' *Reprod. Fertil. Dev.* **6**, 93–104.

Silber, S.J., Balmaceda, J., Borrero, C., Ord, T., and Asch, R. (1988). Pregnancy with sperm aspiration from the proximal head of the epididymis: a new treatment for congenital absence of the vas deferens. *Fertil. Steril.* **50**, 525–8.

Silber, S.J., Ord, T., Balmaceda, J., Patrizio, P., and Asch, R.H. (1990). Congenital absence of the vas deferens: the fertilizing capacity of human epididymal sperm. *New Engl. J. Med.* **323**, 1788–92.

Silber, S.J., Ord, T., Balmaceda, J., Patrizio, P., and Asch, R. (1991). Cystic fibrosis and congenital absence of the vas deferens. *New Engl. J. Med.* **325**, 65.

Silber, S.J., Nagy, Z.P., Liu, J., Godoy, H., Devroey, P., and Van Steirteghem, A.C. (1994). Conventional *in-vitro* fertilization versus intracytoplasmic sperm injection for patients requiring microsurgical sperm aspiration. *Hum. Reprod. (Oxf.)* **9**, 1705–9.

Silber, S.J., Van Steirteghem, A.C., Liu, J., Nagy, Z., Tournaye, H., and Devroey, P. (1995). High fertilization and pregnancy rate after intracytoplasmic sperm injection with spermatozoa obtained from testicle biopsy. *Hum. Reprod. (Oxf.)* **10**, 148–52.

Temple-Smith, P.D., Southwick, G.J., Yates, C.A., Trounson, A.O., and de Kretser, D.M. (1985). Human pregnancy by *in vitro* fertilization (IVF) using sperm aspirated from the epididymis. *J. In Vitro Fertil. Embryo Transfer* **2**, 119–22.

Tournaye, H., Devroey, P., Liu, J., Nagy, Z., Lissens, W., and Van Steirteghem, A. (1994). Microsurgical epididymal sperm aspiration and intracytoplasmic sperm injection: a new effective approach to infertility as a result of congenital bilateral absence of the vas deferens. *Fertil. Steril.* **61**, 1045–51.

Van Steirteghem, A.C., Liu, J., Joris, H., Nagy, Z., Janssenswillen, C., Tournaye, H., Derde, M.-P., Van Assche, E., and Devroey, P. (1993a). Higher success rate by intracytoplasmic sperm injection than by subzonal insemination. Report of a second series of 300 consecutive treatment cycles. *Hum. Reprod. (Oxf.)* **8**, 1055–60.

Van Steirteghem, A.C., Nagy, Z., Joris, H., Liu, J., Staessen, C., Smitz, J., Wisanto, A., and Devroey, P. (1993b). High fertilization and implantation rates after intracytoplasmic sperm injection. *Hum. Reprod. (Oxf.)* **8**, 1061–6.

Weiske, W.-H. (1994). Pregnancy caused by sperm from vasa efferentia. *Fertil. Steril.* **62**, 642–3.

Young, W.C. (1931). The study of the function of the epididymis: functional changes undergone by spermatozoa during their passage through the epididymis and vas deferens in the guinea pig. *J. Exp. Biol.* **8**, 151–62.

Manuscript received 5 April 1995

Open Discussion

Simon Fishel (Nottingham):

Have you done antibody assessments on these MESA patients?

Silber:

We did antibody studies (immunobead tests) when we were doing conventional IVF on these patients and we didn't find any correlation between antibodies and fertilization. We also did computerized motion analysis with Russell Davis and Jim Overstreet, but no matter how carefully we studied these patients, we found nothing that we could measure that was predictive of fertilization after conventional IVF. We've lost interest in the antibodies now that we use ICSI and we haven't studied them with the patients currently undergoing ICSI.

Harold Bourne (Melbourne):

The cleavage rate in one of your slides was only 79%. Does that mean a lot of the embryos arrested at the pronuclear stage?

Silber:

Yes. On average, we achieved 46% two pronuclear fertilization instead of 60–65% as you would expect with ejaculated sperm, but this was very predictable with either testicular or epididymal sperm. The average cleavage rate was only 60–70%.

Bourne:

Any ideas why?

Silber:

No, I don't even know why we should have such consistently lower two pronuclear fertilization rates with epididymal and testicular sperm compared with ejaculated sperm.

Herman Tournaye (Brussels):

Your definition of Sertoli cell only syndrome seems to be exactly the same as hypospermatogenesis. As soon as you find some gonadal cells, then by definition it's not Sertoli cell only syndrome.

Silber:

Hypospermatogenesis is defined by most pathologists as a condition in which you see many tubules with only a small amount of spermatogenesis in them. We traditionally think of Sertoli cell only as a condition in which you look all over the slide and all you see is Sertoli cells, but then you might see one isolated tubule making sperm. David Page found that deletions in all these cases occur at the same location regardless of whether they're complete Sertoli cell only syndrome or there are occasional tubules which appear to be making sperm. This is an example of what geneticists call a 'leaky gene'. So I think it's probably fair to call it Sertoli cell only as long as I define carefully what I mean.

In most cases of hypospermatogenesis, most of the tubules are producing small numbers of sperm and sperm can be found in the ejaculate after it has been centrifuged, and these cases don't even come into consideration for testicular sperm extraction (TESE). But in many cases of Sertoli cell only in which there is an occasional tubule producing sperm, there are no sperm in the ejaculate even after centrifugation at 1800g. We have gone back over Sertoli cell only cases carefully and it's amazing how many of them have one or two tubules that are making a few spermatids.

David de Kretser (Melbourne):

It shouldn't be called Sertoli cell only syndrome. It really is a question of what the aetiology of the material is and we don't fully understand that yet.

Silber:

We can debate terminology, but the interesting thing is that, if we see that picture rather than classical hypospermatogenesis, we consistently find the same gene defect on Yq (78 patients). They have isolated the gene and they're about to start sequencing it.

Alan Trounson (Melbourne):

Are you saying that ΔF508 is genomically imprinted for congenital absence of the vas (CAV)?

Silber:

Every patient with CAV is presumed by geneticists to have a CF deletion, but in 30% of cases you don't pick it up since we routinely screen for only 36 mutations and there are certainly over 300 mutations that we don't screen for.

Whenever we found a ΔF508 heterozygote, for example in a male with CAV, there was a ΔF508 either in his mother or in his father. If it was in his father it was obvious his father had bilateral vas and was fertile. Furthermore, if the male with CAV had ΔF508, then there was a 50% chance that the offspring from MESA would have ΔF508, and if it were a male offspring with ΔF508, he would have the vas deferens present bilaterally. So therefore the mere fact of carrier status for CF does not cause congenital absence of the vas. We presume it requires either compound heterozygosity, homozygosity or something from both parents.

Trounson:

Two years ago, you said that IVF fertilization rates with MESA were about 30%. Now it's only 7%. Is this radical difference due to the patients or techniques?

Silber:

In the first 100 MESA cases that we did with conventional IVF, we reported 16 pregnancies with live births. We were pretty excited about that. But in the next 67 cases we had only 9 pregnancies and half of those miscarried (4·5% live birth rate per cycle). The fertilization rate was always low though, 17% in the first 100 cases and only 8% in the next 67 cases. I don't know whether it was a different group or whether we did repeat cycles on people that were less likely to succeed. I really can't explain why it got worse, but frankly it was never very high.

Technical Discussion

Panel: Harold Bourne (Melbourne), Gianpiero Palermo (New York),
Dianna Payne (Adelaide).
Chairman: Simon Fishel (Nottingham).

David Edgar (Melbourne):

One major difference which emerged concerns the use of polyvinylpyrrolidone (PVP) for immobilizing sperm. Harold Bourne showed some very consistent results without using PVP. I wonder if the people who are still using it would like to comment on that?

Palermo:

PVP is not necessary for immobilizing sperm. It just slows down the sperm, making it easier to pick them up with a narrow injection pipette, and it also gives finer control when the spermatozoon is in the pipette. It can also be of benefit if you deal with semen samples which contain other cells and debris. I use a 5 μL droplet of PVP and add 1 μL of sperm at 6 o'clock so that the moving sperm swim up into the cleanest area of the PVP droplet. In this way you avoid contamination. If you use normal medium, you will pick up all the other debris.

Payne:

We find PVP to be very useful for controlling sperm in the injection pipette and for control during the injection procedure. We have correlated the volume of PVP injected into the oocyte with fertilization rates, embryo development and pregnancy rates and found there was no influence. So PVP is essential for good control of sperm during the injection procedure and it doesn't seem to harm the oocyte.

Fishel:

Sometimes we use extremely good sperm with very rapid motility for ICSI and it's much easier to slow them down using PVP. But the most important thing is to immobilize the sperm. If slowing them down helps, that's fine, but if you can immobilize them without using PVP then it actually doesn't matter.

Bourne:

A few comments on the non-use of PVP. When we started our ICSI programme we were unable to obtain the correct PVP so we started without it. In reference to Simon Fishel's comment about chasing highly motile sperm, if there are a large number of sperm and they're moving randomly, it's quite easy to just hold your pipette in one place and when you find one that's moving in the right direction, move the pipette there and it goes straight up. So we don't have any problems dealing with that.

Gianpiero, in reference to testicular sperm samples which contain a large amount of residual debris, PVP didn't seem to prevent debris sticking to things. Any comment?

Palermo:

The molecular weight (MW) of PVP is the key point. If you use PVP with a MW of less than 360 000, then there is no benefit in using PVP at all. It is also important to use the right amount of protein to avoid sticking. I use 0·5% BSA.

Robert McLachlan (Melbourne):

Harold, with regard to the hypo-osmotic swelling (HOS) test which you suggested might be useful for selecting viable, immotile sperm, have you actually compared the fertilization rates with and without HOS selection? In other words, is the 27% fertilization rate you report better than having not performed any selection in the first place?

Bourne:

There have only been a small number of cases so far. As I said there were two cases in which we did the HOS test to select the sperm but there was no comparative study done in those patients. There was another case in which we did not select sperm using the HOS test and they did very poorly. However, I suspect that there was a high percentage of dead sperm and the HOS test probably wouldn't have helped us find any live sperm anyway.

Fishel:

We've done a number of cases now in which we did supravital staining. If approximately 20% of the sperm were alive we would proceed with ICSI. We split the cases up into sibling oocytes in which we had our vitality value for the ejaculated sperm and then we did a HOS test. The fertilization rate doubled when we selected sperm with the HOS test.

Yvonne Du Plessis (Stockholm):

How do you pick up sperm with curled tails after you've done the HOS test?

Bourne:

I was just doing one sperm at a time and it was fairly easy. The samples we were dealing with had a reasonable number of sperm in them and we'd aspirate a single sperm from the suspension, expel it into the hypo-osmotic medium, see if the tail curled, and if it didn't, go and pick up another one. In those cases, up to 50% of the sperm were live.

Du Plessis:

After you'd done that, was that the sperm that you straight away injected into an egg?

Bourne:

Yes, as soon as it had been expelled into the medium its tail curled. We aspirated that sperm, transferred it to the injection medium, aspirated and cleaned the injection pipette to make sure that we didn't have the wrong osmolarity solution in it, and then picked up the sperm and injected it.

Herman Tournaye (Brussels):

I have a comment on the use of the HOS test. We don't have a large series, but we have done it on a few cases and apparently in some patients it doesn't work at all. In a few of those patients we had the results of ultrastructural assessment by electron microscopy and in the patients having 100% immotile sperm cells due to ultrastructural problems, the HOS test doesn't work at all. So we probably need to do more research to define subgroups of patients with 100% immotile sperm.

Fishel:

Did you immediately inject the sperm or did you allow them to reconstitute before you injected them?

Tournaye:

They were allowed to reconstitute.

Bourne:

One of the patients that I mentioned had a structural defect and they achieved fertilization, but as you said, there may be subgroups which do not behave in that fashion.

Alan Trounson (Melbourne):

We need to define what we mean by dead sperm, because I think what you're saying, and I agree, is that a dead sperm is one which is incapable of reacting to the conditions in the egg. If an egg has the capability of forming a male pronucleus, there are sperm which cannot react to that. I don't think we know why that is, but I think that's what we ought to look for, rather than just calling them dead and alive. We need a better definition of what is dead and alive. I think it's important for selecting sperm from men who have completely immotile sperm as well as for animal conservation work.

Bourne:

I totally agree with Alan Trounson. It depends on how we define live and dead sperm. Just as a comment, in all of the frozen epididymal sperm samples that we used, we only selected motile sperm so we did not need to select immotile sperm from the frozen epididymal samples.

Trounson:

But it even works with those immotile sperm. Often you can't get any motile sperm back after freezing epididymal sperm, but if you use the immotile sperm, they form pronuclei at high rates and embryos develop normally.

Fishel:

I think what's very important in this discussion and what we've really got to focus on in the next few years is what we mean by 'works'. We need to look at live births and perhaps even do follow-up studies on the sperm that were injected and the outcome. We can get mislead by overall data which shows that we can get successful fertilization, embryos and occasional pregnancies. But I think we're really honing in on the status of individual sperm.

Sherman Silber (St Louis):

I've heard reference to a 45° bevel and a 28° bevel on the injection pipette. What angle does Dr. Palermo use?

Palermo:

In Brussels I used a 50° bevel but now I use a 30° bevel. A 30° bevel makes it easier to penetrate the oolemma, although this still depends on the kind of oocyte you get. I still prefer to have a spike on the injection pipette because if you don't need it you can always break it off.

Fishel:

I think it's a bit like 'which catheter do you use for embryo transfers?' We have used 6–8-μm outer diameter injection pipettes and various bevel angles. The most important thing is to understand the tools that you have and know your technique.

Sean Flaherty (Adelaide):

Would the panel or anyone else like to comment on the instrumentation that they use and what they find is suitable or unsuitable for ICSI?

Payne:

When you manufacture instruments, I think it's important to be able to clearly visualize the end of the pipettes, particularly the injection pipettes. The optics that were supplied with our microforge included $10 \times$ eye pieces and we changed them to $20 \times$ eye pieces so that we could actually see what was happening.

Fishel:

I think it really is a matter of getting familiar with the instrumentation that you've got. However, the angle of your holding and injection pipettes is important and you have to go in at 180°. So you need good optics. The whole range of instruments that I've tried are good enough, but it's good to have microscopic observation while you're bevelling (grinding).

Bourne:

I'd like to comment on the joy stick manipulators that are available. Perhaps it's our non-use of PVP, but I would not like to try collecting and immobilizing sperm without the responsiveness of the Narishige joystick manipulators.

Palermo:

When I joined the Cornell group in September last year, it took me one month to be able to do ICSI there because I was used to a certain system and I didn't know any other. I think that the Narishige microforge makes things easier and I make the holding pipettes on it. It takes no time and they are all reproducible. You don't need any special ability to make them and any technician can learn to make them in 3–4 days. I think the Narishige joystick, hanging type micromanipulators are safe and avoid damage to the oocyte. When you are in a unit which has a high number of cases, you need many people that inject equally well, so you need to have safe instruments and standardized material. The best puller is the Campden 753 which is now out of production. They have a new model (773) which is not as good as the 753.

Rohini Edirisinghe (Perth):

I find that the new model 773 Campden puller is inconsistent and doesn't always work the same way when pulling injection pipettes. My question to the panel is, what type of oil could we use to obtain better control during injection?

Palermo:

Concerning the Campden, I agree, it is not a very reliable machine. I am working with the company to try and design a good programme on the 773 so that it will reliably make pipettes with the right shank. I think it will take a few months and then we'll be able to have the right programme for making ICSI pipettes. Regarding the oil, what kind of injection system do you use?

Edirisinghe:

It's a Narishige micrometre syringe set-up.

Palermo:

That's another problem. Narishige stopped making the right syringes. The syringes were 800-μL stainless steel syringes but they're making glass ones now. They insist that people had difficulty seeing when they filled the stainless steel syringes with oil. But they delivered the highest pressure for the small size of the pipettes we use for ICSI. I always use BDH lightweight paraffin oil with the metal syringes because it gives the best result after you shorten the tubing.

Fishel:

Just one point which nobody has mentioned yet, and that is the system for controlling the sperm which I think is quite important. I used to use oil but I found that it was very messy and unnecessary, so now we just use a pneumatic system. We find that it is extremely important to make sure that the injection pipette is equilibrated first. Once it is equilibrated then you can have extremely fine control of the sperm. And getting that control is very important for ICSI, regardless of which system you use.

Du Plessis:

What's the best and cheapest way of securing a microinjection system that is disturbed by vibration?

Palermo:

I work on the 8th floor in Manhattan and it's quite shaky. I found that there is a table made in Newport, California which uses air pressure as a suspension. You have to be careful when you touch the manipulator or everything moves, and the noise of air discharging can be annoying too. But it's the only way to have complete isolation from the floor. It is very expensive.

Bourne:

We work on the 6th floor in Carlton, but we're very lucky that our hospital is fairly stable and we don't encounter much vibration. We just had an extra strut put under our bench and that has been fine. But at Melbourne IVF, I think they do have some problems and I believe they use a pneumatic table.

Fishel:

We have a concrete slab which is tiled. This is not perfect but it actually does offer a significant amount of resistance to vibration. I know some people that set their microscopes into table tennis balls or polystyrene beads.

Payne:

We work on the 4th floor of a fairly shaky old building which sometimes vibrates rather dramatically, and the cheapest and most effective way we've found of stabilizing the table is to use half court tennis balls (soft) and miniature wheelbarrow tyres on a wooden platform. That works quite well.

Silber:

We use a pneumatic table and at first I hated it, but now I realize it's spectacular and I really recommend it. It really makes a difference.

Michael Tucker (Atlanta):

Just a quick comment to Harold Bourne. He mentioned that harvesting testicular sperm can be difficult because of all the other tissue. I use a 10-μm blunt ended-needle and just suck up sperm at random and then expel them into a clean droplet so that I can then harvest them for injection.

Bourne:

What sort of biopsies were they?

Tucker:

We've used both types. We started off with fairly hefty chunks of testis but we have started to use needle biopsies. It's amazing how the sperm wake up.

Bourne:

In the open biopsies that we did there was a considerable amount of tissue and it was easy to isolate motile sperm from that. But in the fine needle biopsies, the amount of tissue was quite small, perhaps a 0·5-cm plug from a 20 G needle. Often we only found a few sperm in the original dissection, but in a 35-mm Petri dish we would find enough to count them.

Silber:

I would like to say that the testicular biopsy is another, maybe novel solution to the immotile sperm. We've used this for Kartagener's syndrome with fertilization and successful pregnancy. One approach with immotile sperm is the assumption that if you go directly to the testis you're more likely to find sperm that have not yet undergone senescent changes and we believe that you can get more sperm from a testicular biopsy. It's remarkable how few sperm stay in the seminiferous tubule. They're transported immediately to the rete testis, so in most testicular biopsy specimens you'll find very few sperm. However, they will be almost 100% alive.

Final Discussion

Chairmen: Lars Hamberger (Göteborg), Colin Matthews (Adelaide).

Matthews:

Are there aspects of the physiology of gametes or indeed any of the laboratory aspects which need further discussion?

Hamberger:

I would like to discuss reactive oxygen species (ROS) and how important it is to protect the sperm and eggs from ROS using different scavengers. There have been some reports on the use of catalase and dismutase during sperm preparation. Any comments? Could ROS be responsible for fragmentation of embryos?

Matthews:

Some established ICSI programmes have better implantation rates per embryo than their conventional IVF systems and it has always seemed to me that sperm by-products and ROS may be having an adverse effect on the embryo which is not evident during the early stages of embryo development but may be detrimental to implantation. If we are reducing the number of inseminated sperm, or with ICSI reducing it to single sperm, then in effect we may be taking preventative measures.

Robert Edwards (Cambridge):

The fetal karyotype results from the Brussels group were astoundingly good because the trisomies they reported could have been due to sperm defects (XY sperm). Despite going into the egg with a needle and perturbing the cytoskeleton and the systems in the egg, this still has not affected non-disjunction as far as we can tell. It is a very positive point because they have shown a very low rate of trisomy and monosomy compared with published data on the general population and after IVF.

Alan Trounson (Melbourne):

I think the challenge is to use ICSI to look at some of the underlying mechanisms involved in infertility and fertility. Henry Sathananthan can't find any ultrastructural evidence for the acrosome reaction after ICSI. Perhaps we can treat the sperm in better ways in order for them to always decondense and thus produce 90% fertilization rate. And what about sperm that do not have centrioles? There are a lot of those sperm in the 100% immotility cases.

Simon Fishel (Nottingham):

Could I ask a question about HEPES. For cases in which we use testicular sperm and it takes a while to isolate individual sperm for injection, are the eggs sitting in HEPES longer and could that be the cause of reduced fertilization? We got much better fertilization and cleavage rates when we only kept one or two eggs at a time on the heated microscope stage. So could HEPES have a detrimental effect?

Trounson:

One of the problems with HEPES is that once you inject it into the oocyte, it's like PVP and can't come out. I wondered if it would interfere with the delicate pH balances that must occur, but I've never seen an experiment that examines it.

Dianna Payne (Adelaide):

Our micromanipulation has all been done with bicarbonate-buffered medium and not HEPES-buffered medium because we use a CO_2 and temperature-controlled environmental chamber on our microscopes. Our fertilization and cleavage rates are no different than the results of groups who use HEPES routinely for microinjection.

Harold Bourne (Melbourne):

I'd like to comment on the use of HEPES with our testicular samples. It takes about 1·5 h to prepare the sperm by the time the tissue is collected, dissected etc., and the sperm are in HEPES-buffered HTF all the time. For the data I presented, the eggs were transferred into the injection chamber in groups of 3, and they would stay in there for 15 min and then they were transferred back into bicarbonate-buffered HTF. So we weren't leaving the eggs in the HEPES for an extended period in those cases. Is that different to what Sherman Silber was doing in Brussels?

Sherman Silber (St Louis):

They collect the good sperm, put them in the PVP and then put the eggs in and get ready to do the injection. So they are not in HEPES very long.

Gianpiero Palermo (New York):

When I started ICSI, I first used PBS, but then I switched to HEPES and I thought the results were better.

Now I think it's better not to use HEPES if you have a choice like Dianna Payne. But HEPES makes it easier and apparently there is no real reason not to use it. When you have a very difficult sperm sample to work with, it's better to work on the sperm while the oocytes are in the incubator. So when you have clean spermatozoa, you can place them singly in the PVP, ready for injection and then get your oocytes. At Cornell, we usually don't put more than 4 oocytes in one dish. I'm a little faster, so I put 5 or 6, but if it's a bad sperm sample we only put 2 oocytes in the dish.

Lou Warnes (Adelaide):

Does anyone have any views on how we can decide when oocyte defects are causing fertilization failure after ICSI?

Palermo:

Van Blerkom described oocytes with a central dark cytoplasm after superovulation, and claimed that these oocytes either did not fertilize, or if they did, they cleaved poorly. We have seen that various oocyte abnormalities (vacuoles, granularity, central dark cytoplasm) do not affect the fertilization rate, which is surprising. So oocyte morphology is not very useful for identifying an oocyte factor.

Bourne:

There are differences between batches of oocytes, and Gianpiero Palermo mentioned the syndrome of sticky or elastic membranes. We do find fragile membranes in some batches of oocytes whereas at other times they're like chewing gum. They're very different. I don't know whether that's related to age or to something else.

Palermo:

If the egg membrane breaks right away, you have a very high chance of destroying the egg. I found a way to overcome this problem. When you have 2–3 eggs and the first one breaks right away, you can try to avoid this problem by going through the zona at 12 o'clock or 6 o'clock as in partial zona dissection (PZD), then you release the oocyte from the holding pipette, roll it and then you just push the injection pipette directly through the oolemma. That's the only way to avoid oocyte damage. It's tricky to do.

Trounson:

Is it related to patient age or stimulation?

Palermo:

I think it may be related to the stimulation.

Fishel:

We need to concentrate more on the eggs, because we're doing so much with the sperm. There are clearly a number of differences and we can't really go solely on anecdotal cases. There are patients who are clearly affected by Buserelin or desensitization and their egg quality is certainly affected. There are patients who have an egg problem whether they are on different stimulation regimes or even natural cycles, their eggs are difficult to inject. I think there is a whole series of effects which can give you problems with eggs. We have a group of women that have an intermittent egg problem and we can't seem to overcome that.

Bourne:

A comment about egg membrane elasticity. In a number of patients, we've had some eggs which were immature on the day of collection and we've allowed them to mature and injected them the following day. That was usually as a rescue attempt, meaning that if a patient had a large number of immature eggs at collection, we tried to get a few more fertilized eggs by injecting some on the next day. And I think there's a noticeable difference between the mature eggs that you inject on Day 0 and those that you inject on Day 1. The membranes on Day 1 tend to break very easily.

Matthews:

Are there any clinical aspects of ICSI that you would like to discuss?

Rob Norman (Adelaide):

I'd like to raise an issue that we haven't looked at so far and that is, whether we should reconsider natural cycle IVF with ICSI. This came from a case that we had in Adelaide in which a patient who needed ICSI refused all drugs completely (including hCG) and recently become pregnant after the transfer of one embryo derived from ICSI. We've had results presented today that range from a 30% implantation rate downwards. If we were able to pick up a single egg in 80% of patients and get fertilization in 70% of those eggs, then we should have a very real chance of getting significant pregnancy rates in natural cycles. Does anyone have any experience with natural cycle IVF and ICSI in this situation or in the 70% of female patients that Lars Hamberger told us have no discernible abnormality? Can we re-invent natural cycle IVF?

Hamberger:

Yes, that could be very exciting. On the other hand, I don't think everyone feels safe about dealing with just one oocyte, even with high fertilization rates. But it would be very tempting, and as you said, we should have a much higher implantation rate in normal healthy women compared to the infertile female population. So if we do natural cycle IVF, why not also include ICSI.

Herman Tournaye (Brussels):

If the fertilization rate is quoted as 70%, in fact it's only 70% per successfully injected mature egg. So I think with patients undergoing natural cycles, there is the risk of first not having a mature egg, and second, damaging the egg. In our experience, cases with less than four eggs after stimulation are the ones most susceptible to failure so I really don't think that you will have good success rates in that group. In ICSI you have some loss of oocytes at every stage, so if you have one egg retrieved it must be a mature one, it must not get damaged, and it must fertilize and cleave.

Trounson:

I wanted to endorse Rob Norman's suggestion about natural cycles, basically because I've been developing the immature oocyte programme in which we try and average 6 or 7 mature oocytes which we always inseminate by ICSI. If we can collect a single mature egg, I strongly endorse the use of ICSI because I think ICSI clearly raises the chance of a successful outcome and there is no reason why it shouldn't be used, because how long does it take to do ICSI on one or maybe two eggs? It is sensible to offer that option to women who don't want to have fertility drugs.

Janina Michalowska (Chicago):

All the centres here are performing intrauterine transfers. Does anybody have any information on intratubal transfer of ICSI embryos?

Hamberger:

The attitude in northern Europe is that we prolong culture more and more so that we can select the best embryos for replacement. And it is even more important if we really do have a problem freezing ICSI embryos, which we haven't really determined yet. The longer you culture the embryos, the less indication there is for tubal transfer.

Silber:

We have looked at the data and I don't think there is any evidence that a tubal transfer will increase the pregnancy rate or the implantation rate of an embryo compared with a uterine transfer.

But what is very dramatic is the outcome if you look at the age of the patient or at the age of the egg so to speak, and the embryos that derive from them. Can we rejuvenate these older eggs by doing pronuclear transfers into the eggs of a younger woman or is this just an inevitable genetic aging process?

Trounson:

You could take an embryo from an older woman, take out the blastomeres and fuse them with enucleated oocytes from a younger woman. However, we should do those experiments in animals first. Is this a limit to the technology that we would be prepared to deal with for the sake of repairing infertility? If most of the problems are chromosomal and genetic then we're not going to repair them by putting the DNA into surrogate cytoplasts.

Matthews:

Does ICSI offer better prospects for older woman (> 40 years) compared with conventional IVF?

Fishel:

There is no evidence of any oolemma or zona pellucida problems in the older women so it's probably a genetic or chromosomal problem. We certainly see the same reduction in success rates with age after ICSI that we see with conventional IVF.

Palermo:

Our patients range from 31 to 44 years old and 20–30% are ≥40 years old. There is, of course, a difference in pregnancy rate. A study on the incidence of aneuploidy in these older oocytes has also been done at Cornell. I think that ICSI will be of benefit because the older patients often have poor pregnancy rates because they have fewer eggs, and a technique which guarantees a higher fertilization rate will increase the chance of pregnancy as well. At Cornell, we often have patients who produce only a small number of mature eggs after stimulation, so that we only inject 2–3 eggs or sometimes only a single egg.

Matthews:

Are there any ethical issues to discuss?

Jeff Persson (Sydney):

I have an ethical question for Sherman Silber. We had a number of pubescent boys who were about to undergo cancer chemotherapy but weren't able to obtain a semen specimen. It's tragic for them and for their parents. Is there anything from your testicular biopsy work that might provide a mechanism for gamete preservation for them?

Silber:

That's a fantastic question but I don't have the answer to it. We see many patients of all ages who want to have sperm frozen because they're about to undergo chemotherapy and they may never get a return of spermatogenesis. I think it's crucial that we no longer freeze up to 10 samples and then plan on doing inseminations at some later date, because there are many stories of men that were cured of Hodgkins or a lymphoma and then, after a couple of inseminations the wife isn't pregnant but they have run out of frozen semen. So I think we should just take one specimen before they undergo chemotherapy and divide it into 40 straws and freeze it, and they should have enough sperm so that they are able to have children in the future using ICSI.

John Tyler (Sydney):

If you've got someone who's only got one sample and you thaw it and use it for ICSI, does anyone have any experience of re-freezing that sample for future use?

Hamberger:

Yes, we have done that successfully at least 3 times. When you re-freeze the sample, it is wise to separate it into different straws, so that you don't need to recycle it again.

Trounson:

I don't think that this information is in the minds of urologists and the community. I think it's very important that if there is a possibility of preserving some sperm now for these boys or men, that it be well known in the community. I believe the same will apply to cortical ovarian tissue for young women. We should make that known to all the specialists and people that work in the cancer field, and make sure the community knows it as well.

Sean Flaherty (Adelaide):

I think that what Sherman Silber said is quite correct, that we certainly can use ICSI for these men who freeze samples. But I disagree that we should just store one sample. There are many cases in which you get very poor post-thaw motility, but you also get samples which are not that bad. If you have the time and the patient has the inclination, you're much better off freezing a number of samples, because then they do have the option of, for example, stimulated intrauterine insemination (IUI). So, if you can't get enough sperm or it's a really poor sample then ICSI is the obvious way to go. But I think if you can get a good sample, then you still should look at simpler treatment options.

Silber:

I'd be very cautious and not use all the sperm on IUI.

Matthews:

Ladies and gentlemen, I think the time has come to close this wonderful Symposium. Clearly, we are witnessing an ICSI revolution and the bringing of hope to couples who have been, to this time, without much hope of ever having their own genetic children. We do need to take care that these same couples have access to the very best technology and therefore the very best chances of conception. A symposium such as this, with virtually all of the world's proponents of the ICSI art present, must reflect the cutting edge of reproductive technology as 1994 closes. We are most grateful to all the overseas contributors for coming to Australia and to Serono for their enterprise in supporting this meeting so well.